It's Your Body:
A Woman's Guide to Gynecology

"Dr. Spock spoke to our mothers, this man speaks to us.... This book is knowledge that can only enhance the great joy of being female."

Gael Greene,
NEW YORK MAGAZINE

"Dr. Lauersen has been willing to break through the doctor mystique, climb down from the godlike throne, and treat women as people who can and must make informed decisions about their own bodies. That such a man is already teaching a whole new breed of obstetricians and gynecologists to thus respond to the personhood of woman—her body, her self—is what the woman's movement hardly dared to dream could happen so soon."

Betty Friedan

"Offers women a virtual textbook of gynecology translated into readable, sensible, practical information."

Barbara Seaman,
author of FREE & FEMALE

"...a sane and sensible book dedicated to making every woman a full partner in the care of her own body. IT'S YOUR BODY is one book to lean on for the facts."

THE NURSE'S BOOK SOCIETY

"Within the context of medical guides, Lauersen's book is impressive. He covers everything from abortions to orgasms in a manner that's unusually contemporary, sensible, sympathetic and detailed."

THE NEW YORK POST

Berkley books by Niels Lauersen, M.D.

IT'S YOUR BODY, A WOMAN'S GUIDE TO GYNECOLOGY
(with Steven Whitney)
LISTEN TO YOUR BODY: A GYNECOLOGIST ANSWERS WOMEN'S
MOST INTIMATE QUESTIONS (with Eileen Stukane)

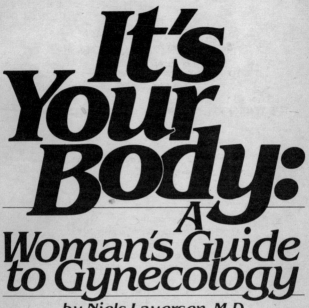

It's Your Body:

A
Woman's Guide
to Gynecology

by Niels Lauersen, M.D.,
and Steven Whitney

BERKLEY BOOKS, NEW YORK

This Berkley Book contains the complete
text of the original edition.

IT'S YOUR BODY: A WOMAN'S GUIDE TO GYNECOLOGY

A Berkley Book / published by arrangement with
Grosset & Dunlap, Inc.

PRINTING HISTORY
Grosset & Dunlap edition published 1977
PBJ Books edition / June 1980
Berkley edition / January 1983
Second printing / May 1984

ISBN: 0-425-07504-4

CONTENTS

ACKNOWLEDGMENTS

There are many friends, colleagues, and patients who stimulated and encouraged us throughout the preparation of this book. To each and every one of them, we offer our gratitude.

The research, drafting, and critical analysis done by Kathleen H. Wilson, Jeffery Wood, and Craig Buck were invaluable in the completion of the manuscript. Our most profound thanks go to each of them. Without these three, this book would not be.

Others who helped immeasurably with research, verification, analysis, and drafting were Joel Surnow, Suzanne Grace, Mark Jacobsen, and Flansy Lewis.

The entire manuscript was typed by Lynn Scalla. The drafts, transcripts, and research notes were typed by Lori Leeds, Linda Elmore, Debbie Butler, Susan Donovan, Robin Fegley, Marsha Stein, Joann Froner, and Sue Janssen. Each of them also gave us insightful comments at every step.

The original art was done by Enrique Senis-Oliver, and the medical illustrations are the work of Pauline Thomas and Peter Ng. We also express our gratitude to Tom Saltarelli for photographic work and to Barry Cummings for photographic artwork.

So many others helped in so many ways, we can do little more than list them by way of saying thank you: Rob Morris, Janet Green, Phyllis Keitlen, Clair Sater, Allen Ralston, Harvey Rubin, Barbara Sater, Diana Davis, Jane Toonkel, Stafford Morgan, Tara Cole, Barbara Karpf, Laura Roth, David Schwartz, Vicki Till, Adrian Rothenberg, Steven Kriegsman, Tom Barad, and Cindy Boscowitz.

And a special thank-you to Gael Greene, who guided the project to success.

ILLUSTRATIONS

All drawings, graphs, diagrams, and photographs have been created solely for use in this book, except where noted by a credit line, and are the property of the authors.

NOTE

For the purpose of simplicity, the authors have chosen to designate the hypothetical gynecologists in this book with the male gender pronouns—he, his, him, etc. This gender rendering should not be viewed as a political or chauvinistic choice; rather as a means to greater clarification—making it easier to distinguish between the patient, who is always a *she,* and the doctor. It is true that more than 90% of all Ob.Gyn. specialists are men, but it is obvious to everyone that this field can only benefit by the increasing number of women who choose it for their profession. Hopefully, this future sexual balance in personnel will bring a greater closeness and understanding between doctors and patients.

INTRODUCTION

Today's woman is increasingly concerned with the well-being of her body. Consequently, she is determined to know more about her normal bodily functions and her medical care. The controversial effects of various drugs (such as the birth-control pill) and the epidemic proportions of certain illnesses (such as venereal disease) rightly concern every responsible woman. Too often, widespread media reports emphasize the more sensational aspects of medical findings, causing patients to be greatly confused by the apparently endless deluge of conflicting information. There is a need for practical and relevant information about a woman's body and the medical procedures relating to it. *It's Your Body* was written to fill that need.

We hope this book will help women realize the wonderfully complex functions of the female body. The normal functions are explained so that any abnormal functions that are symptoms of illness can be recognized in time to seek appropriate professional help. This should help inform and prepare a woman who does have an illness or malfunction become a partner in her own medical treatment.

However, our book was not written as a guide to self-treatment, but as a thorough encyclopedia of all aspects of a woman's life, from menarche to menopause, including a guide to sexual terminology and problems. The theory behind the book is simple: The best patient is an informed patient. We hope *It's Your Body* will help women understand their physicians' instructions and recommendations more completely. Through both its written words and its many illustrations, this book should lead women to a better understanding of a particular condition or a suggested treatment.

The data is the most recent available. For this reason, we hope our work leads women to the latest developments in the field of gynecology.

—NIELS H. LAUERSEN, M.D., NEW YORK
—STEVEN WHITNEY, LOS ANGELES

chapter 1

SELF-EXAMINATION

GROWING UP AFRAID

A little four-year-old white boy is standing nude after taking a communal bath in his nursery school. He looks at the nude four-year-old black girl standing next to him. An expression of great puzzlement crosses his face as he continues staring at the black girl. Finally, he calls the teacher over to him and whispers in her ear. "Teacher, I didn't know there was such a big difference between white kids and black kids!"

A charming story, but, sadly, it is all too true. This statement and others like it are heard again and again at this age level, even between sisters and brothers. The reason is simple: a shocking lack of early education.

Most of us remember the time we first noticed the difference between penises and vaginas. Freud felt (and this is still a widely held opinion) that this was a traumatic event for little girls. His reasoning was this: Upon seeing a penis, the little girl was seized with jealousy and feelings of castration and inferiority.

> They notice the penis of a brother or playmate, strikingly visible and of large proportions, at once recognize it as the superior counterpart of their own small and inconspicuous organ, and from that time forward fall a victim to envy for the penis . . . She has seen it and knows that she is without it and wants to have it. [From *The Complete Psychological Works of Sigmund Freud,* The Hogarth Press.]

This statement, more than anything, seems to shed light on Freud's own phallocentricity. Today, "penis envy" has been called into question by many leading psychiatrists, who feel there is nothing superior or inferior in the way of genitalia; that everyone is equal.

11

They feel Freud never considered the idea that little girls may have been jealous of the preferential treatment given to boys. The Victorian era was particularly repressive to women, and it is very possible that little girls of the time would have liked penises so that they, too, could have enjoyed the privileges bestowed on boys.

The girl who has enjoyed equal standing with boys and who has observed mutual respect between her parents should, upon viewing her first penis, notice merely that boys are different. If she has been allowed (mostly through example) to be proud of her body, she will probably be very happy with her streamlined build. Indeed, why should she envy the little boy his excess baggage?

Fortunately, there is a natural biological curiosity to discover and explore one's own body. A little girl discovers her opening and also discovers the pleasant sensation she derives from touching it. This

Fig. 1-1: The reproductive organs in men and women have the same genetic origin. The sex of every child is determined at conception, but it cannot be discerned until the end of the eighth week after conception, or the tenth week after the mother's last menstrual period.

A small bud develops on the groin area of the fetus. If the child is to be a girl, this bud will form into the clitoris. Likewise, the bud will become a penis if the child is to be a boy. The tissue surrounding this bud folds back into the labia with girls, while it forms the scrotum in boys.

This tissue, which is called *genital tubercle*, begins to develop five weeks after conception, or seven weeks after the last menstrual period. This is shown in the top picture, where the genitalia is seen in the undifferentiated state. At this point, the bud appears as a phallus-like organ, but it is still too early to determine the sex of the fetus.

Ten weeks after conception, or twelve weeks after the last menstrual period, the development of *specific* sexual determination can be seen (see middle set of drawings), although a complete development of the penis or vulva does not occur until the fourth month (see lower set of drawings).

The illustration clearly demonstrates how the glands of the penis and the glands of the vulva both develop from the genital tubercle. The clitoral and penal foreskins are also developed from the same tissue in the undifferentiated state. The *labia minora* and the *raphe* (the tissue on the underside of the penis) are developed from the same tissue. Because of this, the *raphe*, like the *labia minora*, is extremely sensitive to touch.

THE DEVELOPMENT OF THE EXTERNAL SEXUAL ORGANS

UNDIFFERENTIATED

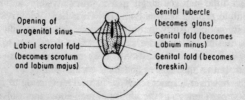

Opening of urogenital sinus

Labial scrotal fold (becomes scrotum and labium majus)

Genital tubercle (becomes glans)

Genital fold (becomes Labium minus)

Genital fold (becomes foreskin)

MALE

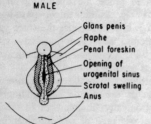

Glans penis
Raphe
Penal foreskin
Opening of urogenital sinus
Scrotal swelling
Anus

FEMALE

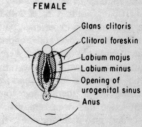

Glans clitoris
Clitoral foreskin
Labium majus
Labium minus
Opening of urogenital sinus
Anus

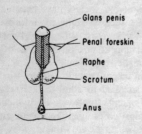

Glans penis
Penal foreskin
Raphe
Scrotum
Anus

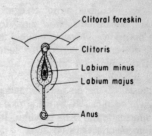

Clitoral foreskin
Clitoris
Labium minus
Labium majus
Anus

pleasure is all too often offset by her parents' stern warnings not to play with anything "dirty" or of a sexual nature. This results in enormous anxiety and guilt concerning the exploration of her own body, an exploration that is the most natural urge of humanity.

Instead of having a knowledgeable feeling of comfort about their vaginas, then, little girls are caught in a complex mystery, and no one seems willing to explain what is going on. Girls hear old wives' tales and horror stories that fill them only with fear. They are told not to touch boys, not to bathe in the same water as boys, not to touch themselves, and not to ask questions. They grow up suspicious not only of men, but of themselves and their own sexuality.

Most girls, however, cannot resist the natural temptation to explore their own bodies. They go to the library to read about themselves and their vaginas. They even begin to probe the opening with their fingertips. Here they meet with trouble. As their fingers push against the hymen, they experience pain, which underlines the scare tactics used by their parents and grandparents. "Keep your fingers away from that, it is dangerous," they were told. And when they experience the pain on their own, those warnings seem warranted.

Of course, in recent years, attitudes toward sex education have become more liberal, and some of the stigma surrounding self-knowledge has been removed. Ironically, in many of the world's so-called primitive societies, the exchange of sex information between generations is considered an early responsibility of the tribe elders.

As liberalized as some segments of our society have become, the fact remains that *most* girls do not receive sufficient information. Confusion and mystery cloud the early years. When a girl gets her first menstrual period, the sudden appearance of blood is often a frightening, and sometimes a traumatic, experience.

It has been consistently shown in recent years that many—indeed, most—of the emotional traumas attached to adult sexual behavior have been caused by the refusal of parents to provide enough *correct* information to their children. In most cases, girls receive even less information than boys, so it follows that, as women, they must overcome even greater fears. Not surprisingly, many women come to regard the opposite sex with fear, suspicion, and confusion. And emotional friction between men and women serves no one.

The solutions are so simple.

First, there must be an open and honest communication between the girl and her parents. The differences between boys and girls should be examined, as should any other questions that arise in the girl's mind. Perhaps most important, every girl should be infused with the excitement and joy peculiar to becoming a woman.

Second, every girl should be given access to books which will help explain her budding sexuality. These books should show all the functions and relationships of the sexual organs. They should also provide clear illustrations, either drawings or photographs. (Be very careful in selecting the books you give to your daughter. Surprisingly, many of the new sex education books for children merely reflect the sexist attitudes of their authors. For example, there are many books that have no mention of the clitoris. Diagrams of the vaginal area *should* include graphic representation of the clitoris, followed by an explanation of its function.)

Third, girls should be given freedom to explore their own bodies without incurring the disapproval of their elders or their peers. Every child has a normal urge to explore her body, and this should be encouraged, not discouraged. As an adult, the more a woman knows about her body and its functions, the more she can appreciate the impulses constantly in motion within her. The more a woman knows about sex, the more she will be able to enjoy it.

EXPLORING YOUR VULVA

Many women mistakenly believe the vulva is itself an organ. They have heard their friends and physicians refer to it, and they have read books in which the word *vulva* is frequently used but never explained. The vulva, though, is not one specific organ. Instead, it is the name given the *entire outer area* of a woman's genital-urethral organs. The vulva comprises the *labia majora* (large lips), *labia minora* (small lips), the clitoris, the urethral opening, and the vaginal opening. The anus and the pubic hair are not, technically, considered part of the vulva, even though most discussions of the vulva inevitably mention them because of their close proximity to the vulva.

Mirrors

Throughout history, mirrors have been used to do more than can be described in this book. If ever there was an object whose development arose from insatiable curiosity, it is the mirror. From the beginning of time, men and women alike have enjoyed seeing their images reflected in a piece of glass. Unfortunately, in many minds, the mirror became to vanity what food was to gluttony; unfortunately, because

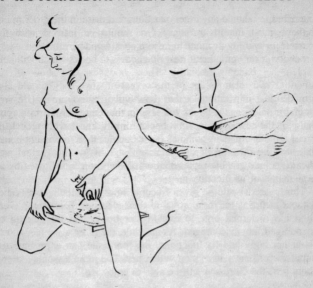

Fig. 1–2: Pictured here are two positions that are easy for most women to achieve in self-examination of the vulva.

At left, a woman is standing on her slightly separated knees with a mirror between her legs. This mirror is tilted, allowing the woman a clear view of her vulva through its reflection in the mirror. If the reflection is too dark, focus a beam of light against the vulval area.

At right, the self-examination is shown as it occurs in the lotus position. Here, the mirror is resting on the legs, giving you two free hands to spread the vulva apart, which will allow you to examine more specific portions of the vulva.

the mirror is one of the world's most useful tools, and to confuse healthy curiosity with vanity is a sad mistake.

Unless you are a skilled contortionist, the mirror will be the most valuable tool at your disposal in examining your vulva. Certainly it will help you examine the outside region, but it will also, to a certain extent, allow you to look inside yourself.

Many physicians feel that mothers should use mirrors to show their daughters the exact location of the pelvic organs. Whether or not one subscribes to that theory, it must be admitted that a mirror, per se, is neither evil nor morally wrong. To use a mirror to learn more about yourself and your body could hardly be considered harmful; indeed, it can and will do you a great deal of good.

Position

In using a mirror to examine your vulva, there are two easily attainable positions. You may either sit in the lotus position with your legs comfortably crossed, or you can simply kneel with your legs spread. In either position, you can lean backward or forward to reach the most comfortable state.

Regardless of which position you have chosen, place the mirror underneath you, between your legs. This will give you a relatively good view of the general area. To get a more specific view, though, you should use a flashlight, aiming it at the specific organs you wish to examine in detail. When you are doing this, you may also want to move the mirror closer to the specific organ you are examining.

Some women prefer using a mirror with some degree of magnification. This is certainly understandable, but it would probably be best to start with a mirror that will reflect the exact size of the organs. Once you have done that, though, you should feel free to use whatever sort of mirror you desire.

Labia Majora

Now that you are in a comfortable position and examining yourself with a mirror, the first organ to come to your attention will probably be the *labia majora*, or large lips. The *labia majora* contain deposits of fatty tissue and are covered with hair. As women get older, these lips become more flaccid and will contain less fatty tissue. In very old women, the large lips usually become just atrophic membranes, or shapeless pieces of skin.

These large lips may appear useless, but in fact they are extremely functional. The fat and the hair combine so that the large lips completely cover the vagina. In this way, no dirt or sweat can work its way into the vaginal opening. It might be said that the large lips are nature's contribution to preventive medicine. By protecting against dirt, the lips prevent a great deal of infection and disease.

Labia Minora

As the large lips are pulled aside, you will have a clear view of the *labia minora*, or small lips. These small lips are without hair, but they

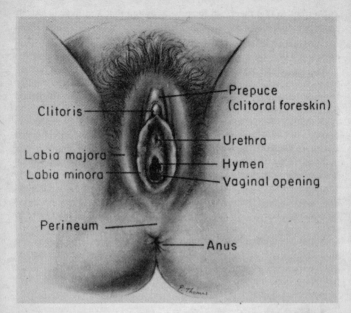

Fig. 1–3: Above is a drawing of a vulva showing the normal anatomical relationship between the various parts of the vulva and the pubic hair and rectal opening (the anus). Every woman is slightly different and so is each vulva. Because of this, during self-examination, you shouldn't be disappointed if the anatomical parts of your vulva are not as easy to recognize as those in this drawing. The *labia majora* are here separated to allow a better view of the outer part of the vagina, locating the urethra and the hymen ring surrounding the vaginal opening.

serve the same general purpose as the large lips—protection from dirt. They are the backup system, the secondary covering.

The small lips also play an important role in sexual activity. During any sort of sexually excited state, blood rushes to the small lips, filling and enlarging them in the same way blood causes an erection in the male penis. When a woman engages in intercourse, this sudden growth of the small lips creates a tighter grip around the penis, resulting in more pleasure for both parties. This enlargement also gives more cover to the vaginal opening, and so can help keep the sperm in the vagina after intercourse.

During masturbation, the small lips are incredibly sensitive in their enlarged state. This, of course, should give greater physical pleasure.

The small lips are completely covered by the *labia majora* during early childhood, but as a girl becomes a woman, the small lips usually begin to protrude past the large lips to varying degrees. The small lips do, indeed, become larger for a variety of reasons.

First, the genetic factor undeniably influences the entire physical structure of each human being. Just as genes are responsible for the size and shape of the nose, they are equally responsible for the makeup of the *labia minora*. Some women will naturally have more pronounced *labia minora* than other women.

Second, extensive sexual activity, be it intercourse or masturbation, will also cause the *labia minora* to protrude beyond the large lips. Sexual activity stretches the *labia minora*, just as it stretches, to some extent, the penis. For example, women of African tribes usually have very pronounced *labia minora,* a fact sometimes attributed to the encouragement of early sex play in these tribes. Generally speaking, the more a woman masturbates or has intercourse, the larger her small lips become.

It follows that childbirth and abortion also stretch the small lips, though probably to a lesser extent, due to the relative infrequency of such events.

In rare cases, the *labia minora* might become so large that they cover the vagina to an extent that interferes with intercourse. If this happens, the excess skin can be surgically removed, restoring the *labia minora* to a more functional state.

The Clitoris

When one sees an early-developed fetus, it is impossible to determine whether it is a boy or a girl because the stemlike area in the pubic region could be either a clitoris or a penis. If it is a boy, this stem will grow into a penis; if it is a girl, the stem will open up into a vulva and vagina, with the clitoris remaining as what was the base of the early stem.

As you pull the large lips apart, the clitoris will be seen at the top of the inside folds where the large and small lips come together. The *prepuce*, or clitoral foreskin, is the name given to the additional folds which sit on the small lips at an angle and look like a triangular hat. The clitoris is directly in the middle of this small hat. In girls, the

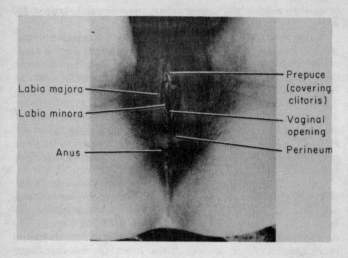

Fig. 1–4: Shown above is a photograph of the vulval area of a twenty-year-old woman. One can clearly see hair covering the *labia majora*. As in the majority of women, the clitoris is not completely visible and is covered by the *prepuce,* or clitoral foreskin. To see the clitoris, the prepuce must be pushed up. The *labia minora* are seen protruding between the *labia majora.* Notice also that the *labia minora* is without hair. The size of the *labia minora* varies from woman to woman. This difference can be traced partially to genetic factors and partially to sexual activity. The vaginal opening is visible between the *labia minora.* The area between the lower portion of the labia and the anus is called the *perineum.* Most women who have borne children will have scars in the area of the perineum. This scar is from the *episiotomy*—the cut made to enable the passage of the baby during delivery.

prepuce covers the clitoris very tightly, but it loosens its grip on the gland as the girl becomes a woman. If it does not loosen its hold, a portion of the prepuce can be removed, a process akin to circumcision.

When you get the head of the clitoris between your fingers, you can feel it as a small mass and that is what it is—a small mass, or a gland.

When you play with the clitoris, you will find that, like a penis, it is an extremely sensitive area, and it will become stiffer and larger with manipulation. By extensive clitoral play, you will usually bring on an orgasm.

It is important to bring on this sensation by self-manipulation, and you should train yourself to do it for two major reasons. First, it will enable you to recognize an orgasm when you have one, and second, the more these organs are trained to reflexive action, the easier it becomes to have an orgasm.

Unfortunately, the clitoris is in a rather inconvenient position for intercourse. It is, sexually speaking, too high up in the vulvar region. When the penis enters the vagina, it will not usually rub against the clitoris. The lack of stimulation to the clitoris is, perhaps, the main problem in intercourse. Because of this, it is often necessary for either a woman or her partner to stimulate her clitoris during intercourse.

Orgasm is not caused merely by clitoral sensation, but by the nerves of the entire, sensitized vulvar area. Each woman must explore and manipulate each organ to find out which one is the most sensitized and most likely to bring orgasm.

The clitoris becomes larger with extensive masturbation or manipulation. The size of the clitoris is also genetically factored. Some women have larger clitorises than others. But the size of the clitoris has no influence on the facility to reach orgasm. What is influential is the training and learning of the reflexes of the nerve endings.

SEEING INSIDE

The Hymen

When looking inside the *labia minora*, it is usually a good idea to insert a finger into the vaginal opening, using the finger to stretch the opening to allow a better view. About half an inch inside the vaginal opening, you will see a small membrane or rudiment of a membrane. This is the *hymen*. The hymen is usually broken after the first intercourse, but fragments of it exist throughout a woman's life. When it is broken, the hymen looks like small pieces of flesh sitting along the half-inch circumference of the vaginal wall. Occasionally, the hymen lingers as a long piece of flesh, and this can be surgically removed if it is bothersome.

Some women are born with extremely small hymens. These women will have little problem or pain upon first intercourse, and sometimes the hymen does not even rip.

Other women are born with hymens almost completely closed. Sometimes the hymen is so tight it is almost impossible to penetrate during intercourse. In such an event, the hymen might have to be opened by surgery *(hymenectomy)*. In most cases, though, patience and a slowly induced finger can break the closed hymen, even one that will not allow the penetration of a penis. With some women, an emotionally or physically traumatic event will open the hymen.

Of course, the hymen can open during horseback riding, or bicycling, or even because of a simple fall. In cultures where virginity is prized above all else in brides, many a tragic horseback ride has been confessed in many a bedroom.

The Vagina

If you have not yet had intercourse, it might be impossible to explore deeper into yourself with a mirror and a light. The hymen might obstruct a clear view.

On the other hand, even if you have had intercourse, it might still be difficult for you to see into the vagina. The reason is simple. Although many people (women included) think of the vagina as a sort of hole, it is, in fact, a *collapsed space surrounded by muscle*. Some physicians and women prefer the term *muscle tube* in describing the vagina.

Being comprised of muscle, the vagina is controllable. You can train yourself to contract and/or expand these muscles. The effect is obvious—it increases sexual pleasure. During intercourse, a woman tightens the muscles around the penis, giving not only the man, but herself as well, more sensation, since more friction is created between the penis and the vaginal walls.

Under certain physical and/or psychological situations, the muscles of the vagina will tighten to the degree where it becomes difficult for the man to pull out. This can, of course, be desirable if planned and controlled, but if it is an accidental reflex, the woman must train herself to relax and train her muscles to respond to her desires. If this happens and the woman has not yet learned to relax, nature still compensates. At the moment of orgasm, the upper part of the vagina balloons out, almost like a silent explosion, after which the muscle tension naturally decreases and the man is able to withdraw.

Vaginismus is a more serious problem. Again, for either physical or psychological reasons, this condition occurs when the muscles of the vagina tighten so much that nothing, much less an erect penis, can enter the space. This problem will be explored fully later in this book.

The length of the vagina has been the topic of discussions ranging from the *Kama Sutra* to the locker room. Just as men and women

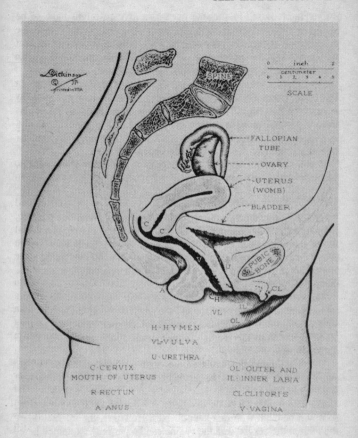

Fig. 1–5: This picture shows the relationship in position and size of the pelvic organs in a standing woman. The uterus in this drawing is in the *anteverted,* or front, position. It should also be clear that the vagina is not a hole, but a collapsed space directed backward and connected to the uterus by the cervix at an almost right angle. Notice that the clitoris is located at least an inch from the opening of the vagina. For this reason, during normal intercourse, no direct rubbing of the clitoris takes place. (Dickinson Anatomical Chart—reproduced by permission of Educational Department, TAMPAX Incorporated, Lake Success, New York.)

believe many myths concerning the length of a penis, they are apt to be just as silly about the length of a vagina. In general, black women have longer, deeper vaginas than their white European counterparts. However, unless a woman has hang-ups about this, the length of the vagina has no bearing on either productivity or enjoyment.

Most surface abnormalities in the vagina, like warts or discharges, will be seen through the mirror. With discharges, it is very important to note the coloring. This can aid in the diagnosis of an infection. Venereal warts, brought on by a sexual virus, are in the back part of the vagina and drain out with a discharge. The warts sometimes spread all the way down to the rectal opening.

If you see either warts or discharges, or any other abnormalities that worry you, see your physician.

The Cervix

By sitting down on your heels or by standing up with one leg on a chair or toilet seat, you can merely bend down and insert your index finger or middle finger into the vagina. As you push your finger deeply into the vagina, you will feel something like the tip of your nose. This is the *cervix*. It is a hard area with a small depression in the middle at the top of the vagina.

The cervix serves as a valve between the vagina and the uterus (which lies behind the cervix), and the small depression that you feel with your finger is the tiny hole through which sperm enter the uterus, blood flows from the uterus during menstruation, and babies come during birth.

The area around the cervix on the vaginal side is called the *fornix*, and it not only surrounds the cervix but serves as the outer, protective wall of the uterus.

The uterus will not be accessible to you during a self-examination, so it will be dealt with in a later chapter. However, the interaction of the uterus, the cervix, and the vagina can be partially explained here.

During intercourse, the penis may push hard against the cervix, hitting the uterus and throwing it higher up inside you. Certainly this will be more frequent when you are in the superior position, because the muscles push down on the bladder, shortening the vagina. You should not worry about this, unless, of course, there is unusual pain during or after sex. If you have an intrauterine device, your partner may think he is hitting the IUD and he might complain. Although this is possible, it is much more likely that he is, instead, pushing against the cervix.

In some positions, the uterus is tilted into an abnormal position, and this may cause some pain. This depends on the length of the vagina, and may be avoided by knowing that the vagina achieves different lengths in different positions. You may feel how this happens by moving from one position to another by yourself with your finger in the vagina. You will notice how the vagina expands and contracts as you move. This is, of course, an interaction with the uterus, which is pushing against or away from the top of the vagina. Because of this tendency, the knee-chest position is a favorite of many women, especially those with shorter vaginas. In the knee-chest position, the vagina is stretched to its greatest extent, usually allowing the greatest degree of pleasure.

Obviously, when examining the vagina and the cervix with your fingers, if you feel a lump or something that you think is irregular, you should ask your physician about it. In fact, if you have any questions concerning any part of your self-examination, you should not hesitate to bring it up with your gynecologist.

With your finger, you will probably be able to palpate, or touch, the cervix. If you have an IUD, this palpation is particularly important (see Chapter 9), but even if you don't have an IUD, it is useful to be able to judge the depth and the breadth of your vagina by such a palpation.

EXTRA TEXTURES

Usually considered a part of the vulva are the anus (rectal opening) and the pubic hair. In fact, they are separate from the vulva, but their close proximity makes it convenient to examine them at the same time as you are exploring your vulva.

Pubic Hair

The hair covering the *mons pubis* is another dirt-collecting agency, protecting the orifice below. It also absorbs a great deal of sweat.

Pubic hair should generally be in a triangle, the top of which is usually a fairly straight line. Orientals generally have less pubic hair, and do not necessarily have a straight upper line. In blacks and white European women, however, if the upper line of the pubic hair moves in a triangular direction toward the navel, it usually indicates a higher than average presence of male hormones in the system. If this is true, the hair itself will also be of the male hormone type, and there will

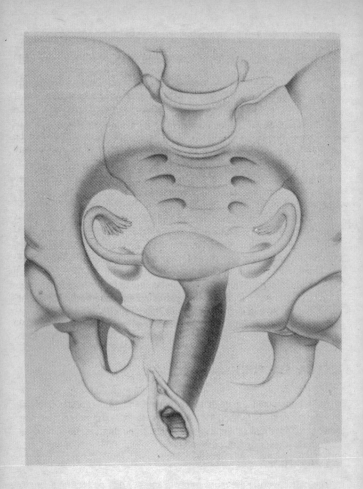

Fig. 1–6: A frontal view of the female reproductive organs, showing their relation in size and position to the pelvic bones. The vulva and the vaginal opening are clear. The muscular tube of the vagina is pointed to the back and the cervix can just be seen in the upper portion of the vagina. The uterus is tilted forward, antiverted in the normal position, and the fallopian tubes lead away from the uterus toward the egg-shaped ovaries. (Reproduced by permission of Ortho Pharmaceutical Corporation, Raritan, New Jersey.)

probably be more hair on the legs, arms, and even perhaps on the face.

Possessing more male hormones in no way affects your femininity or your womanhood. It is probably just a genetic happenstance. But if you recognize this tendency, you should be aware that it is often associated with a condition known as polycystic ovaries, or Stein-Leventhal disease, discussed in Chapter 14. This condition can be evaluated by your physician, and he should be able to answer any questions you have.

The Anus (Rectal Opening)

Approximately one or two fingers'-breadth below the lower end of the vagina, you will see the anus, or the opening to the rectum. This is usually a very tight area, but if you engage in frequent anal intercourse, it will appear more relaxed. Also, the area around the rectal opening is usually very smooth, but after childbirth there might be external hemorrhoids, which are seen as pieces of flesh sitting on the outside.

Any lumps, warts, or other irregularities that you see around the rectum should be reported to your doctor, who can check them out. If these irregularities are not serious (such as prickly heat), be sure you can recognize them the next time around. It will save you needless, but normal, worry.

chapter 2

HOW TO CHOOSE A GYNECOLOGIST

Many women have more trouble finding a good gynecologist than Stanley had tracking down Livingstone. Some women, trying to avoid the dilemma of a search altogether, give the matter little thought. They quickly settle either on someone in the neighborhood or become loyal, if dissatisfied, patients of their mother's gynecologist. Other women realize they must shop around to find a doctor they like, just as they must shop around for any good buy. The trouble here is that many of these women are insecure about judging doctors (it is something they have been taught by society not to do), or they are not sure they could recognize a good gynecologist if they saw one.

The easiest way to begin this search is by eliminating certain doctors who don't fulfill even the simple basics of the profession.

If a gynecologist is cold or unsympathetic, he probably won't be able to support your emotional needs. If the physician is rushed during your first examination, or if he is terribly disorganized, you will probably have to look elsewhere. You want a gynecologist who doesn't resent the time spent with patients, and you want one organized at least to the point that it is your file he's reading when he's with you. For most women, unusually high fees are another basic that sends them elsewhere. It must always be remembered that high fees do not necessarily guarantee good medicine.

These are basics that everyone knows. Still, they must be repeated time and again. Unfortunately, even these do not provide sufficient information for choosing a gynecologist who is right for you.

This book cannot offer a definitive list of competent gynecologists, but it can give you some basic guidelines for finding a good one. In following these guidelines, you must be as tough and as critical as you would be in any other area of your life. It is a very important *personal* decision, but it is also a hard *business* decision; you are paying money and you should get the very best value for your dollar. We live in an age of consumer activism; and choosing a gynecologist should be approached, at least in part, as a *consumer* decision.

Although you must find a physician with complete technical competence, he must also fit your specific psychological and emotional needs. The human element is very important—a technically superb gynecologist may be right for your neighbor's emotional needs, but wrong for yours. It is essential to find a doctor with whom you can relate easily. Such a doctor will make you feel as comfortable as possible and will gain, as well as earn, your trust and confidence.

After all, you and your doctor are engaged in the healing process. To accomplish this, you will be working closely together. If there is little or no rapport between the two of you, the healing process will suffer.

Of course, you should have alternatives from which to choose. To settle on the first doctor you hear mentioned would be unfair to both you and the physician. Neither should you rely solely on the advice of family or friends. A doctor who is good for your mother, your sister, or your best friend still may not be good for you.

If you are a young woman and your mother's doctor is older, as is often the case, his opinions about birth control or his knowledge of the latest techniques may not be compatible with your needs. His practice, in this case, would probably consist mostly of older women, contemporaries of your mother, whose problems, illnesses, and emotional needs would be different from those a younger woman would have.

Usually younger women want a doctor closer to their own age, not only for his more recent medical training, but also because it may be easier to relate personally to someone more contemporary. Such a physician will also be able to tend the younger woman throughout her lifetime, just as her mother's doctor tended her for years.

Some younger women are concerned also that their mother's doctor might, as a gesture of innocent friendship, tell the mother more about the daughter than the daughter wishes her to know. Whether this is classified as spying or as motherly concern, the problem is avoided by finding your own doctor.

HOW TO FIND A GOOD DOCTOR

The selection process begins by seeking advice from trusted friends. As different doctors are discussed, you should discover how long your friend has been seeing the gynecologist she has recommended. A woman who has seen a doctor for years is undoubtedly more qualified to judge than a woman who has been seeing one for only six months.

You should also find out the recommended doctor's opinions on such matters as abortion, birth control, estrogen therapy, or any other topic which concerns you. Regardless of a physician's skill, most women prefer gynecologists to share at least some of their beliefs. Again, get the name of more than one doctor—you may have to visit quite a few before finding one who is compatible with your beliefs.

If you have moved to a new town or if your friends fail to supply you with satisfactory choices, you might get the information you need from the nearest good hospital, preferably one associated with a medical school. The chief resident of the hospital should be able to help, as should a hospital administrator or any other knowledgeable staff worker. Such a person should give you three or four names to consider. This can be particularly valuable when you are seeking a second opinion.

You may wish to visit a nearby hospital to seek advice. Nurses and interns, both of whom work closely with a number of doctors, can often give well-grounded opinions about the better doctors on the staff. Better yet, interns and nurses often are not caught up in the medical game of protecting other doctors.

A local Planned Parenthood chapter or the county medical society can usually provide the names of a number of well-qualified gynecologists in the area.

If you are specifically looking for a woman gynecologist, you should contact the American Medical Women's Association in your area for their recommendations. Be advised, though, that as a medical association, they cannot recommend one doctor over another; they can only supply a list of women gynecologists, from which you will have to do further study. In many areas, the National Organization of Women (NOW) can refer you to a women's health organization.

Certainly one of the most common methods of choosing a gynecologist is to ask your own internist or family doctor, if you have one, particularly if you are pleased with him. Good doctors tend to associate with other good doctors, and should be an excellent source of referrals.

HOW TO EXAMINE YOUR GYNECOLOGIST

After you have the names of several recommended gynecologists, you will want to find out more about them for yourself. You may be justifiably concerned about not having the medical background to decide which doctor is most qualified for your needs. The average person is not expected to have medical training, but there are still some simple ways to evaluate a doctor.

Start by looking up the doctors who interest you in the *Directory of Medical Specialists,* available in medical libraries, many public libraries, and at local county medical society offices. The directory lists a physician's birthdate, medical school, and the hospital where he took his residency. This information is a good point of departure. An older physician may be more traditional in his outlook and perhaps less involved with the latest ideas or techniques. Perhaps a younger doctor's practice may not be as large, allowing him more time per patient.

Although medical schools are not all alike, they all provide a basic standard of education. Because of this, the medical school a particular doctor attended is not, by itself, grounds for determining a doctor's qualifications. More important is where the physician took his residency, because this is the institution where he received training in his specialty. Hospitals or medical centers associated with medical schools are usually the best places to serve a residency. These are teaching hospitals, in which doctors become familiar with a greater variety of cases and conditions than is possible at smaller or nonteaching hospitals. A residency lasts a long time, generally three to five years. A longer residency training usually produces a more qualified physician, so you should take special note of the length of residency. Taking residency at a good hospital associated with a medical school generally indicates a high-quality physician.

There are other factors you may wish to consider. If a woman favors abortion, for example, and she notices that a doctor was trained in a Catholic medical school or hospital, she would probably do better to find someone else. This is not merely a philosophical problem, but can be one of practical experience as well. As Catholic hospitals perform very few abortions, the doctors trained there are not nearly as experienced in this procedure.

The directory also provides a physician's hospital affiliation. Good hospitals are your best assurance of quality medical care, and a doctor's ability is strongly indicated by which hospital has appointed him to its staff. The best physicians are usually affiliated with the best hospitals, and the best hospitals are those associated with medical schools. Remember, this is the hospital where you, as a patient, may be admitted, so it bears serious consideration. The hospital reflects the care you may receive, as well as the doctor's standing within his profession.

Another important consideration that is sometimes overlooked by the general public is that of a physician's board certification. Board certification indicates a true specialist in a particular field; in this case, gynecology. To become board certified, a doctor must train in residency for three to five years and pass several difficult examinations in his specialty. These examinations have a failure rate of nearly 40 percent. Passing these boards indicates a doctor of top professional standing in his specialty. The doctors who complete these requirements are known as board certified, while physicians completing all but the final examination are board eligible, which is almost as significant. Studies have shown that specialists holding board certification provide a significantly higher standard of medical care. A doctor may call himself a specialist even without passing these boards, so it is your responsibility to examine this fine point. Whenever possible, especially if you have a complex problem, you should seek a doctor who is board certified. This information is available from the *Directory of Medical Specialists*, local medical societies, and some libraries. You might even ask the gynecologist or his secretary in which specialty he holds certification.

After you have checked out a number of physicians and narrowed your list on the basis of their qualifications, you should call their offices and compare fees. A polite question to the secretary about the doctor's fee for your initial visit and examination is completely proper, and you should not hesitate to ask. It makes no sense to pay one physician significantly more for the same services provided by another, equally qualified, physician.

It is also an excellent idea to talk with the gynecologist and discuss your personal needs. This is a good way to determine if the two of you are emotionally and philosophically compatible. If he is too busy to talk to you or fails to return your call, he probably is not the man for you. You may have a particular problem (infertility, for example), with which you want special help. Doctors often have subspecialties within their specialties. In this case, you would want to consult a gynecologist whose subspecialty is infertility.

Contrary to popular myth, studies have shown that doctors who are members of group practices usually provide a better standard of care than single or "solo" doctors. The environment of several doctors consulting and checking one another's results naturally keeps doctors at peak performance.

THE GYNECOLOGIST AS PRIMARY PHYSICIAN

The changing life-styles of women have led to changes in the role of the gynecologist. More women than ever before see their gynecologists for problems unrelated to the reproductive organs. In many cases, the gynecologist has replaced the family doctor or general practitioner as the primary physician. Consequently, it is likely that you will see your gynecologist for many reasons, and he should perform routine checks for high blood pressure, diabetes, and similar illnesses.

There is a faction of the American College of Obstetricians and Gynecologists which feels a gynecologist should be educated in the fields of gynecology, obstetrics, family planning and abortion, endocrinology (the study of glands, such as the thyroid or pituitary), and surgery. He should have widespread education in medicine and medical diseases, so he can serve as a primary physician, able both to treat a woman for minor illness and to make knowledgeable referrals to specialists in more serious cases. Gynecologists themselves are accepting this new responsibility of becoming the primary physician.

As with any physician, you certainly should not wait for an emergency to try to locate a gynecologist. This is especially true if he is to serve as your primary physician. Find yourself a doctor *now*, when you can think slowly and logically. Do not wait until you are under the stress and emotion of an emergency, when you must take whomever you can get.

A MAN OR WOMAN GYNECOLOGIST?

While most women realize the necessity of gynecological examinations, it is, nonetheless, an uncomfortable experience. Some women are uneasy because the examining physician is male; others are reassured by that very fact. Many women seek women gynecologists, feeling they are better able to relate to a woman doctor, while others feel no need to do so. This is perhaps the single most personal decision you must make in finding a gynecologist who is right for you.

Medicine is still dominated in this country by men, and there are far more male gynecologists than female. In fact, only 9.4 percent of American, board-certified gynecologists are women. There has been, however, a recent influx of women into gynecology residency programs, and this male dominance may eventually come to an end.

Still, this does not indicate any difference in ability based on sex. Given the same training, men and women should be of equally high caliber. In Russia, for example, nearly 65 percent of all physicians are women. It is probably the traditional American sex bias that is responsible for the small percentage of women in medicine, as well as the feeling that women doctors are somehow inferior to their male counterparts. There is certainly no room in the medical profession for such opinions, nor for jealousy between men and women gynecologists.

As a matter of practical consideration, however, men have been given greater opportunities, especially in the past, to receive medical training. Residency programs have provided many more men than women with opportunities for advanced work. It stands to reason that more advanced training produces better physicians. So, while many women are excellent physicians, others have not been afforded the opportunities for equal training, especially in surgery and other complex specialties.

Gynecology is a relatively new field. Many of the older gynecologists were general practitioners, or perhaps surgeons, who went into gynecology. Their training in advanced or developing fields, such as endocrinology, may not be the latest, be they male or female. You may find some older female gynecologists with a strong antimale bias, or older males with strong feelings on what is proper conduct for a woman. While each physician certainly has an individual identity, points like these should be considered when you are personally evaluating a gynecologist.

Some women feel they can more easily identify with a female gynecologist, and this transference of identity eases their fears and apprehensions during examinations. Or you may simply feel more comfortable being examined by a woman. Perhaps it is easier for you to relate to a younger, woman gynecologist, finding you have a lot in common socially and philosophically. If you think you would best relate to a woman of your own generation, then you should find such a doctor. Conversely, many women believe they can be more honest with a doctor of the opposite sex. They are more at ease asking questions and more comfortable during the examinations, sometimes to the point where they do not even wish to have a woman nurse in the room during the examination.

What is really being discussed is the association between you and your physician. If you are looking for a young woman doctor whom you can treat as a friend as well as a physician, then find one. If you feel more comfortable with a male, that's fine, too, and you will have a few more to choose from. You are seeking an honest, open, and therapeutic relationship with your gynecologist, so consult whichever sex best helps you fulfill this relationship.

GAMES NOT TO PLAY

By now, you should be able to identify a physician who is highly qualified. There are, however, several popular but ill-conceived notions about what makes a good doctor. This folklore has absolutely nothing to do with the quality of medical care. For example, many people are concerned with the social status of a physician or the status of his patients. A wealthy society doctor with patients of high social standing certainly indicates a high fee, but says little about the caliber of the physician. It is easy to see how such a notion developed, but it is equally clear that there are better considerations for choosing a gynecologist than simply "all the best people use him." The same can be said for doctors in exclusive neighborhoods or for those who charge significantly higher fees. It is entirely possible in the case of a specialist or an exceptional physician that high fees are indeed appropriate, but fees *themselves* say nothing about the quality of care. The quality of a physician is determined by his education and expertise, not his fee. Doctors in the most exclusive neighborhoods with higher office rents must pass these high rents on to the patients. You are paying for medical care, not a classy address, and should act accordingly.

You should not be greatly influenced by the size of a doctor's practice. A large practice is no guarantee of a fine physician. Perhaps the physician does not refer enough patients to other doctors, or maybe he has not solved the problems of his own patients. Also, consider that while a younger doctor may be equally skilled, it normally takes several years to establish a sizable practice. It can be to your advantage to catch a new doctor when he is young and eager, and you may receive less hurried and more personal care. Then, of course, you will find the physician who cannot possibly see you for at least a month. Usually even the best specialist can see you within two weeks. If you have to wait much longer, perhaps the physician already has more patients than he can handle, or perhaps he plays a lot of golf. Either way, a long wait for an appointment, unless it is for something quite specialized, tells you nothing about the caliber of the physician. The same can be said for a gynecologist who consistently

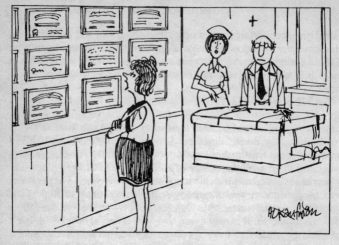

*"No wonder you don't know what's wrong with me. You spent
half your life in school!"*

Fig. 2–1: Reproduced by permission of the artist, Al Kaufman, and
Ob. Gyn. News, Rockville, Maryland.

keeps you waiting for long periods in his office for your appointment.
Maybe he feels you have nothing better to do with your time or thinks
you really enjoy reading those health magazines all afternoon.
Occasional delays and reasonable waits are to be expected, but there
seems no logical reason why you should select a gynecologist who
schedules too many patients in too short a time, unless you enjoy
being examined by an overworked physician.

THE DOCTOR'S PERSONAL SIDE

Besides seeking someone who is medically well qualified, you are
also looking for a physician with whom you can establish a personal
relationship. It is important for your medical care that you be able to
communicate easily with your gynecologist, and to do so, you must
have a comfortable relationship with the physician. Each woman
naturally seeks a different psychological and emotional relationship
with her gynecologist. To accommodate the patient, a gynecologist
must often fulfill somewhat different roles for different patients. Some
women prefer a gynecologist who is somewhat paternalistic, who acts
like a reassuring father. Other women wish to keep the relationship on

a strictly matter-of-fact basis, or perhaps even prefer a gynecologist who is aloof and more of an adviser. Gynecologists are usually aware of their patients' varying psychological needs and try to act accordingly. It is most important that the two of you are satisfied with the nature of your relationship.

You certainly should expect the gynecologist to treat you personally and to sympathize with your problems and concerns. Being rushed through a doctor's office makes any woman feel slighted, as well as indicating the physician's lack of personal concern. There are any number of qualified physicians, and you need not tolerate being tossed about by a gynecologist who is consistently too busy.

Women should not allow their gynecologists to hide behind the mystique and prestige of the medical world. Physicians who adopt rigidly medical postures or who frequently confuse you with endless medical jargon may be intentionally building a barrier between you, the lowly patient, and him, the seer of science. This mystique makes it all the more difficult to communicate with him and to establish a comfortable relationship. Gynecology has made many advances in

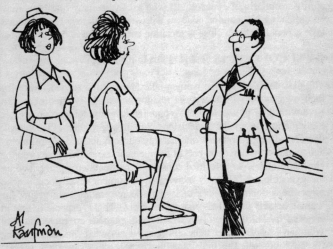

'I can't explain it in laymen's terms.
I don't know any laymen's terms.'

Fig. 2–2: Reproduced by permission of the artist, Al Kaufman, and *Ob. Gyn. News*, Rockville, Maryland.

recent years, but a doctor who insists on acting like a mystical and inscrutable Merlin is ignoring the fact that he is treating intelligent women who want hard talk, not a Latin lesson.

As a patient, you should not tolerate a doctor who treats you in a condescending manner, shields you from reality, or assumes you cannot make your own decisions. The discussions between the two of you should be open and honest. You have the right to expect a physician to take time to answer your questions thoughtfully and sympathetically. You want somebody who understands your concerns and answers your questions in plain English. It is not difficult for a physician to explain a problem or procedure to you in language that you can understand, and it certainly helps your peace of mind to know exactly what is happening. A physician who constantly answers your questions with, "Don't worry, it will be all right," or, "Why don't you just leave that to me," is not giving you the consideration you deserve. He is violating your right to know, and shows little respect for your concern and intelligence. Physicians should not regard questions, if they are properly put, as challenges to their medical authority or ability. Similarly, a gynecologist who asks you many questions may be indicating his genuine concern with your problems. This give and take is beneficial to a close association between you and your doctor.

GYNECOLOGY IS A MUTUAL EFFORT

The past decade has seen women take more active responsibility for their own lives. This affects the relationship many women expect to have with their gynecologists. Women are rightly demanding greater participation in medical decisions which affect them. They seek doctors willing to present alternative solutions to medical problems and to allow women to be part of the medical team. This gives you the chance to offer your informed consent to the treatments prescribed by the gynecologist. There is increasing resentment of physicians who prescribe a treatment more or less by decree, rather than giving the woman herself several alternative solutions. This is especially true in areas such as birth control, in which some methods are more suited to you than others. Rather than telling a woman what she will be using for birth control, the understanding gynecologist describes several methods and their respective advantages, allowing the woman to participate in the selection of the method most suited to her own life-style. This gives you more active control over your medical and sexual life. The gynecologist is your *partner,* not an omnipotent medical seer. As a team in active partnership, you can proceed for your mutual benefit.

If you are partners, a doctor cannot simply tell you what to do. You want a doctor to inform you of your options and state a medical opinion. To remain independent, however, you cannot allow the gynecologist to impose his morality or opinions upon you. As often as is possible, a doctor should be a neutral observer, giving you the opinions and information necessary for both of you to reach decisions. There are obviously times when a doctor must not remain neutral, and he would be negligent of his medical responsibilities if he did not insist on a specific course of action. This, however, is a matter of medical expertise, and not a decision based on personal moral codes. If, after informed discussion, you disagree with your doctor's course of treatment, by all means seek a second opinion from another physician.

What we must realize is that gynecologists are, or should be, healers. They are not philosophers or moral leaders. Gynecologists have no business deciding the moral· or sexual standards of their patients. A doctor has no right to deny you the ability to make judgments which affect your life.

If you are an unmarried woman who wishes some manner of birth control, you should expect a doctor to give it to you without a lecture, snide remarks, or other opinions that have nothing to do with medicine. Your life and sexual activity is your own business, and you should not be subjected to a lecture by a physician with ideas on how you should be living.

Abortions are now legal throughout the United States. There are, however, certain doctors, clinics, or hospitals which still refuse to perform abortions. An individual doctor has the right to refuse to perform abortions, according to his own ethical convictions, but such a doctor should refer you to a physician who does perform this procedure. In the case of hospitals or clinics, especially those supported with public funds, the right to refuse abortions is, at this time, an open question. Although abortions are legal, there are areas of the country in which certain individuals opposed to them are powerful enough to prevent physicians otherwise willing to perform abortions from doing so. It is unfortunate that women are made to feel that they are seeking a disgraceful or illegal solution to a common problem. If a physician does not wish to perform an abortion, a woman needing one should seek another doctor.

A gynecologist's personal morality can also cost you money.

Encouraging you to have more children or to have children sooner than you planned can simultaneously increase the doctor's income. You should not be pushed into anything a doctor feels is good for you because it fits his personal wishes.

Treating the "Total" Person

A good gynecologist understands the complex emotional nature of his patients. When a woman is feeling anxious, insecure, or suffering from emotional strain, these feelings are often manifested in her pelvic organs, causing physical dysfunctions or so-called psychosomatic illnesses. Many physical illnesses do, indeed, derive from emotional stress, so a doctor must treat the mind as diligently as he treats the body.

The gynecologist must consider your background, desires, physical capacities, and life-style, and place these into proper perspective for both of you. The doctor should assist you in feeling comfortable about yourself and should help you live happily with who and what you are. Feeling good about who you are and comfortable about your life as a woman is the most important aspect in maintaining good emotional and physical health. The good gynecologist brings all these factors together.

Your Duty as a Patient

The more you know about the nature of your body or your illness, the more you are able to help yourself. Seek information. Have your questions written down in advance—*and ask them*. Get to understand what the doctor is doing with your body. Don't hesitate to speak up when there is something you don't understand. Offer the gynecologist the best information you can about your condition. The more accurately you describe your symptoms and their occurrence, the better they can be treated. Your physician needs feedback, and hiding conditions or symptoms makes the doctor's work more difficult.

At the same time, be human and do not hesitate to express your emotions honestly. In order to treat the *total* person, a doctor must know what you are thinking and feeling; you cannot expect him to rely on guesswork.

Whenever possible, see that the doctor gives you a choice in the course of your treatment. Do not hesitate to ask for alternative methods for dealing with problems, and have confidence in your ability to help make these decisions. The more knowledge you have, the better decision you can make. In addition, refuse to be bullied or intimidated into something you do not want. Remember, if you have any doubts about a course of treatment, seek a second opinion.

If you believe the relationship between you and your gynecologist is no longer beneficial to you, have the confidence to leave him. An antitherapeutic relationship does no good. The sooner you realize this, the sooner you will seek more satisfactory care.

You must look for mutual participation, a situation in which you and your doctor work together for your good health. By selecting a well-qualified gynecologist—one who meets your emotional and philosophical needs—and by upholding your responsibilities as a patient, you can achieve good health care.

WHEN TO BRING YOUR PARTNER

Even at the best of times, a visit to the gynecologist is an anxiety-provoking experience. You should never hesitate to bring your husband, lover, companion, or even just a friend to join in your discussion with the doctor. Two pairs of ears always hear more than one. Your gynecologist should be receptive to this arrangement. His goal is the accurate transmission of information, and if having a second person hear his remarks helps to achieve this goal, he should have no objections.

Your examination, on the other hand, is a private matter between you and your physician. It is the time to concentrate on the physical manifestations of your problem and the presence of your partner could be a distraction.

THE GREATEST BARGAIN ON EARTH

If you have any doubts about the value of becoming an active participant in your health care, you should think twice about your priorities. The average American spends more money each year on the purchase and maintenance of automobiles than on health care. This same American spends countless hours, days, and weeks looking for the best buy or the best repair shop. Prices, standard equipment, warranties—everything about a car is usually carefully researched before purchase.

Yet the topic of discussion here is not your car—it's your life. Is there anything more important to you? If you ask hard questions and have high standards when buying a car, shouldn't you have even harder questions and higher standards when dealing with your life? If you refuse to buy a car that doesn't meet the standards you set, don't you think you should refuse to see a gynecologist who does not meet your standards? Remember, when you choose a doctor, you are selecting someone who might one day be the difference between your life and your death.

Isn't that worth a little work on your part?

chapter 3

THE PELVIC EXAMINATION

Two women are talking quietly in a department-store cafeteria. The second woman has been summoned by the first, and tension fills the air.

ANN: Susan, something happened the other day that has been bothering me.
SUSAN: What is it?
ANN: It's . . . it's . . . it's damn embarrassing, that's what it is.
SUSAN: That's all right. What is it?
ANN (is silent for a moment, then makes an inner decision to tell all): Susan, how long does it take to do a pelvic examination?
SUSAN: Why? Is something wrong?
ANN: I don't know. I went to my family doctor yesterday and it took him forty-five minutes to complete the pelvic exam!

A Broadway play? Hardly. But the dialogue is representative of a real-life drama that is played every day somewhere in the world. Unfortunately, it has too many repeat performances. The exact question may not be the same, but the questions, doubts, and fears surrounding the pelvic examination affect almost every woman.

Until recently, it was the rare patient who had any idea at all what her gynecologist was doing during her pelvic exam. Even today, the majority of women have no notion whatsoever about what is going on inside them.

Part of the blame, of course, must be placed with doctors. Sadly, many physicians feel that any explanation of procedure would only confuse their patients and open the door to what these physicians would consider needless questions. The correct method, particularly during a woman's first pelvic examination, is clearly and patiently to explain the whats and whys of every step of the pelvic exam. A physician who does not have the time to explain these things may also not have the time to perform the examination correctly.

On the other hand, women must take some of the responsibility. Unlike a surgical procedure, where the patient is anesthetized, a pelvic examination is a two-way street. A woman who is completely ignorant of her own body certainly will not be able to ask the right questions during the pelvic exam, nor will she be relaxed, and an anxiety-ridden patient makes the pelvic exam much more difficult.

What are the right questions? Simply, those that relieve your worries and help you toward understanding the procedure.

And why should you be relaxed? After all, doctors are paid, and some are paid very well, to perform the procedure no matter what your condition. First of all, a woman who is relaxed responds much better than one who is tense. That in itself is a good reason for relaxation. Second, the pelvic organs are extremely difficult to outline when the patient is abnormally tense.

One of the most difficult tasks for medical students is merely to understand the location and shape of the pelvic organs. The pictures and drawings in medical textbooks are not adequate substitutes for the real thing, and since each patient exhibits individual differences, it is only upon the examination of the actual pelvic organs that understanding dawns. Even then, it is no easy task to determine the exact location of the organs. If a woman exhibits extreme tension, these organs become almost indistinguishable and a good examination is hard to accomplish.

Obviously, communication is of prime importance during the pelvic examination. A relaxed patient and a relaxed but alert physician can go a long way to remedy the mistakes of the past.

THE PRELIMINARIES

Communication is one of the oldest, yet still one of the best, tools of medicine. For that reason, your first visit to any gynecologist should begin with a complete medical history. Ideally, this should be conducted with your doctor, but many times the exigencies of a medical practice dictate that the nurse review the patient's history. In either case, you as a patient should be totally honest in giving information. You should also consider the method used by your interviewer, whether it is the doctor or the nurse. If the interviewer makes you feel uncomfortable at this stage, the discomfort often increases as the examination progresses to more personal aspects.

The gynecologist's medical history will pay specific attention to your menstrual record—the onset of your first period, its regularity or irregularity, and the duration and quantity of blood flow. Another important factor to discuss is how much pain, if any, you experience, and its direct or indirect relationship to your period.

During the history, you must be *totally honest* about yourself and your medical history. Your doctor knows how embarrassing certain disorders, infections, or diseases are. But your doctor will not be embarrassed nor in any way judge you (aside from medical judgments) because of your history.

It is important to stress here that if your doctor does make any moral or personal judgments, or makes any disparaging remarks about your present condition or history, this physician will probably not be suitable for you. Doctors are medical practitioners, not philosophers or moralists. If you are seeking moral, religious, or philosophical guidance, you would be better advised to find counsel in a church, in a university ethics department, or with a good friend. Your doctor's task is to understand you and your world, and any doctor who refuses to offer that understanding will very likely be a destructive influence on your general mental and emotional health. Since there is great interaction between physical and mental or emotional health, finding a physician who understands this interaction, and who understands you, is vitally important.

As vulnerable as telling your medical history makes you feel, it is necessary. Your doctor cannot be blamed or held responsible if he or she makes the wrong decision when it is based on an incorrect history. More than that, if a serious condition does develop, you want to know that your physician's decisions are based on correct information.

There are many women who have qualms about relating their medical histories. These qualms run so deeply that these women will not be likely to reverse themselves just by reading here that they should be honest. Still, a good physician should be able to recognize this problem and should be able to help. A big part of any gynecologist's job is to make the patient feel at ease. Commonly called the bedside manner, this quality should be apparent in the office as well as in the sickroom.

If you have made the appointment with some specific questions in mind, the time to ask them is during the history or the first part of the examination. In that way, if your doctor does not have an immediate answer, he will at least know what is troubling you and be able to check it during the actual examination. Many women make an appointment with several questions in mind and then forget those questions when they get to the office. This is a human foible—none of us has a perfect memory—yet it is annoying for the patient as well as the doctor. For this reason, you should write down in advance all the questions you want to ask your doctor and take the list with you to your appointment.

It is likely that questions will arise during your examination, and you should feel free to ask them when they arise. It is also important to remember the name of any pills or medication you are or have been taking prior to your examination. A drug of any sort will influence or alter your chemistry, and the doctor has to know what it is to make a proper diagnosis. Here, again, you should write down the name of any medication of this sort and bring it with you to the doctor's office. Or you may want to bring in the bottle itself. Describing the pills will not provide sufficient information; either bring the medication with you or have its complete, exact name.

So relax, be honest, and come prepared with questions and information. If you do that, any doctor will turn somersaults to treat you—although he will still send you a bill. About that, nothing can be done.

The Physician's Observations

While taking the patient's history, the doctor should observe the patient's entire appearance. The patient's color is important; so, too, is the mental state of the patient. These things should tell a well-trained observer a lot about the patient—whether she is nervous, happy, unhappy, tense, or depressed. This type of observation often helps the physician reach the final diagnosis which enables him to give the patient the best treatment.

This initial observation will also tell the physician the most simple aspects of the patient's general health—whether she appears too fat or too thin and, further, if she looks tired or healthy. If the patient is extremely pale, she might be anemic, which, in turn, might account for all her health problems. If the patient is yellowish, it may indicate jaundice secondary to liver damage, or it might be that the woman just eats too many carrots. It might even be due to genetic coloring.

From these examples and many more, it is easy to see that the initial observation is very important in ferreting out a woman's health problems. Appearance is always a good indicator, and the physician follows these indicators like a detective tracking down a bad guy. In this case, the bad guy is any abnormality that affects your health.

The gynecologist who finds any medical problem outside his special domain should refer you to the proper specialist. The gynecologist should, of course, explain to you exactly why he is referring you to another doctor.

Medical Checks

Since a gynecologist is often considered the primary physician to attend a woman, it is now a commonly accepted practice for this doctor to care for the woman's entire health. Because of this, your doctor should probably perform a complete physical examination on each visit. This includes a breast and pelvic examination; a blood-pressure check; examination of the head and neck, heart and lungs, and abdominal and pelvic organs. The gynecologist should further check the patient's weight and encourage diet if the weight is outside normal limits. A urinalysis should be performed, and if the patient complains of extreme fatigue, a blood count should be taken. In short, a total examination.

Preparations for the Pelvic Examination

After the history has been taken, your gynecologist should instruct you to empty your bladder. Although a urinalysis will be taken on the specimen during your examination, there is another important reason for this procedure. When the bladder is full, it pushes the uterus backward. This makes the pelvic examination more difficult both for you and your doctor.

The urinalysis is a test for sugar and protein. If there are traces of sugar in the urine, it might indicate that you are developing diabetes. If any protein is present, it might indicate kidney damage or malfunction. If either of these checks is positive, it will, of course, be further investigated.

At the same time as you are collecting the urine sample, you will be asked to undress completely for your examination. Many women are uptight about this, but it is necessary. No one can perform an honest and good examination through clothing, and as uneasy as it might make you, you should realize that when you are asked to undress completely, it only means that the physician intends to examine you thoroughly.

Regardless of the need to undress, though, you should be given a private room in which to undress or, at the very least, a curtain or screen behind which you may disrobe. You should also be given a loose gown to wear during the examination so the doctor is able to examine specific parts of your body without exposing your whole body.

If the gynecologist does not have a special gown for you to wear during your examination, you should be properly draped by sheets. Usually two sheets are used, one to cover the body and one to cover the legs.

Unfortunately, some physicians have abused women by not having them dressed in gowns or draped in any fashion. The reasons are numerous and are better dealt with in a separate book. Suffice it to say that if your doctor examines you while you are completely nude, you are well within your rights to object. If this happens, and if the doctor does not pay any attention to your objection, you have the right to end the examination at this point. Indeed, you probably should, for this treatment of you by the doctor will probably create tension and thus will not be conducive to a good examination. Apart from the issue of decency, this is totally unprofessional behavior on the part of the physician. Many women have gone along with this sort of treatment in the past, mostly because of the indoctrinated social training we all receive about the doctor-patient relationship. But the patient is also a consumer engaging the services of a professional, and if those services make you feel bad or uncomfortable, you should probably find a doctor more in tune with your personal preferences.

Once you have given your urine sample and been gowned or draped, the nurse or the doctor will probably take your blood pressure before you rest on the table. Since most people live their day-to-day lives on their feet—walking, running, and so forth—the blood pressure should also be taken in that normal state. If the test is taken while you are lying down, it will not accurately reflect the blood pressure that you normally have; it will only reflect the pressure at rest.

Your weight will be taken at this point, and your urine will be checked. In that way, the doctor will begin the actual physical examination with these tests completed and, therefore, with a better idea of your general health.

The doctor is now ready to begin the physical part of the examination.

THE PHYSICAL EXAMINATION

Now that the preliminary work has been done and you are gowned or draped, your physician will probably ask you to get on the table.

Although this table should be relatively comfortable, you shouldn't expect it to rival your favorite chaise lounge, unless your favorite lounge comes equipped with stirrups. Still, the table should not be a torture rack.

Since your gynecologist should be sensitive to the vulnerabilities inherent in any examination, he will begin his general and well-established check of all organs with an area commonly overlooked —the skin. The covering of your body is just as much an organ as any other and, accordingly, your doctor should examine it thoroughly for any major abnormalities. If any are found, you should be referred to a specialist, but actually, starting with the skin is a doctor's method of psychologically easing you into the sensitive areas of the examination.

It must be stressed that any doctor who goes immediately to the pelvic examination is probably insensitive to your feelings. There are no concrete medical arguments against starting in the pelvic region; rather it is an issue of human understanding. A doctor without compassion and sensitivity is a little like a lawyer with no sense of justice—they might both be good technicians, but it would be difficult to call them complete professionals. Certainly compassion and sensitivity are not salable commodities—no more than is justice—but you as a consumer *have a choice*. You can choose any gynecologist you wish, and you may choose one for whatever qualities you desire in your physician. Most women want the human touch added to the technical proficiency, and they should get it.

The physician will next probably look at your hair and examine your entire head, checking the condition of your hair and whether there is any change in it, either in structure or in amount. Loss of hair might indicate a hormonal imbalance or malnutrition, or it could simply be caused by a lack of vitamins such as vitamin B complex. A decrease in thyroid-hormone production could also cause this condition, and if the doctor suspects this, it should be checked by a blood test to determine the blood-thyroid concentration (a PBI or a T_4 test).

Your eyes should be examined to see if they have a normal appearance. Protruding eyes usually indicate a thyroid gland condition in which too much thyroid hormone is produced. The mucosal coloring underneath the eyelids should also be checked. If the mucous membrane is extremely pale, the patient is usually anemic.

If you complain of "buzzing," the doctor will examine your ears for obstruction and discharge. Naturally, if a serious abnormality is found, the gynecologist will refer you to a specialist.

Your nose will also be checked for any obstruction to the nasal passages; bleeding or abnormal discharge should be investigated.

The doctor will examine the condition of your teeth, gums, and tongue. If there is any unusual bleeding, that should also be noted. The doctor will also examine your throat for the size and condition of your tonsils and/or pharynx.

Next, the doctor will examine your neck for enlarged lymph glands indicating infection, in which case the nodes will be very tender. In rare cases, enlarged lymph glands might also indicate a malignant blood disease such as leukemia or Hodgkin's disease.

The thyroid gland is located in the middle of the neck and is formed like an H, with the bar of the H located one to two fingers beneath the Adam's apple. The gland's arms are located on each side of the bar of the H. This gland produces thyroid hormones, which are extremely important for metabolism. One common function of the thyroid is regulation of weight. If you have a low thyroid function, you might have a slow metabolic rate and will tend to be fat even with minimal food intake. On the other hand, if your thyroid is overactive, your metabolic rate will be high and you will be constantly hungry and able to eat without gaining weight. If that sounds too good to be true, it is; people with overactive thyroids also tend to feel hot and sweaty most of the time, whereas people with slow thyroid functions tend toward fatigue and are extremely sensitive to cold.

The thyroid gland is also closely associated with ovulation pattern. Since the gonadotrophic hormones, produced by the pituitary and regulating the ovarian function, are influenced by the thyroid hormones, a slow or fast thyroid function might interfere with ovulation through interaction with the pituitary hormone.

The thyroid gland can be checked by a blood test to examine the blood content of the thyroid hormone, or it can be checked by a basal metabolism test. This blood test has to be taken on an empty stomach, since food intake containing high amounts of iodine can upset the real values. Infertility (the inability to conceive) has often been corrected just by giving small amounts of thyroid medication to the patient with a slow thyroid function.

Enlargement of the thyroid gland can occur from many causes. It might be due to an overproduction of thyroid hormone by the glands, or it could be caused by a tumor or cancer of the thyroid gland. Of course, there can always be a simple explanation as well. Insufficient iodine intake will cause enlargement of the thyroid gland. This causes the thyroid to enlarge in order to increase the production of thyroid hormone to keep pace with need. This condition is called *goiter (struma)* and is corrected by increasing iodine intake or by adding thyroid hormones to the diet. Goiter is more common than you might imagine and is the reason that many cities and towns add iodine to their drinking water. If you live in an area with an uncontrolled water supply, an iodine supplement may be needed.

The physician should next examine the heart and lungs. This is done by listening, either through a stethoscope *(auscultation)*, or through percussion (palpation or knocking on the area with fingers). The breathing sounds of the lungs will change when conditions such as asthma, bronchitis, or pneumonia are present. Excessive cigarette smoking will also change the breathing sounds. If the physician finds any suspicious symptoms, he might want to send you for a chest X-ray or to a lung specialist.

The heart is examined for size. Normally, the higher your blood pressure, the bigger your heart is. The doctor will also listen to the heart to detect any murmur or other abnormality that might warrant an electrocardiogram (ECG) or a referral to a heart specialist.

The breast examination is the next step in the procedure. Remarkably, this is a relatively new aspect included in your visit to the gynecologist. Just a few years ago, the breast examination was often overlooked: The general practitioner felt the gynecologist should do it, while the gynecologist felt the general practitioner should do it. However, it is now firmly entrenched as a part of the gynecological examination, again because the gynecologist is becoming the primary physician for many women.

The breasts are examined individually. First, each breast is checked for abnormalities in configurations and skin coloring. Cancer, for instance, is often shown by abnormal skin coloring in the area where it is developing, and the skin will often pull down a bit in that area.

Thereafter, the physician should feel each breast with both hands to be sure it is freely mobile to all sides. At the same time, obvious lumps will be felt.

During the breast examination, the physician mentally divides each breast into four quadrants—upper outer, lower outer, upper inner, and lower inner. Generally speaking, the breast is divided in this fashion by intersecting two invisible straight lines at ninety-degree angles, the center of the intersection being at the nipple. Each quadrant is examined by the gynecologist, both visually and by touch, for extra masses or any other irregularities.

In the middle of each breast is the nipple, and behind the nipple is the milk gland. During the menstrual cycle, the milk gland will be influenced by hormonal changes, commonly resulting in cystic enlargement of part of the milk gland or enlargement and tenderness of the entire milk gland. The physician will thoroughly check the breast for any abnormalities.

If there are any suspicious lumps in either breast, a biopsy might be needed. This, of course, is usually performed by a surgeon and is not considered part of the gynecologist's routine procedure, even though it is often done by the gynecologist. Before a biopsy is done, though, if a suspicious mass is found, the gynecologist should send you for an X-ray examination of the breast by mammography or xeroradiography, or by thermography. The thermographic examination picks up abnormal heat patterns in the breast. Since a carcinogenic lesion will be more virulent, it will also vary in color from the rest of the breast on a thermographic X-ray (see Chapter 18 on Breast Examination).

After the examination of each breast, the corresponding axilla (armpit) is carefully examined. This is to check for cancer metastasis, since the lymph nodes in the axilla are the first place the cancer will spread. Each axilla should be explored carefully.

If there are any suspicious abnormalities of the breasts up to this point, your gynecologist should have you sit on the edge of the table with the lower part of your legs dangling over the side. The physician will then reexamine your breasts from this perspective. Your hands should first be at your side, then placed behind your neck to reexamine the axilla.

Following the breast examination, the physician will examine the abdominal region to make sure there are no visible abdominal masses or lesions protruding from the abdominal cavity. The doctor will also ascertain if there are any abnormalities of the skin in this region. The abdomen should then be systematically palpated for abnormalities. The area underneath the right rib cage will be explored for any possible enlargements or abnormalities of the liver. The physician usually should not be able to feel the liver's edge. This is important, since if you do have an enlargement of the liver, a tumor, or even hepatitis, you should not use birth-control pills. As soon as the doctor has finished exploring the right side of the rib cage, you should raise your hands above your head so the left side under the rib cage is exposed. This permits the doctor to ensure that the spleen is not enlarged. This is done both by touch and by sound; as the doctor palpates the area, he naturally feels any abnormality. Percussion, the sound which occurs when a physician knocks on a finger placed on the

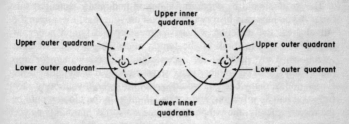

Fig. 3–1: While conducting a breast examination, the physician mentally divides each breast into four parts, or quadrants. The above illustration describes the area of the quadrants. By doing this, a physician can more easily diagnose the location of any mass and also can more easily monitor such a mass on subsequent examinations.

skin, will be high if there is no mass and low if there is a mass present.

At this point, the doctor will examine the right and left flanks for pain or possible enlargement of the kidneys. If either is present, it may indicate tumors or infections in that area. Again, palpation and auscultation are employed. In this case, auscultation equates with listening through a stethoscope to the sound of the peristalsis of the intestines, a sound which changes if there are any intestinal obstructions or abdominal infections present. Although you need not know the normal sound of the peristalsis of the intestines, it might make you more comfortable just to know what your doctor is doing.

The physician should next examine your pubic hair. The hairline should be almost straight, although this is somewhat dependent on race. If, however, the hairline is triangular moving toward the navel, this may indicate a higher concentration of male hormones than is usual. This in itself is not dangerous, and you certainly should not worry if your hairline is not straight. However, a high concentration of male hormones is sometimes a symptom of ovarian tumors or, more commonly, of a condition called ovarian polycystic disease (also called the Stein-Leventhal syndrome).

The doctor next examines the lower portion of your abdomen by feeling just above the symphysis (the major pubic bone just beneath the hairline). The gynecologist will be able to feel your uterus and will be able to ascertain if there are any tumors present or if there is a pregnancy beyond the three-month stage.

The groin should be checked for lymph node enlargement at this time. If you have any history of infection on your legs, toes, or in the vulval area, the infection will have spread to the lymph nodes. It might be useful to think of the lymph nodes as soldiers that fight infections. They catch all the bacteria and either kill them or stop them from spreading to other parts of your body. If it weren't for the lymph nodes, many bacteria would spread throughout your body each time you had an infection, and sepsis infection in the blood would be the result. Luckily, the lymph nodes create a sort of immunity as you grow older. By the time you are an adult, you will have had many infections of different types, and the lymph nodes created to fight the bacteria of these infections have increased in number. These lymph nodes give the body more time to fight the infection, but as they increase, you will be able to feel them in your groin. Tenderness in the lymph nodes indicates an active infection, either in your vulval area or in your legs and/or feet. This condition should be checked. On the other hand, an enlarged lymph node that is not tender merely indicates that you have had a past infection. Of course, if there is a marked increase in the size of the lymph nodes, it should be examined, since most cases of leukemia and some other diseases start in the lymph nodes. In these cases, a biopsy might be the best procedure to follow, especially since cancer also spreads through the lymph nodes. The physical examination, although it seems complicated, need only take a few minutes.

THE PELVIC EXAMINATION

Up to this point, you will usually have been in the supine position (flat on your back) on the examining table. Now it is time to get into the gynecological position. This is one that makes many women nervous, mostly because of misconceptions and exaggerated horror stories. It should not, though, be an uncomfortable situation if you are seeing a gentle and competent physician who cares enough to put you at your ease. Some women find it embarrassing, but the internal examination should be seen strictly as a necessary medical process and not as a procedure to embarrass you. It is the only way to examine you internally and to obtain a Pap smear. Because of this, you should try to relax as much as possible.

In the gynecological position, your legs are spread and your knees are bent as you lie flat on your back. In most examining rooms, the doctor will have a table equipped with stirrups, and you will be asked to place your feet or knees in these to control your position. It is important that your hips are all the way down at the edge of the table. This ensures that the doctor can work very close to the area under examination. The physician stands or sits between your legs, facing the vulva.

Before the internal pelvic examination is started, the gynecologist should be sure that the sheet or drape is covering you completely so that only the vulval area is visible. This makes the examination much less embarrassing for you.

However, if you are interested in observing the procedure, feel free to remove the sheet. Many women feel that watching the doctor's moves lessens the fear of the unknown. Familiarizing yourself with the pelvic examination should also remove the notion of the doctor being in control of your body.

Many people wonder if the internal pelvic examination is a sensual or sexual experience. Suspicions that the doctor performing the examination relates to the patient sexually worry many, and some husbands and boyfriends even wonder if their partners enjoy the examination. It should therefore be stated that even though the pelvic examination should not be an unpleasant experience, neither should it titillate or excite. It is a medical examination—a piece of work that has to be done thoroughly and carefully. If you receive any hints that your doctor is deriving anything but scientific pleasure from your examination, you will obviously feel a little uncomfortable. Again, if this happens, do find another physician.

Sitting or standing between your legs, the gynecologist points a light at the vulvar area. The surface examination includes almost exactly what you can examine yourself with your own light and mirror. The doctor will inspect the entire vulvar area, checking the pubic hair first for lice and growth. He will then see if there are any profuse discharges from the vagina or if there are any obvious lesions or growths such as venereal warts, syphilitic lesions, herpes sores, or abscesses in the area. The physician should then inspect the clitoris and the *labia majora,* spreading the large lips and looking for any lesions or tumors. At the same time, the doctor will usually insert a finger into the vagina and palpate the two Bartholin's glands that are located in the lower aspect of the vagina. These are the glands that produce hormonal secretion to the vagina, and sometimes the ducts leading to these glands will be clogged due to infection. Although most often a gonorrheal infection partially causes this condition, any type of mixed infection can clog these ducts. If they are clogged, the doctor will feel an enlargement on each side.

If you ever feel what seems to be a lump between your legs or in the lower aspect of your vagina reaching toward the rectum, it is probably a Bartholin duct cyst. It might become inflamed and may cause an abscess. This is an extremely painful situation and usually warrants an operation to correct it. If, though, there is an enlargement not accompanied by pain, it will sometimes disappear just with the use of sitz baths and/or with local treatment advised by the gynecologist, which may clear the Bartholin's ducts and drain the cyst.

Immediately inside the vulva underneath the clitoris is the urethra, the short channel from the bladder that drains the urine. The physician will look to see if any glands, cysts, or other abnormalities surround the urethra. Because urine will sometimes dribble down into the labia, it is not uncommon to have a slight irritation in this area.

The Speculum

For some women, the internal examination is a frightening experience. There might be logical reasons for this, but still, these fears can be corrected by a gentle and competent physician. Most of the fears involve the speculum, an instrument which the gynecologist inserts into your vagina.

Part of the fear surrounding the speculum comes from a careless, and mistaken, nickname the instrument has received. Many women actually call the speculum *clamps,* and the image this word provokes is indeed frightening. To correct this, your gynecologist might give you a quick explanation of the speculum, telling you that it doesn't clamp anything. Just the reverse is true—it opens the vagina so the doctor can get a clear view of the inside. The insertion of the speculum should not be painful, though admittedly it might be a little uncomfortable.

The most common complaint in this area is the temperature of the speculum. Many women will swear their doctors keep the speculums in a block of ice, and, indeed, too many physicians thoughtlessly keep these instruments in cold places, though few actually freeze them in ice. In winter, drafts or a lack of heating in the examining room can result in a cold speculum. Women are right to complain—there are few things in life worse than an ice-cold speculum entering your vagina.

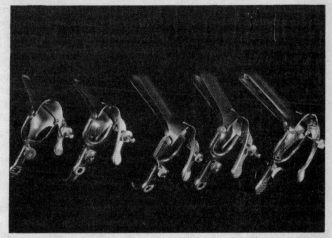

Fig. 3–2: This photograph shows the different sizes of vaginal specula. While the following photograph shows just the different size of the blades, this one shows how the two blades on each speculum open and close by pushing on the handle.

The solution here is simple, and up to the gynecologist. Either the speculum should be kept in a heated cabinet (readily available in the medical marketplace), or the doctor should be careful to place the instrument where it will remain warm. The doctor might hold the instrument under hot water or even heat the instrument with his hand before using. As a consumer, you should insist on a warm speculum. Remember, if your gynecologist is so inconsiderate as to insert a cold speculum, this same physician might also be insensitive to you in other important areas as well.

The problem of pain associated with the speculum is more complex. The patient should be as relaxed as possible, especially since any tension just increases the possibility of pain. A woman who is anxious might make sudden, jerking movements, causing pressure when the speculum is in her vagina. Her muscles will also tighten and perhaps even clamp around the tool. All of this causes pain, and the only remedy is relaxation. That, of course, is easier said than done, but the woman in this situation should ask herself why she is so anxious. If it is because she does not trust her doctor, perhaps she should switch doctors. If it is a more general fear associated either with all doctors or with anything having to do with medicine or penetration of her body, she should certainly try to resolve the conflict by discussing it with her doctor.

The doctor, too, can cause the pain, and for many reasons. Primarily, the doctor might be too rough during the examination, and this is certain to cause discomfort. Supposedly some very progressive medical schools have instituted a policy where every male student is placed in stirrups while a strange woman doctor enters the room, squeezes his testicles, then leaves without saying a word. Although this is perhaps an extreme example, if it teaches these young men to be more sensitive to their patients, it has probably helped some women. One would hope that extreme teaching methods such as this would not be needed to make young doctors more sensitive to women, but that sensitivity, especially when it comes to handling the speculum, is necessary.

If you do experience pain on the insertion of the speculum, it might also be caused by the doctor using the wrong size instrument on you. Speculums are available in different sizes, and if the gynecologist inserts one that is too big, it will cause pain. If it is your first visit to a particular gynecologist, the doctor may have to discover what size instrument should be used. Although this is sometimes an uncomfortable process, it should never be excessively painful. A physician should always use a very small instrument if you are a virgin or have only infrequent intercourse. If, however, you have regular intercourse, the doctor will probably use a medium-sized speculum and then increase or decrease the size of the instrument until finding the appropriate one for you. In this manner, an oversized speculum is avoided. Once the right speculum is found, you should ask what size it is for future reference; remembering the size will save testing if you switch doctors.

Once you know the size speculum you should use, don't lie about it. Many women feel that it is more ladylike to have the smallest speculum, and they even insist their doctors use this. In such a situation, the doctor has difficulty performing the examination. Certain prostitutes insist on a small speculum to minimize their sexual activity, and thus prevent the physician from performing an adequate examination.

If your gynecologist is using the right size speculum but is using it too roughly, ask him to be more gentle. If your physician is offended by this, you should look for a gentler doctor. However, before taking

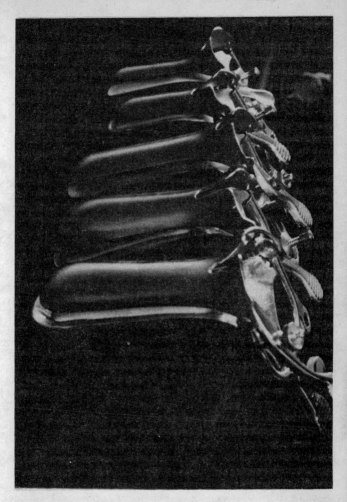

Fig. 3–3: This photograph shows the different sizes of vaginal specula, also referred to by laypeople as clamps. The speculum is available in various sizes, from the small "virgin" type with very small blades to very large speculae to be used for women who have borne several children. The physician should perform a cursory examination of your vaginal opening before inserting the instrument to determine which size is right for you.

this step, be sure it is the gynecologist's rough handling of the instrument and not your anxiety that is causing the pain.

The gynecologist should place a finger on the lower part of the vagina before inserting the speculum. The finger should be pressed gently down so the speculum, inserted sideways, can slide into the vagina on the top of the finger. This prevents the instrument from scratching any part of the vagina. The speculum should be moved slowly into the depth of the vagina, then turned to the right position and opened, again slowly. This avoids pinching any part of the interior. When the physician opens the speculum, it should be opened only to the point where the doctor has a good, clear view of the cervix and the mucosa of the vagina. Opening the speculum any more than this is needless, and sometimes causes pain as the speculum presses against the vaginal wall.

When the speculum is inside you, there might be some occasional pain, but it should not be excessive or anything but occasional.

THE INTERNAL EXAMINATION

After the speculum has been inserted, the doctor will check the wall of the vagina to be sure it is the right color. If everything is in order, the vaginal wall will be pink and clean. If, though, there is any type of discharge, the physician will notice its color. In several cases, the color of the discharge indicates exactly what type of infection is present.

Often, there is a cheeselike discharge, which indicates a *Monilia* infection. If *Monilia* is present, the patient will usually come into the office complaining of a discharge and some type of burning sensation.

If a discharge is greenish yellow, it usually points to a *Trichomonas* infection. If this is suspected, the gynecologist will swab the vaginal wall, smear the discharge on a glass plate, mix it with a saline drop, and examine it under a microscope. If it is present, the doctor will see the *Trichomonas* organism, with two or three small tails, on the slide. This organism is extremely mobile and will move constantly on the slide. There are other methods of determining *Trichomonas*, but this is the most common.

A gonorrheal infection will usually show up as a profuse yellowish discharge originating from the opening of the cervix. If gonorrhea is suspected, a culture should be taken and sent to the lab for immediate examination. The gonorrheal bacteria is very sensitive, so if this specimen is not examined immediately, it will be of no use whatever (this is often the case in offices that are not close enough to laboratories). Once the specimen has reached the lab safely, it usually takes about two days for the bacteria to grow on the culture medium before the bacteria can be diagnosed. Even if the bacteria is not gonorrheal in nature, this method will produce the correct diagnosis.

The gynecologist will next inspect the cervix and the area around it. As you noticed in your self-examination, the cervix feels like the tip of your nose and is in the very back of the vagina. As the physician looks at the cervix, there is a small hole in the center of it, which is the passageway to the uterus. Your doctor might, with the aid of a mirror, let you observe the cervix for yourself.

Occasionally there will be an irritation on the edge of the cervix, which is called *cervicitis*. One cause of cervicitis is a chronic inflammatory reaction, particularly common during pregnancy. When a woman is pregnant, the blood supply to the cervix changes. This in turn increases the probability of irritation and infection to the mouth of the womb. Most often this manifests itself as a sore or an erosion, and is called cervicitis.

Another cause of cervicitis is too high a concentration of the female hormone, estrogen. This most often occurs in women on the high-estrogen birth-control pill. Again, this concentration of estrogen causes an increased blood supply to the cervix, resulting in more breakage and infection in the cervical area.

There are many ways to treat cervicitis. If the birth-control pill is the cause, it would be wise to place the woman on another type of pill with less estrogen. In some cases, antibiotics alone will clear up the infection. Sometimes the doctor will coagulate the cervix with silver nitrate. These treatments clear up most minor cases, but if the infection persists, electrocauterization or cryosurgery might be the solution. Although most women are familiar with the technique of cauterization, cryosurgery (wherein the area around the cervix is frozen) is a relatively new procedure which has been found effective in the treatment of chronic cervicitis.

If you have an IUD (intrauterine device), the gynecologist should see the tail of it. The body of the IUD should not be visible, but the visibility of the tail will enable your gynecologist to determine if the IUD is in the right location (see diagram).

At this point, the physician will obtain a Pap smear (more completely, a Papanicolaou smear). This test consists of swabbing cells shed from the vaginal pool and the cervix, and examining them for any abnormalities. For this reason, you should not douche for at least twenty-four hours prior to an internal examination (even though we are brought up to be clean before going to a doctor, douching might, in this instance, wash away and, therefore, cover up the trace to an accurate diagnosis. You should still wash the outside of your vulva before an examination). With the Pap smear, three samples are taken—one from the vaginal pool, one from the inside of the cervical canal (the *endocervix*), and one from the area immediately surrounding the mouth of the cervix. All three samples are placed on a slide and sprayed with a special solution to fix the cells so their contents will not be altered in the transport to the lab. In the lab, the samples will be treated with a special Papanicolaou stain or color and then examined for cell content. The lab physician will be able to detect if the cells are normal or abnormal. If there is a malignancy pending, it will be spotted early and treated properly. Along with aiding in the early detection of cancer, the Pap smears can also be examined to

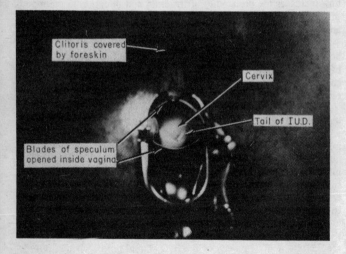

Fig. 3–4: This photograph shows what a doctor sees through a medium-size speculum inserted into the vagina. The cervix is clearly visualized at the end of the vagina. The tail of an IUD is seen protruding through the cervical mouth. The body of the IUD cannot, and should not, be seen, since it is positioned inside the uterine cavity. If a part of the IUD body *could* be seen, it would indicate that the IUD was not in the correct position.

ascertain the estrogen index and can detect other infections of the cervix, including *Trichomonas*.

Following the examination of the vagina and the cervix, the doctor will withdraw the speculum. Reversing the process of entry, the gynecologist closes the speculum, turns it on its side, and slowly removes it from the vagina. Again, this avoids any pinching of the vaginal wall.

The Bimanual Examination

The physician will next conduct a bimanual pelvic examination. It is important for this part of the examination (of the uterus, the fallopian tubes, and the ovaries) that you have emptied your bladder and that you are not constipated. If you appear at the gynecologist's office on a day when you are constipated, the doctor might send you home with a few enemas and ask you to come back another day. There is a good reason for this.

It is very easy to confuse a mass or a cyst with an ordinary fecal mass. Don't forget that the intestines are right next to the ovaries and the pelvic organs. Any sort of lump will come under suspicion, and it is not the doctor's fault if you had a large meal the night before. If, though, your pelvic organs are easily palpated, constipation may not cause a problem. In this case, the physician might have to insert a finger in your rectum to examine you thoroughly.

The bimanual examination begins when the gynecologist slides one or two fingers (with jelly) into the vagina. If you are a virgin or if your vagina is inordinately tight, only one finger should be inserted. This is a procedure to examine you, not hurt you; however, it is again important that you are relaxed. If you are tense, the examination will be infinitely more difficult. If you are worried about the fingers entering your vagina, you should think of the logic of the situation. Certainly your physician's finger will be smaller than your sex partner's penis. If your vagina can receive an erect penis, it will be able to withstand the penetration of your physician's fingers, even though the sensation will be less pleasurable.

With his finger(s) inside your vagina, the doctor puts the finger on the cervix and slowly moves it. The doctor will then place his other hand on your abdomen. As he presses slowly on your abdomen, he slowly rotates your uterus by pushing the cervix from the inside. This helps determine the position and size of your uterus.

The most frequent position of the uterus is forward, or anteverted. Occasionally the uterus will be in a posterior, or retroverted position, or even in what is called the midposition. Many women are frightened if the uterus is not in the forward position, and this is reinforced by many ignorant or dishonest physicians. The "tilted uterus" syndrome is one of the most destructive myths of gynecology. In the earlier part of the century, it was the source of many needless surgical operations. The belief then was that a woman with a tilted uterus could not have a baby, so an operation was performed to rotate the uterus into the "correct"—that is, forward—position. This was all nonsense. The position of the uterus is determined by genes. If your mother had a retroverted uterus, the chances are you will also have one. But your mother gave birth to you, and you can certainly have children, all other factors being equal. Unfortunately, the operation on the tilted uterus provided these doctors with a good source of income, and today, even though we know better, there are still many operations of this type performed.

It cannot be overstated: *The position of your uterus does not make any difference to your health or to your ability to have children.*

This does not mean you shouldn't know the position of your uterus. This knowledge sometimes eases an examination. As the doctor is rotating the uterus, he should tell you exactly what he is doing and the position of your uterus. If your uterus is in the posterior position, the examination will be a bit more difficult, but that is only because the uterus will be more inaccessible to the gynecologist.

The physician outlines the uterus while holding it, and should let you know what he is feeling. If there are any abnormalities, such as fibroid tumors, the doctor should outline them and tell you their exact size. It is extremely important to explain these things to the patient, because when she is examined the next time, she will know if the tumor has grown. To a certain extent, and surely with women who jump from one gynecologist to another, women have to monitor their own health to make sure the correct treatment and attention is given to each infection or abnormality. With tumors, it is important that women know the approximate size of each tumor, for it is the patients who will have to monitor any growth in the tumor, especially if they have changed physicians.

In rare instances, when an IUD has penetrated the walls of the uterus, it may cause a problem. In this case, nature has its own remedy. The *omentum* is a fatty membrane which hangs from the upper portion of the colon like a curtain. If there is a localized infection in the abdomen, the omentum encapsulates the infection, almost like glue, preventing its spread. When this occurs with an

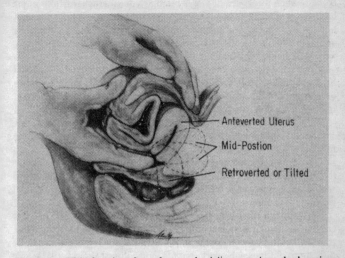

Fig. 3–5: This drawing shows how a physician examines the location and size of the uterus. The doctor here has inserted two fingers into the vagina against the cervix. The other hand is placed on the abdomen. The gynecologist then slowly pushes the cervix with his fingers, forcing the uterus up against the abdomen. This enables him to palpate the uterus. By rotating the cervix, the doctor can get an approximation of the size and location of the uterus. He will also be able to determine most abnormalities of the uterus.

The uterus in this illustration is in the anteverted, or front, position. This is not only the most common position, but also the one most accessible to the doctor, particularly in thinner patients.

The broken lines show the two other possible uterine positions—the mid-position and the retroverted, or tilted, position. As can be discerned, the physician will need to push much harder against the abdomen to get an exact description of either of these two positions. With a retroverted uterus, the physician often must insert a finger into the rectum, the canal lying just beneath the vagina in this picture, to diagnose any abnormality in a tilted uterus.

IUD, the omentum will cover the penetrated part of the IUD. Of course, this will sometimes result in the omentum sticking to the area which the IUD has penetrated. This, in turn, causes a pelvic adhesion, which decreases the mobility of your uterus. In such a case, there can be pain when the gynecologist is rotating your uterus. It is important here that you are not stoical, telling the doctor that something does not hurt when it does. The most common symptom of many infections and abnormalities is pain. If you do not complain, the doctor may very well bypass the area.

If there is pain when the physician moves your uterus and it cannot be connected to an IUD or some other foreign object, an infection or disease should be suspected. Every movement and pain is important in diagnosis, and you the patient cannot afford to forget this.

With his fingers still in your vagina, the physician will move his free hand to either side of your abdomen and try to find the area of the fallopian tubes. These tubes are normally slightly tender when squeezed, but if there is *extreme* tenderness or pain when the doctor touches them, it may indicate an infection. If the tubes are enlarged with a mass, it might be due to an *ectopic* (or tubal) pregnancy, a tubal abscess, or a tumor.

Even though the ovary is usually just the size of the end of your tongue, a good physician will be able to outline it for you while moving up from the fallopian tubes. If a patient is obese, it will be difficult to outline each ovary, but the gynecologist should still be able to feel any uncommon masses.

When the physician squeezes an ovary from the inside and out, it will hurt, just as when one squeezes a man's testicles. That is because there are more nerves in this area.

This process is repeated on both the right and left sides, outlining the fallopian tubes, then the ovaries. If your uterus is in the retroverted, or posterior, position, it will probably be more difficult for the physician to find the tubes and he will necessarily have to press a little harder. At the same time, the doctor should engage in an almost constant flow of conversation, telling you exactly what he is feeling and why.

Following the examination of your uterus (including the tubes and ovaries), the physician withdraws his hand from your vagina. It is at this point that some gynecologists insert a finger into the rectum to be sure there is no abnormality behind the uterus. This is not always done. Some physicians feel that if the pelvic examination has been done on a slim and relaxed patient, they need not put a finger in the rectum unless they suspect an abnormality there. If you are over-weight and/or uptight, though, you will probably be subjected to a rectal examination. But—take heart—it lasts only a few seconds.

That completes the pelvic examination. The rest of your appointment should deal with what the gynecologist has found and with any questions, general or specific, that you may have concerning your examination. The doctor may schedule various tests for you; and should tell you the exact reasons for such tests. If the doctor does not explain adequately, ask.

Do Some Women Achieve Orgasm during the Pelvic Examination?

Word of mouth has it that some women really look forward to their pelvic examinations, supposedly because they get a kick when the gynecologist is holding the uterus between his hands. This has to be a very rare response, but then some people are turned on by plum pudding.

The vast majority of women do not come anywhere close to orgasm during the pelvic examination. Of course, during the insertion of a speculum, the vagina will, in many cases, balloon up just as it does during orgasm. This creates a feeling of well-being, but it is no more erotic than a licensed masseur working a kink out of your neck.

Without a doubt, what turns most women on is when the gynecologist tells them they are perfectly all right and that they need not come back until their next physical.

Do Some Gynecologists Achieve Orgasm during the Pelvic Examination?

No. If so, change gynecologists.

A gynecologist does not look at your sexual organs as anything but medical organs or scientific problems. When something is wrong, the doctor has a problem and is looking for a solution. Being human, it pleases a gynecologist when he solves a problem, but the pleasure is ego-gratifying, not libidinous.

Certainly there are horror stories of gynecologists or general practitioners who love to look at nude women. One story told of a doctor who asked his patient to stand nude on one leg while he looked at her for about half an hour. Another patient recently reported an unethical incident which occurred while she was vacationing in a New York hotel. Feeling ill, she visited the hotel physician, a distinguished-looking older man. She was asked to undress in his lavish office while he went elsewhere to make a phone call. After she disrobed, the woman realized there were no sheets or gowns to cover her. When the doctor reappeared, she was standing in a corner of the office, shivering. The doctor asked her to parade back and forth in front of him while he observed her movement. He then asked her to sit on the examining table, where he interviewed her and performed a lengthy examination. He spent an excessive amount of time examining her breasts and conducting the internal examination. By this time, the patient suspected the doctor's professionalism. While she was still in the stirrups, he told her he had diagnosed the problem. Leaving the room, the doctor announced he would return in a few minutes to start treatment. When the doctor returned, he was completely nude. Moving to the table and positioning himself between her legs, he told her she needed "an internal massage." Panic set in, and the woman jumped off the table, grabbed her clothes, and ran from the office. Because she was not an American citizen, and was therefore unfamiliar with the country's laws, she did not report the incident until recently. By then, it was too late. The doctor had left the hotel and the charges made by the woman would not hold up after the enormous lapse of time.

This type of behavior belongs in the massage parlors, not the gynecological examining room, and physicians of this type should be barred from practice. Both as a consumer and as a patient, it is important that you report any behavior that you feel is unprofessional on the part of your doctor.

Do Women Make Advances to Their Gynecologists during the Pelvic Exam?

This is a question many husbands and boyfriends ask, or want to ask. The answer is a qualified no.

Generally speaking, women do not make advances to their doctors, especially during the examination. Interestingly enough, it has been found that women who do play up to the gynecologist during the internal examination are usually frigid. There are many reasons why these women might release their desires only during the pelvic examination, but that is better dealt with in a book on psychological disorders.

Suffice it to say that those are extremely rare cases.

How Long Does a Pelvic Examination Take?

The internal exam takes no more than two to five minutes. If it takes longer, the doctor should tell you exactly what he is doing and why he is taking the extra time.

HOW MUCH SHOULD I KNOW
ABOUT MY GYNECOLOGICAL HEALTH?

Everything you can. And your gynecologist should be patient and understanding. There should always be an open and honest communication between doctor and patient. If you have trouble understanding something, the doctor should perhaps implement his explanation with a simple drawing to help you understand.

If the gynecologist has to tell you bad news, it should be broken slowly. It should also be explained *in full*. In such a case, the gynecologist should be sure you leave the office knowing exactly what is wrong. Fear does not help any patient on the road to recovery.

chapter 4

THE STORK
AND OTHER MYTHS

Since the creation of humankind, conception has been one of life's greatest mysteries. Amazingly, it has only been in the last two centuries that facts concerning the reproductive process have been scientifically proven. In the countless centuries before this understanding of conception, many myths compensated for the lack of knowledge. Even now, a surprising number of people still cling to these stories about where babies come from.

Human beings were aware at a very early stage that there existed some mysterious connection between the menstrual period and conception. These people realized that pregnant women did not bleed. Unfortunately, this connection was misread. Bleeding was associated with sickness and the lack of bleeding was associated with good health. Obviously, then, the normal, healthy state for women seemed to be one in which they did not bleed. Therefore, it followed that woman's natural state was pregnancy.

The ancient Hindus believed there were three essential components needed for the formation of a baby. First, the father provided white semen, which formed the bones, the brains, and the whites of the eyes. Second, the mother provided the red semen, which produced the skin, the hair, and the iris of the eye. It was left to God to provide the expressions of the face, sight, hearing, speech, and movement.

Another belief concerning the mystery of conception was offered by the Koran. A man was created from "a choice extract" of clay, then placed as semen in "a sure place." The semen was created in a clot of blood, and the clotted blood was formed into flesh. In simple language, humans were clots of various seeds developed into coagulated blood.

Very often the power of conception was linked to animals and birds. Since these beliefs dealt in more metaphorical terms, many of them passed into legend and folklore, where the answers they provided satisfied many people for ages.

Usually these legends concerned beings possessed with supernatural powers and the birds that surrounded and protected them. Ancient Hindus and Egyptians thought the ibis (a cranelike bird) brought children. Young couples would accordingly offer prayers to flocks of these blessed birds. The crane and the butterfly served this purpose in Japan, while early Mexicans honored the red spoonbill.

It was left to ancestral Teutons to develop the most lasting myth of all. This ancient people believed the stork brought children to young married couples, and the familiar picture of a stork flying to its destination carrying a small infant has remained with us to this day. Teutons also believed that to prevent any additions to an already large family, they had only to keep the stork away. When this proved an unsuccessful method of contraception, it gave rise to the theory that the stork flew only in the dark and that babies were born in the hours of darkness.

Belief in the stork was widespread—people in England, the Scandinavian countries, and Germany, as well as in great portions of eastern and western Europe, gave credence to the story. Some of the details of the stork myth were confusing and even contradictory. For instance, it was believed that the stork flew to a hot climate, usually thought to be Egypt, for the winter, and then returned in the spring. Obviously, some babies were born in the winter, and this fact would not support the stork legend.

Yet there might have been a cyclical variation in the nature of those people that could explain this apparent fallacy. At that time, the majority of children were conceived in the late summer. Early explanations reasoned that winters were long and people were more tired. Later researchers found that the energy given off by summer heat was greater than in winter and this caused increased fertility. Since a late-summer conception would result in spring birth, most babies were, indeed, born in the spring, when the stork supposedly returned.

Belief in the stork was strong. A new family would build a stork house on the roof in the hope that they would be given many children. The first children in the family were given the task of luring the stork to the house by placing sugar on the windowsills. Modern-day Scandinavian postcards still commemorate this tradition.

In present-day cultures where the legend of the stork continues, it does so as a children's fairy tale. The stork as a bird is seen as a figure of joy—unthreatening and sometimes even graciously silly. It is a comfortable image for children, and actually not harmful—as long as the truth is eventually told to the children.

Another basically Scandinavian legend concerned the spirit child who lived in lakes, streams, springs, and in the fruits of trees. If a woman happened to bathe in the waters or eat a fruit that was inhabited by a spirit child, she would become pregnant. This myth had its origins in primitive tribes who believed that all children came from the spirit world. These early tribes made no connection between sexual intercourse and pregnancy. The reproductive power of semen was completely unknown.

People in Papua were closer to the actualities of conception. Although ignorant Papuans thought pregnancy was caused by bathing in streams inhabited by eels, an enlightened minority believed the seminal fluid ejaculated by men was the prime force of reproduction. The actual flesh and blood of the child was believed to have been formed by an accumulation of semen. It followed that pregnancy could occur only after repeated intercourse. This gave Papuans a socially based motivation for frequent and lively intercourse, so it naturally became a popular belief.

At the same time, many primitive tribes held to the theory of the wandering-room child, a creature who crawled in and out of a woman's mouth in the shape of a toad while she slept. When it was outside the woman's body, this toad-child would eat and drink, then return to the woman.

In approximately 400 B.C., Hippocrates (generally considered the founder of the medical profession) formulated his own theory of conception. This ancient Greek physician felt that pregnancy was caused by combining male and female semen. When conception occurred, menstrual blood flowed into the uterus daily, not monthly. This accumulation of menstrual blood formed the flesh of the new child. Hippocrates believed that ovaries, like testicles, produced semen—a controversial tenet since it stated that a child owed its genetic heritage as much to the mother as to the father. Hippocrates was convinced that a child's resemblance to either or both parents was due to the semen from both. He believed semen was a representative *extract* of the whole body.

One of Hippocrates' most vocal critics was Aristotle, an early chauvinist who strongly opposed all theories implying that women contributed seeds of any kind to the embryo. Aristotle had observed that a woman could become pregnant while remaining absolutely passive (without orgasm). Exactly how Aristotle observed this phenomenon is not known, but he felt it proved that women made no genetic contributions. After all, men were active during sex while women could be completely passive (at least, one supposes, in Aristotle's case), so it was obvious that men contributed the vital elements to the child. Aristotle granted that the menstrual flow was important to creation, but only as a nutrient to the embryo. He also drew a parallel between menstruation in women and animals in heat. Aristotle felt that the dynamic principles—thought, morality, feelings, and so forth—were transmitted only by the male semen. "The mother of what is called a child is no parent," wrote Aristotle, "but only a nurse to the young life that is sown in her. The parent is the male—she is only a stranger, a friend whose fate bears the plant, preserving it until it is put forth."

Aristotle's thinking in this matter was not as original as some of his other, and philosophically sounder, tenets. The early Egyptians believed fathers alone were responsible for lineage, while mothers provided only nourishment to the fetus. This corresponded with a widespread belief in the old world that a woman's body was nothing more than a farmland in which men planted their seeds. If the farmland (woman) was watered and treated properly, it would reward the farmer (man) with a wonderful harvest. This belief can be seen clearly by examining the war practices of the time. Male prisoners were usually killed, while women survived because there was no fear that they could contribute children in the future of the defeated race.

One point on which almost all Greeks agreed, and one that was even taught in medical schools of the time, was that boys developed in the womb much faster than girls because the male fetus occupied the right, and warmer, side of the womb.

Many feel the Greeks had the most advanced culture of their time. That might have been true, especially in their regard for philosophy and humanism. Yet in the matter of conception and childbirth, their knowledge was meager and inaccurate.

One of the problems during ancient times in understanding the woman's role in conception was the invisibility of the uterus. Being an internal organ, the uterus was misunderstood in size, shape, and function. As far back as the Ebers Papyrus, the uterus was regarded as an animal with an independent life. Its form varied—sometimes it was shaped like a tortoise, other times like a newt, and frequently it took the shape of a crocodile. Abdominal palpations and vaginal inspections were sometimes undertaken just to determine the temporary location of the uterus and its temporary animal form.

In the second century, Arateus also thought the womb resembled an animal because it moved about freely. It was Arateus' postulate that the womb moved toward certain odors and away from others. Some of his generation agreed, and Galen even tried to prove that women played some role, even if a small one, in conception. Although Galen could not reconcile the fact that no woman ever conceived by herself, he still clung faithfully to his belief that women had something to do with baby making.

The idea that men are the sole creators is a ploy used in most patriarchal societies. A patriarchal culture, by definition, oppresses women. All too often the oppression reaches the point of denying women their most obvious attribute: the amazing ability to procreate. It is natural for the oppressor to fear the capabilities of the class it subjugates. In the case of patriarchy, man's fear of woman eventually gave rise to the spiteful, damaging myths concerning her body.

Myths and ignorance on the subject reigned for the next thousand years. There were many variations on the theme, but it was generally accepted that only men had any active reproductive power.

In 1520, Paracelsus theorized conception as involving putrefaction. He began a series of futile experiments with this decaying process in the hope that the tests would provide answers to genetic diseases or birth defects. Although a few manuscripts before the tenth century had mentioned the concept of female eggs, it was only in the age of Paracelsus that chemical methods were applied to the ideology.

Fallopius examined the ovaries and vesicles in search of seminal elements. He found none, so agreed with the historical concept of woman's inferior role in conception. A sidelight of this failed exploration was the discovery of the tubes on either side of the ovaries. These were later named fallopian tubes.

In 1621, Fabricus arrived at a new theory of conception. He organized animals into two categories. In the first were those spontaneously produced from eggs. The second category included animals produced internally by mothers and formed from seminal fluid.

In 1676, a medical student named Ham discovered sperm by examining it through Antony van Leeuwenhoek's invention—a tool called the microscope. Leeuwenhoek was Ham's mentor, so it was his honor to present the discovery to the Royal Society of London.

Leeuwenhoek knew this would be an extremely controversial discovery. Not only did it go against the prevailing knowledge of the time, the entire subject was considered offensive to polite society. He made every effort to convince the Royal Society that the semen in which the sperm was discovered was not gotten by any immoral means, such as masturbation. In his paper to the court, Leeuwenhoek wrote:

> What I here describe was not obtained by any sinful contrivance on my part, but the observations were made upon the excess with which Nature provided me in my conjugal relations. And if your Lordship should consider such matters either disgusting, or likely to seem offensive to the learned, I earnestly beg they be regarded as private, and either published or suppressed, as your Lordship's judgment dictates.

Leeuwenhoek's discovery was published in 1677, but his contemporary colleagues fought firmly against it. They thought these sperm to be only "animalcules"—parasites that were totally unrelated to fertility.

The discovery of sperm ranks among the great discoveries of natural science, but, as can be seen, it was not widely accepted at the time. The more popular belief was purely preposterous. Using Leeuwenhoek's microscope, most scientists claimed they saw minute forms of men with arms, hands, and legs swimming around in the semen. Some microscopists said they saw a figure of a miniature horse riding through the semen taken from a stallion. Animals with long ears were likewise seen in donkey semen. This belief was widely held through the middle of the eighteenth century. Many medical books and pamphlets included drawings showing little men living inside sperm. The masses took this as microscopic proof that the male semen was the sculptor, the menstrual blood was the block of clay, and the fetus was manufactured from this reproductive combination. This phenomenon of miniature men floating in semen illustrated that seventeenth-century scientists were as ignorant in their own way as primitive tribes had been thousands of years before. And at least primitive tribes made their conclusions without benefit of the microscope!

Almost a hundred years passed before the next vital breakthrough. In 1775, an Italian biologist named Lazarro Spallanzani performed an unusual experiment. From waxed fabric, Spallanzani fashioned tiny pairs of "trousers" which he put on male frogs. These frogs then mated with female frogs, but the male semen was caught and encased by the trousers. When the females failed to conceive, Spallanzani knew he was onto something. He then collected semen from other male frogs in the same manner and mixed the semen with female

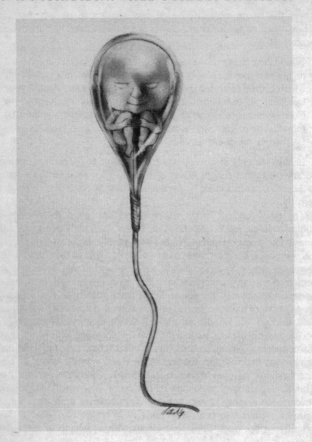

Fig. 4–1: 1976 was the tricentennial of the discovery of the sperm. When it was discovered, though, the sperm was completely misunderstood. Above is an artist's rendition of the human sperm as it was thought to be upon its discovery. Although microscopists never actually *saw* little men in sperm, they believed all new life originated in the male sperm, which they thought contained microscopic entities with all the characteristics necessary to develop into human beings. Women played no role in creation, and the uterus was believed merely to house the growth of the new individual encased in the male sperm.

eggs. The eggs became fertilized and Spallanzani should have been able to link the sperm to conception. Sadly, he did not. Instead, he felt that some vague element in the seminal fluid was the agent responsible for conception.

It was Dr. T. Barrie who finally made the important step in 1843, when he discovered the cellular origin of the sperm-egg union. From that date forward, scientists and medical people have been in agreement concerning the roles the male sperm and the female egg play in conception.

Each person is formed by genetic factors passed on through the mother and father. The sperm is the medium by which chromosomes from the father are taken and joined to the mother's egg, which carries her half of the chromosomes. This union of sperm and egg forms the fetus and, ultimately, the individual.

A spermatozoon is 0.002 inches long. Appearing almost like a microscopic snake, it has a small, oval head and a long, whiplike tail. It would take three billion sperm to fill a thimble. In every ejaculation, a healthy man releases approximately three hundred million active sperm. This high number of sperm is apparently necessary for the journey to the egg, a journey which few sperm survive. Along the way, half the sperm enter the wrong oviduct. Others are stranded in folds and crannies in the oviducts that trap sperm, preventing their contact with the egg. The opposing current which carries the egg down to the sperm also evacuates many sperm traveling upward to the egg. Many sperm die before they swim the distance—about a foot—to the egg. Sperm swim at the rate of about three inches per hour. All in all, only about one hundred of the original three hundred million survive. Even then, ovulation must be occurring for conception to take place.

From the time of Barrie's discovery, science did not adequately explain conception to lay people. For years, the masses continued their beliefs in myths and stories. Even while the correct information was readily available, ignorance on the subject remained widespread. Some old stories even acquired new twists to help them bridge the gap into the modern world.

The stork was one of the birds to survive the leap from the age of ignorance to the age of neglect. In many countries, when a woman was about to give birth, she would leave home to go either to a hospital or to stay with a midwife. If this woman already had children, they were rarely told the real reason their mother was gone. They were usually told only that their mother would be gone for a few weeks and, in the meantime, the stork would come and give them a new baby. When the mother returned to the family, she might still look pregnant to the children because her abdominal muscles would be stretched and her uterus would be hypertrophic, or enlarged. Since their mother looked about the same as when she left, the children actually believed the stork had brought their new brother or sister.

Today, of course, the mother does not leave home for weeks on end, but that is a relatively new treatment. It was recently found that the long bed rest given to women after childbirth was a common cause of phlebitis and related syndromes. Nowadays, the mother is released from the hospital as soon as possible. This has drastically reduced the occurrence of phlebitis due to long bed rest. Modern childbirth methods have also made it difficult for the illusion of the stork to survive in the minds of the mother's other children.

The problem of educating children on the subject of conception today is different. Science knows how conception occurs, and so, generally speaking, do the masses. Yet most people are still embarrassed about the sexual aspects of conception and are either too shy or too uncomfortable to explain it to their children. A modern-day child may believe in the stork for a while, but by the time the child is about to reach puberty, the stork no longer seems logical and the child must look for other answers. If parents do not provide the correct facts, the variety of theories children receive concerning conception is truly astonishing.

Some children are told that babies come from semen, which at least starts with the right premise. But then they are told that the semen is spread out and as soon as the sun's rays touch it, it turns into a child and the semen flows into the mother, where it grows and is finally born.

In the midwestern United States, children sometimes learn that a woman has three vaginas leading to three different uteri. As a man enters a woman, he lodges in one of the three locations. The mother's egg is supposedly in only one of the three uteri, and if the man enters the vagina leading to the uterus containing the egg, the woman will get pregnant. This Russian roulette sort of theory lends a hidden excitement and danger to sex for early teenagers, and perhaps that is the reason this myth has not died.

Of course, modern society encourages complete sexual education. Although this is to be praised, we must be careful not to go overboard in a backlash of past ignorance. A child's psychological attitude toward sex and conception is vitally important, and it is just as vital that the child is given correct information in a comfortable and natural way. Society must not force-feed sex education to three-year-old children; they may not want it, and further, they may not be able to cope with it.

Teaching children about sex and conception should perhaps be handled in the same way children are taught the three Rs—gradually. As each new step is easily and comfortably consumed by the child, another new facet of sex can be explained. This can be done in a variety of ways, such as parental talks, picture books, and even showing parallels in the animal world.

Whatever method is chosen, it should not be one that will shock, upset, or disgust the child. Recently, a well-known psychiatrist told of his ultramodern method of educating his daughter. When the child was eight years old, this man encouraged her to watch him have sex with his wife. The child could not absorb this because the man's wife was, of course, *her mother,* and her image of her mother did not coincide with this behavior. Eventually, the girl would have come to know her mother as a sexual being, but in this case, the experiment was too much, too soon. The child was traumatized and she is now in a psychiatric institution.

If there is a lesson to be learned from the stork, perhaps it is that the idea of conception and childbirth is one that is best related to children in a spirit of love and gentleness. Now is the time for loving, caring, and gentle parents to replace this giant white bird, who so lovingly served children and their parents for so many generations, with the truth, told gently and gradually. No woman can afford not to do this.

chapter 5

THE REPRODUCTIVE CYCLE

LEVITICUS 15

19 And if a woman have an issue, and her issue in her flesh be blood, she shall be put apart seven days: and whosoever toucheth her shall be unclean until the evening.

24 And if any man lie with her at all, and her flowers be upon him, he shall be unclean seven days, and all the bed whereon he lieth shall be unclean.

28 But if she be cleansed of her issue, then she shall number to herself seven days, and after she shall be clean.

29 And on the eighth day she shall take unto her two turtles, or two pigeons, and bring them unto the priest, to the door of the tabernacle of the congregation.

30 And the priest shall offer the one for a sin offering, and the other for a burnt offering; and the priest shall make an atonement for her before the Lord for the issue of her uncleanness.

THE CURSE—A BLESSING IN DISGUISE

If you have ever wondered why the aura of shame surrounds menstruation, look to your Bible. Although most patriarchal cultures have antifemale myths, we can blame Leviticus for our Judeo-Christian menstrual hang-ups. These few lines sufficiently capture the essence of male fear concerning the menses.

The purpose here is to dispel the image of the "unclean woman." Menstruation is a healthy function. Contrary to biblical belief, menstruation is a cleansing process, whereby the uterus prepares itself for the next ovulation.

There have been more nicknames and euphemisms concerning the menstrual period than perhaps any other female function. So much so that the word *menstruation* is hardly even in the everyday vocabulary of many women, who prefer even in these modern times to refer to their monthly bleeding process as a "period." For other women, a period is still only something that ends a sentence, and these women might refer to this quite normal phenomenon as "the curse." Women known for discretion smile sweetly and announce to co-workers that "my good friend is visiting." Others—usually teenage American girls —whisper to schoolmates that "Mary just fell off the roof!" Very rarely does a woman announce the onset of a menstrual condition with anything but embarrassment or irritation.

Men don't help at all in this area. In fact, quite possibly, men are more insensitive to the monthly bleeding pattern than to any other facet of a woman's physical condition. They crudely tell their friends that their wives or girl friends are "on the rag" or "riding the cotton pony," obvious references to sanitary napkins and tampons.

The reasons behind this subterfuge are many but simple. More frightening stories and descriptions have been associated with menstruation than with any other physiological aspect of a woman's life. Like stories concerning conception and contraception, myths and misconceptions on the topic vary from one culture to another. Most patriarchal societies exhibit misogynist tendencies regarding menstruation, while matriarchal cultures reverse the trend.

Thousands of years ago it was thought that the menstrual period was a sign of fertility. Ancient peoples connected the event to the bleeding in animals that aroused sexual excitement. Some cultures even thought menstruation heralded a two- or three-day time in which women were to be fertilized. Now, of course, we realize they were wrong and, conversely, that if there is any time of the month that is less fertile than others, it is during a woman's monthly bleeding.

Ancient cultures naturally observed that this bleeding occurred approximately once a month. Ironically, the Romans gave it the name *mens*, not a sexual designation, but rather a word that translates as *monthly*.

No connection was made in the Greek culture between menstruation and childbearing. Birth was considered a gift from God that happened once every couple of years. Strangely enough, the connection made was between breast-feeding and childbirth. The ancients thought that women would not become pregnant while they were breast-feeding, so the gift of God was thought to be given only to women not breast-feeding a child. Many women, therefore, breast-fed their children much longer than was necessary in the hope they would not become pregnant again.

This fairly common belief enslaved women in a perpetual state of pregnancy or breast-feeding. Since menstruation did not occur in either state, most women did not have regular periods. Therefore when bleeding occurred, it was looked upon as a sign of abnormality. Because of this, every time a woman started to bleed, it was thought she was sick inside or was bleeding from internal scars or sores caused by childbirth or disease. When she conceived again, or stopped bleeding, she was considered healthy. It was a vicious circle, made more tragic by the fact that women of the past often died during childbirth at a young age because of anemia or other diseases which attacked them while they were in weakened states of health.

Another reason women were constantly pregnant was the low rate of survival among their children. In those days, medicine knew few cures for the diseases that ravaged populations. Babies were extremely susceptible to major illnesses, diseases, and viruses. Only a few of the strongest could survive before the advent of modern medicine.

This was an era in which there was no knowledge of the menstrual cycle—a time when it was known merely that intercourse had some vague, but unclear, connection to conception. The belief that men dominated the reproductive cycle was universally accepted, so menstruation was ignored for many centuries.

A true understanding of the menstrual cycle and an exact comprehension of the pattern of ovulation and its relationship to the menstrual period was not discovered until 1930. At that time, two physicians—one Austrian, one Japanese—arrived independently at the same conclusions concerning ovulation. These men established that ovulation occurs approximately twelve to sixteen days prior to each menstrual period. That discovery, coupled with the knowledge of the full twenty-eight-day menstrual cycle, made it possible to determine almost positively the exact days of fertility. The most immediate effect of this discovery was the creation of the "safe period" of intercourse—the time just before, during, and after the menstrual period when a woman could have sex without worry of pregnancy.

Of course, this new "safe period" was completely opposite to prior beliefs. For centuries, the period was associated with animals in heat and was, therefore, considered the proper time for reproduction. At the same time, many women who had sex during the previously regarded safe period when they were not bleeding found themselves pregnant. Now we know that the bleeding function is not only reproductive but sanitary, and that it cleans the internal organs, washing away dead and dying cells with monthly regularity.

Even today, misconceptions about menstrual bleeding run rampant. There are even twentieth-century subcultures which encourage the belief that menstrual bleeding is a sign of unhealthiness.

For a long time, the Jewish heritage, and in particular the Orthodox sects, demanded that a woman be taken from her home during her period because she was considered dirty. These women would be locked up until the bleeding stopped; then they would be washed and their vaginas fumigated before they were considered clean enough to reenter their families and society. This type of irrational belief only traumatized women and gave vent to no true understanding of what it was to be a woman.

Other, more matriarchal cultures taught women that their periods cleansed them. Even so, there were many misconceptions. As recently as twenty years ago, American women were told by many doctors not to bathe or swim during their periods and to get plenty of bed rest. This would indicate that these physicians thought bleeding was akin to the flu or common cold, something which required medical attention. Although the period was considered beneficial to a woman's overall health, the stigma attached to it was difficult to shake.

With the personal and political choices being made by women today to have fewer or no children, the menstrual period is more and more being viewed not as a curse but as a blessing. For women who do not use any form of birth control, and even for those who do, the period signals one more month in which they have not gotten pregnant.

WHAT IS MENSTRUATION?

Stated simply, the uterus is an organ which is under the influence of hormones and which is constantly undergoing changes throughout the monthly cycle. The *endometrium* (the lining of the uterus) increases in thickness throughout the monthly cycle by becoming thicker and more vascular (increasing the blood supply). This readies the uterus for conception, but if conception does not occur, the build-up of the endometrium is essentially wasted. To enable the process to begin for the next month, the build-up of wasted cells in the lining of the uterus must be cleared away. The menstrual blood is the medium by which these waste matters are disposed of, washing them away from the uterus through the cervix and vagina. The blood removes the dead cells from the uterine lining, but it does not clean the lining. The cleaning is accomplished by the endocrine function, in which the hormonal changes are activated and deactivated. It is this endocrine function which affects the entire body, another reason women often feel better immediately following their periods.

Because it is the endocrine function which actually cleans the uterus, the amount of blood flow during the period has no connection to the amount of cleaning accomplished. Some women mistakenly feel that if they have a heavy blood flow, they are cleaner than women who experience a light flow. This is untrue. The amount of flow may affect the speed by which the uterine lining is cleaned, but not the extent of cleaning itself.

The amount of flow would be *increased* in the presence of an IUD or fibroid tumors (see Chapter 13). Moreover, if a woman is obese, the fatty tissue causes higher estrogen levels, which in turn overstimulate the build-up of the lining of the uterus. The result is heavier bleeding. The best treatment for an obese woman would be weight reduction; secondarily, *antiprostaglandins* (such as Motrin or Naproxen) might be prescribed to decrease the menstrual bleeding. The drug would be taken four times per day, starting on the day before expected menstruation and ending on the fourth day of her flow.

Some women express concern that menstrual blood is also evacuating cells which are beneficial to good health. This is a natural and somewhat logical worry, but a needless one all the same. Menstrual periods merely indicate a loss of the *unused* and *unnecessary* lining of the uterus. Nothing that is essential to good health is removed by menstrual blood.

The interaction of these two functions—the removal of the dead cells by the blood and the cleaning of the uterus/uterine lining by the endocrine function—is the *total sanitary process* of menstrual bleeding.

Physical and Emotional Changes during the Menstrual Cycle—Premenstrual Tension

The physical and emotional ups and downs most women experience during the menstrual cycle cannot and should not be overlooked. Most of them are caused by the hormonal changes every woman experiences during her cycle. The basic body temperature rises. The levels of progesterone and estrogen are also higher just prior to the period.

One physical manifestation of this hormonal change occurs because the hormones bind salt, and the salt, in turn, binds water. Because of this, many women retain water and feel bloated immediately prior to menstruation. This bloated condition makes many women feel

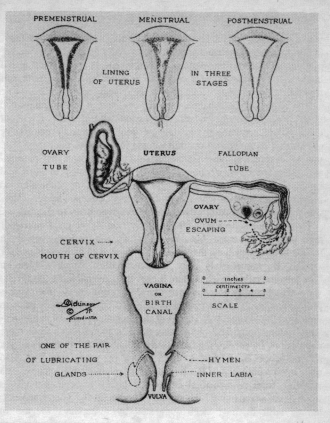

Fig. 5–1: The lower part of this picture is a cross-section of the vagina, the cervix, and the uterus that approximates the relationship of the ovaries and the fallopian tubes to the uterus.

On the right is a further cross-section of an ovary and a fallopian tube. Shown is an egg (ovum) escaping from the ovary and in the process of being caught by the end of the fallopian tube.

At the top is a cross-section of a uterus and *endometrium* (the lining of the uterus) during the premenstrual, menstrual, and postmenstrual phases. Each month, the *endometrium* accumulates a mass of vascular tissue. This prepares the uterus for conception. If conception does not occur, the egg disintegrates and the *endometrium* is expelled via the menstrual flow. (Dickinson Anatomical Chart—reproduced by permission of Educational Department, TAMPAX Incorporated, Lake Success, New York.)

worse and many physicians prescribe diuretics to ease the malady. Other doctors tell their patients simply to avoid excessive salt intake, particularly before their periods. The decrease in salt content in the body will likewise cause a decrease in water retention. Acne and nausea also commonly occur prior to or during menstruation.

The physical disturbances accompany and/or cause emotional upset, such as depression. But depressions can also occur without these physical manifestations and are quite common. Studies have shown that more women commit suicide just prior to their menstrual periods than at any other time. Certain instances of severe premenstrual tension or depression may be directly related to hormonal imbalance—specifically, an excess of estrogen as compared to progesterone. Women with this problem may be helped by progesterone therapy, in the form of a suppository given prior to menses.

Depression has been a justifiable motivation for women thinking of their periods as a curse, but now something can be done even about this. It has recently been discovered that there is an increased need for vitamin B_6 immediately prior to menstruation. Since women on birth-control pills (which contain higher than normal hormone levels) were also found to require an increased amount of B_6, the need is probably a result of the similarly increased hormone levels prior to menstruation. The lack of B_6 has been associated with some premenstrual depressions, and many women have found relief from these depressions by consuming increased amounts of B_6 at that time. An advantage of B_6 is that it often clears up acne, which is also associated with a lack of B_6. It is therefore recommended that women suffering from premenstrual depression and/or acne should take a multivitamin containing high amounts of vitamin B_6. Special multivitamins with B_6 have been suggested by researchers for use in connection with oral contraceptives. These same multivitamins are ideal for the prevention of depression and acne. One can also take a vitamin B complex, as long as it contains a high amount of B_6. Zinc may also be helpful. If vitamin therapy is the solution to your menstrual ills, you will probably find the exact intake for your particular problem on your own or in conjunction with your doctor. In most cases, one multiple vitamin per day is taken throughout the menstrual cycle, and if acne or depression is severe, the vitamin intake is usually doubled or tripled just prior to menstruation.

Although hormonal changes certainly account for some or most of the depressions, research has shown that even these depressions can be caused psychosomatically. For instance, a woman who has been fed frightening stories about her period will dread its onset. Even though her hormonal changes alone would not lead to a depressed state, she psychologically braces herself for the period by sublimating her fear. This fear grows subconsciously and the effect, if not the cause, is the same: depression. This is one very obvious proof of the harm done by menstrual myths, and it should be reason enough on its own for seeking to destroy those myths.

During menstrual bleeding, a woman will lose iron from her body. It is disadvantageous to have a heavy flow, since more iron is lost. If you feel weak or tired after a particularly heavy menstrual flow, the cause may be an iron deficiency. In such a case, you will have to replace the loss with vitamins and iron pills to keep your hemoglobin level up. This should make you feel much healthier. Of course, if you have been placed on some type of hormone pill that prevents iron loss, you should feel consistently energetic.

Manipulators

The few women who abuse their periods should not be overlooked, either. These are women who try to reinforce the myth that a woman's period is a terrible thing to endure and who manipulate people around them by exaggerated displays of suffering. These women get out of dates, business meetings, or gym classes at school on the excuse that their periods are having a devastating effect on their health. Some of these women don't consciously want to manipulate, but just want a little sympathy, and this, sadly, is one of the few ways they can get it. Other women will use their periods to punish their sex partners subtly, saying they can't have sex during their periods. And the small offenders are those women who use their periods to indulge in activities they don't normally support, like smoking or drinking.

In the long view, women who abuse their periods might be getting back at the society which has, from the beginning, perverted the concept of menstruation.

What Happens after Menstruation?

After their periods, women should feel better, both physically and psychologically. Not only have they disposed of uterine waste; the hormonal levels which were high prior to their periods have returned to normal. This causes a lower progesterone and estrogen level. They also dehydrate and lose some of the water they had retained. This would make anyone feel better.

THE FIRST MENSTRUATION—MENARCHE

Because of incorrect histories and scare stories concerning the menstrual cycle, a mother's explanation about the process to her daughter is extremely important. Before the child has her first menstruation, her mother should tell her to expect menstrual bleeding and should explain the entire process to her in a reassuring and positive manner.

If the child is not told, one day she will start bleeding and, not knowing what is happening, she will probably think something is terribly wrong with her internally. The resulting psychological trauma could very well follow her the rest of her life.

Most children begin menstruating at age eleven, twelve, or thirteen. The time of the *menarche* (first menses) varies, of course, and two girls who are otherwise almost totally alike may experience their first bleeding three or four years apart.

However, if a girl starts to menstruate very early, say before ten years of age, she should be seen by a physician, since certain types of hormone-producing tumors could be located either in the adrenal glands or in the ovaries. These tumors sometimes cause early menstruation, and that very menstruation is a signal of the tumors.

Likewise, if a girl does not menstruate until very late, say fifteen, she should also be seen by a physician, since there may be some sort of organic malfunction which is responsible for the late menstruation.

These variations in onset of the first menstrual period may also be due to very simple causes. Genetics is one factor: If a mother menstruated at a late age, her daughter will probably show that same tendency. Variations might also be caused by different nutritional intakes or by psychological strain. It is important to realize that the menstrual period is part of a very delicate process, and almost any upset might delay or speed its onset.

THE MENSTRUAL CYCLE AND IRREGULARITIES

The regular pattern of the menstrual period varies from woman to woman. The majority of women have their periods approximately every twenty-eight days, but other women exhibit irregular patterns of ovulation. When a woman has an extreme weight gain or loss, this likely is reflected in her menstrual cycle and the cycle probably becomes irregular.

It is now known that the menstrual period is closely associated with the hormones LH (luteinizing hormone) and FSH (follicle-stimulating hormone), both of which are secreted from the pituitary gland in the brain. LH and FSH are further influenced by hormones released by the hypothalamus, which is, in turn, influenced strongly by a woman's psychological and emotional state. Because of this, if a woman enters a time of extreme stress (and the definition of extreme stress also varies from woman to woman), *amenorrhea* (a stoppage of the bleeding pattern) will result. It is important for women to know that their menstrual periods are affected by emotional conditions and/or stress. Armed with this knowledge, women might find it easier to cope with stressful situations and their resultant menstrual irregularities.

Certain other medical conditions can cause irregular menstrual bleeding. Polycystic ovaries, which is a cystic enlargement of the ovaries, can cause irregular bleeding. Many other diseases and infections can cause menstrual irregularity, but each abnormal menstrual malfunction should be evaluated individually to find the cause.

Hormonal Changes during the Menstrual Cycle

During the menstrual cycle, there is a close relationship between the pituitary hormones (FSH and LH) and the ovarian hormones (estrogen and progesterone). These hormones are responsible for ovulation as well as for the cyclical change of the endometrium (the lining of the uterus).

Immediately after menstruation, there is an increased discharge of FSH from the pituitary, which stimulates the follicles in both ovaries. *Follicles* are cells in the ovaries that might develop into eggs. As the follicles start to increase in size, their production of estrogen also increases. For unknown reasons, each month one follicle will surpass the growth of the other follicles and develop into a Graafian follicle, which produces the egg for that particular month. In the case of unidentical multiple births, several Graafian follicles produce several eggs for the month. At present, there is no rigid pattern that can be discerned in ovulation, so it cannot be determined if a woman has one or many Graafian follicles in her ovaries at any given time, or in which ovary ovulation might occur.

The increased amounts of estrogen produced immediately prior to ovulation have a feedback to the pituitary, resulting in a decrease in FSH production and a surge in LH production. This will result in ovulation.

After the egg is released from the Graafian follicle (the process of

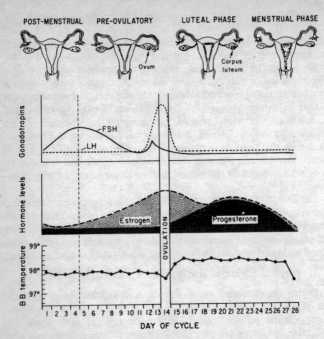

Fig. 5–2: This graph illustrates the close relationship between the brain hormones (gonadotrophins), the ovarian hormones (estrogen and progesterone), and their influence on ovulation, the menstrual period, and the Basal Body Temperature (BBT).

At the top of the illustration, one ovum is seen developed in the preovulatory phase. Note also that the end of the fallopian tube is reaching down toward the ovum to ensure that the tube will catch the ovum during ovulation.

As illustrated, the BBT, which has been steady during the first two phases, usually drops 0.1° to 0.2° at ovulation.

After ovulation, the graafian follicle containing the ovum of the month changes into a special cellular unit called the corpus luteum, shown here in the luteal phase. It should also be observed that the end of the fallopian tube here releases its grip on the ovary.

ovulation), the Graafian follicle changes into a *corpus luteum* (yellow body). The cells in the corpus luteum then produce progesterone Progesterone is a Latin name; *pro* means "for" and *gesterone* means "gestation," therefore *progesterone* means "for gestation." In medical

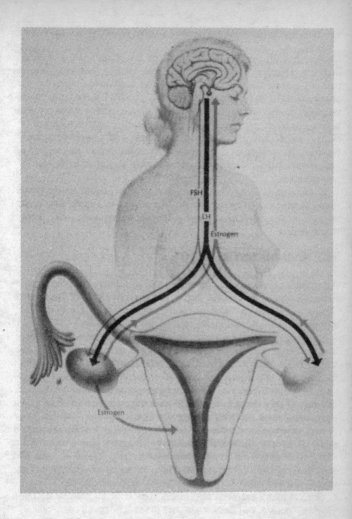

Fig. 5–3: The interaction of the pituitary, the ovary and the uterus during ovulation caused by the secretion and stimulation of LH, FSH, and estrogen. An egg has been released by the woman's right ovary and is about to be picked up from the fimbriated end of the fallopian tube. (Reproduced by permission of the Ortho Corporation, Raritan, New Jersey.)

circles, it is also called the hormone of the mother, since it helps maintain pregnancy. Progesterone is an ovarian hormone that is partially responsible for the changes in the endometrium and for the change in basal body temperature (BBT). The BBT is the temperature obtained in the morning immediately after a person awakens and before any active movement. This temperature is approximately 97.5 degrees for the two weeks after menstruation, with a slight decrease at the time of ovulation; a one-degree increase occurs thereafter, to approximately 98.5 degrees, from the time of ovulation to the time of menstruation.

If conception does not occur, the corpus luteum disintegrates immediately prior to menstruation. This results in a steep drop in the amount of progesterone and in the BBT approximately a day before menstruation.

SEX AND MENSTRUATION

All manner of scare stories have been told to women about the terrible consequences of intercourse during the menstrual period. Like many stories told for shock value, several of these tales start with one fact and then travel into the realm of total fantasy.

It is true that during menstruation the uterus is open and pumping waste through the cervix. Consequently, as the penis goes into the vagina during menstruation, it will push bacteria from the penis into the uterus. If this bacteria is harmful or the kind that spreads easily, such as venereal bacteria, it will probably spread infection or disease. Because of this, it might be wise to have the man use a condom if you have intercourse, at least during the first couple of days of your period, or when the flow is heaviest. As the blood flow decreases to a minimal amount, the uterus will usually be almost closed again and it will not be dangerous to have condom-free sex. This is the one and only danger of sex during menstruation, assuming all other factors are equal, and any other scare stories should not be believed.

Several men have been told that if they have intercourse during a woman's period, and the woman uses the superior position, blood will run into the penis and cause damage. This is patently ridiculous and has no basis in fact. In fact, the origin of this fear is an acceptance of the misogynist myths society has foolishly embraced for such a long time. If you cannot convince your male sex partner of the silliness of this myth, let him use a condom if he wants. He will probably worry less and therefore be free to give you more sexual satisfaction. If this doesn't work, you might be better off finding a less neurotic bed partner.

If you find that a heavy flow reduces the amount of friction you need during sex, you can temporarily halt the flow by inserting a diaphragm. If your partner is particularly neurotic about the presence of blood, you can douche to remove the last traces. Douching should *not* be done if you are using a diaphragm for contraceptive purposes, as the contraceptive jelly will be washed away.

Remember, the presence of menstrual blood is a sign of health. A woman need never be self-conscious about her period during sex. If there is a psychological problem here, it is probably the result of believing the male-originated myths about menstruation.

Sexual Stimulation during Menstruation

A majority of women describe an increased sexual desire during their menstrual periods, particularly in the last few days of bleeding. This is not abnormal, because the blood acts as an aphrodisiac by stimulating, or tickling, the sexual organs of the woman. This aphrodisiac effect of menstruation is usually highest in the last few days of the period, when the flow is light and there is no association with painful menstrual cramps.

Some women feel an increased sexual desire immediately prior to the period, a phenomenon probably due to an increased sensitivity in the nervous system.

As mentioned before, intercourse is not harmful at these times. To the contrary, it might even help relieve the tensions built up at this time.

IS MENSTRUATION NECESSARY?

In recent years, several physicians have investigated the menstrual pattern in an attempt to determine whether or not the period is a necessary or desirable part of a woman's life. The newer birth-control pills, especially the low-estrogen-containing contraceptives, usually retard the stimulation of the uterus or the lining of the uterus which causes the tissue build-up responsible for menstrual bleeding. Therefore, with this type of pill, women experience very little menstrual bleeding.

If it is ever proven that menstrual bleeding is, indeed, unnecessary or harmful, many women will rebel against the proof since they feel their periods are an inherent part of being a woman. If and when this comes to be, a program of wide reeducation may be necessary. Certainly the presence or absence of a single function in a woman has little bearing on her womanliness. Women who have hysterectomies or mastectomies are no less womanly than other women, and this logic would carry through to menstrual bleeding.

Obviously, many women benefit from the low-estrogen contraceptive pills. Women who experience too much bleeding early in life, causing a huge loss of iron, or women who have *dysmenorrhea* (extremely painful menstruation), find many of their physical problems lessened by use of these pills. It is important to teach women that this treatment will not harm them in any way. The glands which produce menstrual blood are not damaged or altered, just put in a state of rest as a natural function of this type of birth-control pill. Some of the new birth-control pills lessen bleeding; others stop it altogether, causing complete amenorrhea (cessation of menstruation).

What is vitally important is that the physician completely explain to each woman what she can anticipate with each type of pill. If you are on a birth-control pill containing a lower level of hormone, you will have very little menstrual bleeding. If you are placed on the minipill, you might have regular bleeding in the beginning and then later on have almost no menstrual bleeding. If you are on the newly researched antigonadotrophic hormones such as danazol, you might have no bleeding whatsoever.

Studies in England have shown there may be an important link between the menstrual cycle and breast cancer in women. Researchers there found that older women who had little menstrual bleeding when they were younger because they were constantly pregnant or were breast-feeding had a significantly lower incidence of breast cancer than the general female population. These test results have sparked concern among physicians and have given new support to the birth-control pill. The results show that the cyclical changes of menstruation, where the breasts change size month after month, might possibly cause cancer. If this is borne out by further research, women might be better off being placed on ovulation-suppressing birth-control pills.

DO MEN HAVE A TEMPERATURE CYCLE SIMILAR TO WOMEN?

Recent investigation indicates that men appear to have a temperature cycle synchronous with the temperature changes of the women with whom they are living. This is interesting, since men do not undergo any significant fluctuations in hormone levels such as women do during their menstrual cycles.

Factors that influence a partner's cycle can, however, secondarily affect the other's cycle. In reported findings, the male cycle ran from seventeen to thirty-five days, which fairly closely coincides with a woman's cycle. Men *seem* to have behavioral changes occurring in the same rhythmic fashion as women.

A typical male pattern shows temperature drop in the middle of the month, near or at the same time as his female partner has the ovulatory mid-cycle temperature drop. A man's temperature then rises to a high level, also compatible with the one occurring in women after ovulation.

A major difference shown in the survey was that a man's temperature usually dropped approximately a week after his female partner's ovulation, where a woman's temperature remains high for approximately two weeks after ovulation.

The type of hormone changes or causes of this male temperature cycle are unknown. It was found, however, that when partners were not in cyclic temperature harmony, there appeared to be more strain and difficulty in the relationship.

OVULATION

Ovulation occurs only once a month, approximately fourteen days before a menstrual period. Even women with irregular bleeding patterns ovulate two weeks before their next period. The egg is released from only one ovary at a time, and there is no way to predict which ovary will release the egg at any given time. Women who have had one ovary surgically removed will still ovulate regularly from the remaining one.

The first day of menstrual bleeding is called *day 1* of the menstrual cycle. The bleeding is accompanied by a decrease in estrogen and progesterone, a hormonal change that might create a tendency toward mild diarrhea, and creates a water and weight loss, making the woman feel lighter and healthier.

During the first five days of the cycle, the decreased estrogen results in a release of follicle-stimulating hormone (FSH) from the pituitary gland. The FSH stimulates the follicles in the ovaries. This matures several of the stored eggs, and as they grow, they produce estrogen.

The estrogen stimulates the growth of the endometrium (the lining of the uterus). The mucous plug of the cervix becomes thinner and more slippery, ready to aid the sperm in their travel through the cervix. During this part of the cycle, one of the still undeveloped follicles (the mass of cells containing the almost-mature egg) begins to outgrow the others, becoming the Graafian follicle that produces the egg of the month. As the Graafian follicle grows to the surface of the ovary, preparing to expel the egg, the fallopian tube on the same side reaches down around the ovary to catch the egg. The increasing estrogen level starts to block the FSH from the pituitary.

As ovulation nears, the Graafian follicle has a higher amount of *prostaglandins* (fatty acids present in many tissues), which cause the ovary to contract and expel the egg. As this happens, the ovary turns to the side close to the fimbriated, or fringed, end of the fallopian tube, which, like a hand with fingers, grasps the egg and its surrounding protoplasm (egg white).

In the fallopian tube, the egg travels slowly toward the uterus, propelled by fine, fingerlike *fimbria*. The ruptured Graafian follicle becomes a corpus luteum, or yellow body, and begins to produce progesterone and estrogen to stimulate the uterine lining to become thicker and spongy. This is accompanied by an increase in basal body temperature (BBT). The temperature decreases slightly at ovulation, while increasing one degree to about 98.5 degrees the two weeks after ovulation.

If conception does occur, the corpus luteum does not disintegrate. This causes a persistently high level of progesterone and the BBT remains about 98.5 degrees. This is the first proof of pregnancy.

CAN A WOMAN TELL WHEN SHE OVULATES?

Ovulation occurs two weeks prior to each menstrual period, but since many women are not sure when their next period will take place, it can be difficult to determine the exact time of ovulation. By taking the basal body temperature for a few months, a woman can get an approximate idea of when ovulation takes place. This, however, is only possible if she has a regular cycle. The temperature usually decreases slightly on the day of ovulation and increases sharply on the day following ovulation.

Some women state that they know exactly when they ovulate because they feel several changes in their bodies. Many women experience mild pain or backache at the time of ovulation. Other

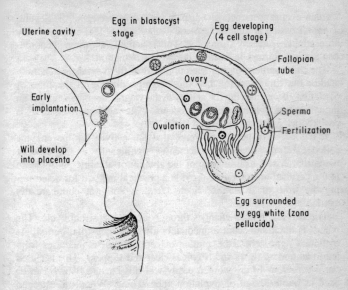

Fig. 5–4: This schematic drawing shows the various stages involved in ovulation and fertilization. In the ovary, the development of an egg into first a follicle, then a Graafian follicle, followed by expulsion of the egg, ovulation, and remaining corpus luteum can be seen. The fimbriated end of the fallopian tube reaches toward the ovary; the egg passes into the fallopian tube. In the tube, the passage of the egg toward the uterus is assisted by the motion of small, hairlike projections called *cilia,* and is nourished during this time by the egg white, the *zona pellucida* that surrounds the egg. Fertilization, the conjunction of the egg with sperm, usually takes place in the mid-portion of the fallopian tube. As it continues its journey toward the uterus, the fertilized egg, called a *zygote,* begins to divide first into two cells, then into four, and then, by geometric progression, into a hollow ball consisting of many cells, called a *blastocyst.* In the blastocyst stage, the fertilized egg enters the uterine cavity and implants in the uterine wall. At the site of implantation, blood vessels develop which provide blood to the developing placenta, the source of nourishment to the fetus. It usually takes an egg 3 to 5 days to make the journey from the ovary to the uterus. If the egg is fertilized and this journey is interrupted due to some fallopian-tube abnormality, the blastocyst might implant in the fallopian tube, resulting in an *ectopic,* or tubal, pregnancy. The egg and sperm in this illustration are not drawn to scale.

women even experience severe pain (called *Mittelschmerz*). Several women say that around the time of ovulation they feel more sexually aroused and erotically stimulated. This is actually a known phenomenon among animals in heat on the day of ovulation.

The environment of the secretion within the vagina is generally acidic, but this secretion becomes slightly alkaline at the time of ovulation. By measuring the acidity in the vagina, a woman can get an indication of when ovulation occurs. The acid-base balance is checked by using a special test paper.

It has recently been discovered that the activity of the enzyme called *alkaline phosphatase* decreases significantly at the time of ovulation. A self-examination of the amount of alkaline phosphatase in the cervical mucus might provide a practical method for determining the time of ovulation. Such a test is still not commercially available.

The cervical mucus changes throughout the menstrual cycle. The mucus is thick and scant immediately after the menstrual period. As ovulation approaches, the amount of cervical mucus increases from ten to a hundred times and becomes clear and slippery. This is called *the wet period.* Many women easily feel this change, which can be used as another sign of ovulation approaching. When the estrogen level peaks and ovulation occurs, the cervical mucus has reached its maximum change. A new device the size of a tampon is being developed in laboratories in Boston. This device, called an Ovutimer, is designed to read the direct change in the cervical mucus and thus indicate the time of ovulation. The device may be commercially available in the future.

MITTELSCHMERZ—INTERMENSTRUAL PAIN

Intermenstrual pain, or *Mittelschmerz,* usually occurs at the time of ovulation. Normally, ovulation causes no pain, or sometimes just a dull cramping. Occasionally, ovulation is combined with such severe pain that a woman cannot walk and is confined to bed. Often a physician is seen because the woman might easily think she has appendicitis or a pelvic infection. *Mittelschmerz* can occasionally be associated with vaginal bleeding. This sometimes scares women, although it is a normal physiological happening. The pain is probably due to intra-abdominal bleeding from the ovulation site. This causes a reaction from the peritoneum in the abdomen, which results in pain from the nerve endings. The vaginal bleeding which occurs is usually due to spillage of hormone, mostly estrogen hormone. The spillage of this hormone can cause a change in the body's mechanism and can alter the contraction pattern of the uterus. Some of the endometrial lining of the uterus is then shed, resulting in bleeding. The pain usually disappears in a few days. There is no treatment save bed rest with a heating pad. The bleeding is usually slight and self-limiting. The bleeding site usually heals and no other problem occurs. However, if pain continues, one should see a physician.

CONCEPTION

Conception occurs when the sperm fertilizes the egg in the fallopian tube. This happens between one and three days after ovulation. The egg remains in the fallopian tube for about four or five days before moving into the uterus.

The round egg cell is the largest single human cell, yet it is smaller than a single dot. The sperm cell is considerably smaller. Though shaped like a comma, it would take about 2,500 sperm cells to cover a comma. In fact, all the sperm required to repopulate the earth would be no larger than an aspirin tablet. Sperm have tails, which they use to propel themselves, much as fish use their tailfins. They move quickly, reaching the fallopian tubes eight to ten minutes after being ejaculated into the vagina.

A fertilized egg implants in the uterine wall six to seven days after ovulation, or approximately three weeks after the last menstrual period. It unites with the blood vessels inside the uterus, and a human being begins to develop. The spongy uterine wall in which the egg lodges becomes the placenta, providing the developing fetus with nourishment.

The exact mechanism enabling the sperm to penetrate the egg shell is unknown, but hormones in the head of the sperm probably effect the fertilization. Though approximately two million sperm cells are present in a normal ejaculation, only one penetrates the egg during conception. If fertilization of the egg does not occur, the egg disintegrates and is slowly expelled from the uterus.

Fertility drugs containing LH and FSH in abnormally high doses overstimulate the follicles, and several eggs may be released as a result. This can result in multiple births if several eggs are fertilized.

How Can a Woman Tell if She Is Pregnant?

The first sign of pregnancy is usually a missed period. If you miss a period, you should take your basal body temperature (BBT) every morning to confirm or deny any suspicions of pregnancy. If you are

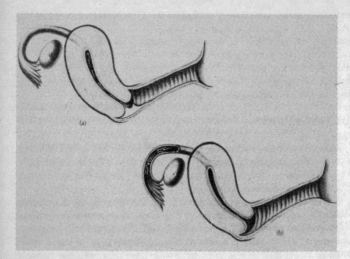

Fig. 5-5: The vagina, uterus, fallopian tubes and ovaries in cross-section, with the approximate angles of these pelvic organs in a woman lying on her back. In picture (a), the ejaculate is lying close to the cervix and sperm have begun their migration through the uterus toward the fallopian tubes. The egg is about to be expelled from the ovary and caught by the fimbriated end of the fallopian tube. In picture (b), the egg and sperm meet in the mid-portion of the fallopian tube, the most common place for proper fertilization. (Reproduced by permission of the Ortho Pharmaceutical Corporation, Raritan, New Jersey.)

pregnant, your BBT does not drop; it remains elevated around 98.5 degrees. A routine urine test for pregnancy will probably not be positive until two weeks after the missed period.

A new and more sophisticated urine test which has been recently developed can detect a pregnancy within two weeks of conception. That test, known as a *radioimmunoassay* (RIA), is expensive, time-consuming, and available only in major medical centers.

The most widely used pregnancy test, called the *slide test,* is cheap, fast, easy to perform, and available in many doctors' offices. But it is not usually accurate until after the first month of pregnancy.

At the Cornell Medical Center, a new blood test has been developed but its use is still limited. It can occasionally diagnose pregnancy even before a missed period. This test is a so-called *receptor assay*, which detects very small levels of human chorionic gonadotrophin (HCG). HCG is a hormone manufactured by the placenta, the organ which nourishes the fetus. If a woman is pregnant, HCG is in her blood and urine. The level of HCG will be so small in the beginning of a pregnancy, however, that it cannot be detected by the available, routine pregnancy tests. This new test enables a woman to know if she is pregnant at the earliest possible date, an important consideration whether she is interested in abortion or in establishing a healthy environment for the fetus.

There has been a recent proliferation of over-the-counter home pregnancy kits which are based on the detection of HCG in the urine, but their ability to detect very early pregnancy is still being tested. The kits range from $9 to $15.

A physical examination by a gynecologist should reveal some blueness of the cervix and a slightly enlarged uterus if you are pregnant. The cervix should also be soft and pliable (positive Hegar's sign), the breasts should swell, the areolas around the nipples should become darker, and the blood vessels in the breast become much more visible. Morning sickness frequently occurs.

Pregnancy Care

As soon as a woman suspects that she is pregnant, she should contact her physician to confirm the diagnosis of pregnancy. If she wishes to bear a child, a proper diet should be started, she should avoid any drugs, and proper antenatal care should be instituted. If there is any abnormal bleeding or pain during this very early part of the pregnancy, a physician should be immediately contacted. Full information on pregnancy and childbirth is beyond the scope of this book, which deals strictly with gynecological rather than obstetrical matters. There are, though, several excellent books on obstetrics available.

Egg Cells

All potential egg cells, or follicles, are present at birth in women. Thus, every month, the egg that descends into the fallopian tubes at ovulation is as old as the woman. When a woman reaches forty, the eggs begin to feel their age. Occasionally, the genetic mechanism suffers, causing possible birth defects or miscarriage. Modern medicine has developed certain tests to analyze the amniotic fluid around the fetus and determine whether the chromosomes are normal. Obstetricians are particularly worried about the possibility of delivering a child with Down's syndrome (sometimes called mongolism), which happens much more frequently in women over the age of forty. Today, women at that age can safely carry a child if the pregnancy is carefully monitored by an obstetrician associated with a modern medical center. To be on the safe side, these women should undergo amniocentesis when they are between sixteen to eighteen weeks pregnant to exclude mongolism or other genetic abnormalities.

Men do not have this problem because sperm is freshly produced. Even if the man does not ejaculate, old sperm cells are automatically expelled.

CAN YOU CHOOSE YOUR CHILD'S SEX?

Much has been written lately about various techniques used to preselect the sex of a child. To date, however, only one method has been proven successful—a method which raises a serious ethical question.

Around the sixteenth to eighteenth week of pregnancy, it is possible to insert a needle into a woman's abdomen, withdrawing some of the amniotic fluid that surrounds the fetus. Laboratory tests can then determine the sex of the fetus. If the fetus is not the desired sex, an abortion can be performed. The moral questions in this type of sex selection are obvious, and the test should be performed only in very special cases, such as when there is the possibility of hemophilia, which is a sex-related disease.

History of Predicting Sex

The Berol Papyrus, written around 1350 B.C., described a method by which both pregnancy could be ascertained and the fetal sex predicted with the aid of urine taken from the potential mother. Barley and wheat in two bags were moistened daily with the urine. If the barley germinated, a girl would be born; if the wheat germinated, a boy. If no germination occurred, the woman was not pregnant.

Doctor Manger, who presumed that estrogen in the urine stimulated the germination of barley but had the opposite effect on wheat, repeated the experiments in 1933 and reported a correct prediction in 80 percent of the cases. Other physicians, however, were unable to find any correlation between the content of estrogens or gonadotrophins in the maternal blood and the sex of the fetus. Nevertheless, pregnancy serum, like urine, does contain one or more substances which stimulate the growth of certain plants.

According to the Egyptian papyri, the sex of the unborn child was also indicated by the color of the mother's face. A pregnant woman whose face had a greenish hue could be sure of giving birth to a boy. The Hippocratic school, on the other hand, taught that a woman with child, if it were to be a boy, had a good color. If she was carrying a girl, her facial color would be poor. Aristotle held that females were on a lower developmental level than males; consequently, a male fetus made more demands on the mother than a female fetus, needing greater body warmth and better circulation.

The sex of the fetus has also been thought to be an influence on the mother's disposition, a male fetus making her cheerful (Arabian), happy (Indian), and untroubled (Jewish).

Similarly, some people believed that a woman's desires reflected those of the sex she was carrying, and that her dreams were equally telling. In India, she dreams about men's food if she is carrying a boy. In Russia, dreams of knives or clubs are associated with boys, whereas dreams about spring or parties signify the arrival of a girl. In Japan during the tenth century, Temba taught that women desiring boys should concentrate on male pursuits, such as hunting. Until recently, it was a Japanese myth that if the husband called to his wife while she was on her way to the toilet, causing her to turn suddenly to the left, the outcome of the pregnancy would be a girl.

How to Have a Girl, How to Have a Boy—Modern Suggestions for Preconceptual Sex Determination

Many gynecologists prescribe programs of timing and douching to determine sex. Unfortunately, these programs have not been proven effective. Some programs even contradict other programs.

One of the most popular methods of sex preselection was developed by Dr. Landrum B. Shettles. Dr. Shettles created two programs —one to produce boys, one to produce girls—which patient couples are to follow with strict adherence. If a couple wants a girl, Dr. Shettles suggests the following procedure:

1. No intercourse for two to three days before ovulation.
2. Since a lower sperm count may increase the couple's chance of conceiving a girl, they should engage in intercourse freely before the two or three days prior to ovulation.
3. Precede intercourse with an acid douche of two tablespoons vinegar to one quart water.
4. The woman should avoid orgasm, since it increases alkaline vaginal secretion.

5. The missionary (male superior) position should be used so the
    sperm can be deposited at the mouth of the cervix.
6. Penetration should be shallow at the time of male orgasm.

For a boy, the procedure is different:

1. Intercourse should be timed as closely as possible to the time of
    ovulation.
2. To ensure the highest possible sperm count, intercourse should be
    avoided from the beginning of the menstrual cycle until the first
    day of ovulation.
3. Precede intercourse with a douche of two tablespoons baking
    soda to one quart water.
4. The woman's orgasm should be encouraged simultaneously or
    before the man's.
5. Vaginal penetration should be from the rear position, in order to
    deposit the sperm at the entrance of the womb where the
    secretions are alkaline.
6. Penetration should be deep at the time of the male orgasm.

This program is questioned by many reputable gynecologists. On
the other hand, Dr. Shettles claims an 85 percent success rate. (David
M. Rorvik with Landrum B. Shettles, M.D.; *Your Baby's Sex: Now
You Can Choose;* Dodd, Mead, Inc.; 1970.)

Whether or not Dr. Shettles's program is effective, research in this
area is accelerating. Even skeptics admit that the days of clearly
proven sexual predetermination are not far off.

What Is the Theory behind Sex Preselection?

The *female sperm*, which carries an X chromosome, is larger than
the *male sperm*, which carries the Y chromosome. The male sperm
seem to move faster because they are smaller. If intercourse occurs at
the time of ovulation, the fastest-moving sperm supposedly reach the
egg before the slow-moving sperm. Therefore, there is a better chance
of pregnancy with a male fetus if intercourse occurs at the time of
ovulation.

The acidity in the vagina is highest several days prior to ovulation.
The larger female sperm has a greater chance of surviving in this
environment than the male sperm. Intercourse several days prior to
ovulation should give a higher probability for a female baby.

It is true that vaginal secretions become increasingly alkaline during a female orgasm. This milieu might be better for the Y chromosomes. However, these changes are so sudden that they may have no influence on the sex.

Recent reports indicate that the X and Y chromosomes can be separated by centrifugation, and artificial insemination can be performed using either female or male sperm. Whether this will ever be a clinically available technique of preselecting a child is unknown.

If You Had the Choice, Which Sex Would You Choose?

Research on sex preference has shown that there is an overall preference for a male child as the first-born child. Eighty percent of the couples interviewed preferred a girl as the second born.

This might be very unhealthy, since it tends to separate the sexes even more. It has been theorized that first-born children of either sex are more ambitious, creative, achievement oriented, self-controlled, serious, and adult oriented. They are also more likely to attend college and to achieve eminence. This is all characteristic of masculine sex-role stereotypes.

Second-born children of either sex have been described as cheerful, easygoing, talkative, popular, practical, likely to seek help, and nervous. These characteristics supposedly resemble female stereotypes.

If exact sex preselection were possible and a majority of couples chose boys as the first born and girls as the second born, this could create even greater dissimilarity between the sexes and further the sexist stereotypes that are so destructive for us all. Perhaps, though, because of the recent examination of sexist values, more couples in the future will choose to have a girl as their first child.

PROBLEMS ASSOCIATED WITH THE MENSTRUAL CYCLE

Premenstrual Tension

Premenstrual tension usually occurs three to five days before menstruation, coinciding with the time during the menstrual cycle when the amount of ovarian hormones, estrogen and progesterone, is at its highest level. One of the most characteristic symptoms is water retention, usually between two to five pounds. This occurs because the hormones bind sodium chloride, and sodium retains excess fluid. Water retention gives a bloated, uncomfortable feeling, and might be responsible for headaches, dull aching or heaviness in the abdomen, and backaches. The high estrogen and progesterone levels give a general feeling of malaise, tiredness, and lethargy. Hormone levels are also responsible for nausea, breast enlargement, and pain. Some women become more irritable, tense, or depressed during this period. Many women also develop acne. This is the time during the menstrual cycle when a woman may have a tendency to be more nervous and irritable. Statistics show that the highest suicide rate for women occurs during the premenstrual period, and that women experience more emotional and nervous breakdowns at this time. The swelling of the pelvic organs and/or pelvic congestion can affect the bowels, resulting in constipation and the bloating or swelling of the stomach.

Premenstrual tension is clearly associated with the increased hormone levels immediately prior to menstruation. Some women have described the same symptoms when they initially start taking birth-control pills, particularly a birth-control pill with a high estrogen level. Researchers have found that women who suffer from premenstrual tension produce too much estrogen compared to progesterone.

It is not the hormone levels alone that determine the degree of symptoms, since many women never experience any premenstrual difficulties. Premenstrual tension depends to a great extent on a woman's mental state. If a woman is well, happy, and in good physical shape, she might have no or very few complaints. However, if a woman is anxious, nervous, and run-down, she will be more affected by premenstrual hormone changes and could develop severe symptoms.

Recent studies show that women who suffer severe premenstrual tension are more likely to react poorly to stressful situations and are more prone to psychosomatic illnesses.

Treatment of Premenstrual Tension

Most women suffer from sodium retention. The elimination of excess water by reducing one's salt intake or by adhering to a no-salt diet is recommended one week prior to menstruation. It is also necessary to drink a large amount of water to wash out the excessive waste products in the blood stream. If this is not sufficient, diuretics should be prescribed.

Recent discoveries show that there is an increased need for vitamin B_6 prior to menstruation, since the lack of B_6 has been associated with premenstrual depression and acne. Women suffering premenstrual symptoms should increase their intake of vitamin B_6 or take a multivitamin containing 50 to 100 milligrams of B_6 prior to menstruation.

Women who have a high estrogen level but a relatively low progesterone level have found relief when they take progesterone suppositories or tablets prior to menstruation. Some women have found relief when on low-estrogen birth-control pills, while others have found that this precipitated the symptoms.

There have been suggestions that spasmodic and congestive discomforts are due to calcium loss. If that is the case, extra calcium intake in tablet form or by drinking milk helps the condition.

Orgasm is the most pleasant way to alleviate the symptoms of premenstrual tension and to realize the origin of the problem.

Many women are riddled with feelings of anxiety, fear, and pain, which are triggered by their menstrual periods. In order to alleviate these symptoms, you should be as open as possible about them. Discuss your feelings with friends and close relatives. Exercise, eat a well-balanced diet, and relax, and keep your body in a healthy state. Most women have learned to live satisfactorily by following the above suggestions. Along with understanding the difficulties, women who know they might not feel well a few days prior to menstruation will not plan important meetings or special events on those days.

Dysmenorrhea—Painful Menstrual Cramps

Dysmenorrhea is the medical term for the painful cramps that accompany the menstrual period. A great number of men probably think that it is merely a woman's monthly excuse for acting bad-tempered and pampering herself, but any woman who has experienced dysmenorrhea knows it is a very real and debilitating condition. The cramps accompanying menstruation, particularly during its onset, can be so severe that a woman must be bedridden with her heating pad, feeling sweaty and at times almost in shock. There is usually a general feeling of malaise, lack of energy, and weakness in the legs; some women describe it as feeling as if their insides are falling out. Although the term "curse" is outmoded and Victorian, dysmenorrhea can be so severe that some women undoubtedly view it as such.

There may be an explanation why cramps can be so severe as to cause this condition. Scientists who have studied uterine physiology have found that the strength of cramps during menstruation is as high, and at times even higher, than contractions during labor. However, it is not the contractions per se that cause the severe pain (although they may cause some malaise); it is the dilation, or opening, of the cervix that results in the pain experienced during menstruation. The cervix is richly enervated and extremely sensitive. Each time the cervix stretches to allow passage of a blood clot, extreme pain results. Prior to the passage of menstrual clots, an increased amount of cramps causes dizziness and sweating similar to that of a woman in labor.

No one knows why some women suffer so much more than others from menstrual cramps, but it may have something to do with uterine anatomy. Some women have longer cervices than others, with tighter openings. If the cervix is tight, dilation is more difficult, often resulting in more severe pain. The cervices of certain women with dysmenorrhea are so tight they allow only a trickle of blood to pass, and the bulk of menstrual waste is instead pumped into the abdominal cavity, where it could grow and lead to *endometriosis* (see Chapter 12, Infertility and Chapter 13 on Uterine Abnormalities). This is more common if the woman is very tense.

Another possible factor in dysmenorrhea is hormones called *prostaglandins*. These hormones are used to induce labor and abortion. A number of studies have shown that women with dysmenorrhea produced and excreted more prostaglandins with the menstrual blood than women with normal cramps. Since these hormones can cause strong cramps, this might be the cause of the dysmenorrhea.

Pain during menstruation is also related to a woman's mental state. A tense person usually complains of more severe menstrual cramps than a relaxed person. It is often noted that highly strung women have a higher degree of dysmenorrhea.

Tolerance to pain varies greatly from one person to another, as it does from one culture to another. Eastern women, such as Chinese and Japanese, are more conditioned to tolerate pain than are Western women. When they are in labor, these women usually require much less pain medication than their Western sisters.

Cultural background and religious upbringing also have some bearing on a person's tolerance for pain. Jewish, Moslem, and Catholic women usually experience a higher degree of menstrual difficulty than Protestants. Several psychologists believe this difference is directly due to religious beliefs. Jewish women are brought up to believe that menstruation is unclean: Orthodox Jewish women must even take a ritual bath *(mikvah)* before resuming sexual relations after menstruation. This same custom applies throughout the Middle East for Arab women. Religious Arab women are not allowed to bathe during their menstrual periods. Catholicism, with its strict emphasis on purity and its rigid rules against premarital sex and birth control, tends to give Catholic women a negative view of menstruation.

Protestant women, on the other hand, are raised to suffer less in this aspect, as the Protestant church is more liberal in its view on women's sexuality.

Occasionally there is a clear pathological reason for severe menstrual pain. Women with pelvic infections sometimes develop extreme pain during menstruation, since the pumping movement of the uterus rapidly spreads the infection. There are several other causes for a painful menstrual period, such as fibroid tumors, which are occasionally located in such areas in the uterus that they interfere with the menstrual flow. A woman with a tilted uterus often has painful menstrual cramps, particularly when the cervical canal is bent backward to an extreme degree. If the menstrual period is delayed a week or two, tissue builds up inside the uterus. This subsequently results in a heavier flow and more menstrual pain.

Cramps tend to decrease in severity as a woman gets older. They might even disappear completely. After childbearing, when the cervix has been opened, many women have fewer or no symptoms of pain. However, some still continue to have severe dysmenorrhea even after giving birth.

At times, menstrual cramps can be so severe that some women feel menopause will be a welcome relief.

Treatment of Dysmenorrhea

There is no specific treatment that completely alleviates the misery connected with dysmenorrhea. Each woman with severe cramps usually finds her own special remedy, but her formula might not work for another woman. Menstrual cramps are often relieved to some extent by heat. A hot water bottle or heating pad placed on the abdominal area or on the lower back often lessens the pain. Some women find relief soaking in a hot bath. This relaxes the muscles and the heat also helps open the cervix, which facilitates the blood flow and subsequently alleviates the cramps. A hot bath is not dangerous. You should not use a tampon at this time, allowing the blood to flow normally. In fact, you should never use a tampon if you have severe dysmenorrhea. Many women find that a few drinks lessen menstrual pain. This can be recommended, since alcohol is found actually to decrease uterine contractions.

Exercises are also recommended to alleviate pain. There are several types of abdominal exercises which should be done a week prior to menstruation. These exercises strengthen the abdominal muscles and keep the body in better physical shape. It is well known that dancers and athletic women have fewer menstrual complaints.

Many women find that lying on their backs with their legs elevated on a pillow, or with their knees bent, often alleviates pressure and pain. Other women find relief by pulling their knees up toward their chests. The "fetal position," lying on the side with the knees pulled up tight to the chest and the head bent forward, is also strongly recommended.

As with premenstrual tension, some women have found that orgasm is the most enjoyable way of alleviating severe menstrual cramps. This is actually in accord with medical research, since the severe pelvic congestion which occurs immediately before the onset of menstruation can also be alleviated by an orgasm. The orgasm drains the pelvis and, therefore, causes relaxation and comfort.

Recent research has demonstrated a clear connection between the severity of menstrual cramps and the blood levels of a hormone called *prostaglandin*. Drugs such as Midol, Motrin and Naproxen are the most effective new treatment for the control of dysmenorrhea. These drugs prevent prostaglandin release from the body tissues and thus prevent propagation of menstrual cramps. It is important to take these agents before the prostaglandin enters the system. A woman might be advised to take two Midol four times a day twenty-four hours prior to the expected onset of menstruation and through the first days. The other antiprostaglandins, Motrin, Naproxen, and Ponstel are also very effective, but can only be obtained by prescription. The compelling evidence on the potency of these drugs in the treatment of dysmenorrhea is recent, and some physicians may not be aware of these new findings.

Like Midol, Motrin, Naproxen, or Ponstel should be started at a dose of one to two tablets four times a day, on the day prior to the expected onset of menstruation. This dosage should be maintained through at least the first two days of menstrual bleeding.

Another possible treatment of dysmenorrhea is the birth-control pill. Actually, the reason not as many women suffer from dysmenorrhea today as years ago is that millions of women take the pill. The hormones in the birth-control pill replace a woman's own hormones and thus prevent ovulation. The pill, particularly one with a low estrogen content, does not stimulate the endometrium as much as the woman's own hormones; therefore, there will be less menstrual flow and less pain. A woman suffering from severe dysmenorrhea should take the pill if she has no contraindication to it. The minipill and a low-estrogen pill are preferred for this purpose, since menstruation on these pills is limited to very little bleeding or spotting.

As previously stated, having a period is not altogether necessary. A woman can take the birth-control pill continuously; this avoids menstruation. If cramping and bleeding occur, she can even double up on the pills.

The newly released medication for endometriosis—danazol (Danocrine)—can also be used successfully for dysmenorrhea. Danazol also stops bleeding. Thus a woman will not experience premenstrual tension or dysmenorrhea.

The menstrual cycle usually renews spontaneously when a woman stops taking these drugs. Because of this, these drugs will prevent conception only while they are being taken.

If menstruation does not begin again after you stop taking these drugs, you should have it induced by other drugs. Here again, this treatment is not dangerous.

If there is a clear medical reason for dysmenorrhea, such as pelvic infection or fibroid tumors, the condition should be treated by antibiotics or surgery. If a tilted uterus causes severe dysmenorrhea, surgery might be indicated to pull the uterus forward. Several physicians perform a D&C (dilation and curettage) which alleviates symptoms due to a very tight cervix. There have even been cases in which all alternative treatments have failed and a hysterectomy has been unavoidable. However, this should be the last resort and done only if a woman does not want any more children.

Sometimes cramps will respond to none of the nonsurgical remedies suggested here and women turn to narcotic drugs, such as codeine. If cramps are that severe, and persistent, consult your physician in order to determine the medication best for you, and remember that narcotic drugs are habit-forming and should be used with caution.

Dysmenorrhea is real. It is important that your colleagues, as well as your husband or boyfriend, understand this and are supportive. Do not be embarrassed or feel guilty about this condition. Instead, be more open and free yourself from the social, cultural, and religious factors that might have precipitated your situation. Try to understand the physiological and psychological factors responsible for dysmenorrhea. This enables you to cope better with the situation. And remember: keep yourself in emotional balance, get plenty of exercise, and learn to relax.

PELVIC PAIN RELATED TO THE MENSTRUAL CYCLE

In addition to dysmenorrhea (painful menstrual cramps) and *Mittleschmerz* (pain on ovulation), a woman may experience pelvic pain at other times during her cycle. The regularity and the timing of this pain throughout the cycle can give a clue to its origin. Pain occurring after the menstrual flow has stopped could be a sign of pelvic infection, because menstruation promotes the spread of bacteria in the pelvic region. On the other hand, the pelvic pain that starts after ovulation, increases as menstruation approaches, and continues month after month could be a sign of *endometriosis*. The presence of severe pelvic pain when the menstrual period is late and the possibility of pregnancy exists could indicate an *ectopic pregnancy,* or a threatened spontaneous abortion. Pain is the body's signal to the brain of some physiological event—a normal event, as in the case of *Mittleschmerz,* or an abnormal event, as in the case of ectopic pregnancy. A woman's sensitivity to this pain is not a sign of egocentricity but an indication of alertness to these important body signals. Stoic endurance of regular, persistent, or severe pelvic pain is not a display of fortitude but a dangerous result of ignorance and misinformation.

ABNORMAL UTERINE BLEEDING

Abnormal uterine bleeding can be any abnormality, from amenorrhea (no bleeding whatsoever) to irregular bleeding occurring either too infrequently (oligomenorrhea) or too often (menorrhagia), and is completely unrelated to ovulation or menstruation.

Most women experience abnormal bleeding sometime in their lives. This could be due to an abnormality, but often it is just a symptom of a hormonal imbalance or even of a stressful situation.

Amenorrhea

This is a condition in which there is no menstrual bleeding. There are two types of amenorrhea: *primary,* in which a woman has never had a menstrual period although she is past puberty; and *secondary*, in which a woman stops menstruating after regular bleeding.

Primary amenorrhea can be caused either by congenital abnormalities (absence or abnormality of the vagina, the uterus, or the ovaries) or by a malfunction between the pituitary and the ovaries. A young girl with this condition should be taken to a gynecologist by the time she reaches sixteen to determine why she does not menstruate. If there are any congenital abnormalities, these should be corrected surgically. If there are no abnormalities, the physician usually administers hormones to initiate the menstruation.

The most common cause of *secondary amenorrhea* is pregnancy, but it can be due to many other reasons. Menstruation depends on a very delicate hormonal interaction between the ovaries and the brain. If this is upset by weight gain, weight loss, poor nutrition, emotional trauma, birth-control pills, or serious diseases, bleeding may not occur. If secondary amenorrhea persists longer than two or three months, you should see a doctor.

Diagnosis and Treatment of Amenorrhea

If you miss more than one period and have been sexually active, you must have a pregnancy test, since pregnancy is the most common cause of secondary amenorrhea. If the pregnancy test is negative, you should have a hormone analysis (to determine the body's estrogen level) and a biopsy of the endometrium (to determine if you have ovulated). This can be done either in the office or in a hospital under general anesthesia. You should also have an X-ray taken of your brain, since a brain tumor could disturb the interaction between the pituitary and the ovaries. Weight gain or loss can also cause the problem, and you must report to your physician if this is the case. Prolonged use of the birth-control pill can, as mentioned above, cause amenorrhea. Therefore, the pill should be stopped until bleeding occurs. There are also certain cases in which these conditions are due to pituitary damage occurring as a result of severe hemorrhage or infection during previous deliveries. This usually can only be treated by hormone replacement.

Amenorrhea is frequently caused by nervousness and tension. Mental mood can influence brain hormones, also called the *releasing hormones* (R-FSH and R-LH), which regulate ovulation through FSH and LH. Bleeding usually reoccurs as soon as the woman relaxes or moves to a more peaceful environment.

Oligomenorrhea

Oligomenorrhea is a condition in which a woman has only occasional periods, perhaps just one or two a year. This is usually due either to a pituitary malfunction or to polycystic ovaries (Stein-Leventhal syndrome). In this condition, the ovaries are enlarged. This prevents regular ovulation and development of the corpus luteum, inhibiting menstruation.

This condition can be treated with birth-control pills or other hormones. Bleeding is usually initiated after progesterone administration, either in the form of injection or Provera tablets of 10 milligrams, administered twice daily for five days. If the estrogen level is sufficient, the progesterone results in a sloughing off of the endometrial lining a few days after the injection or the last tablet. The condition can also be regulated by Clomid administration or after a surgical procedure called a *wedge resection of the ovary,* in which a part of the ovary is removed so the size of the ovary is reduced to normal and ovulation resumes. If untreated, a woman with oligo-menorrhea *can* conceive, but it is more difficult since she does not know when she ovulates. This condition can also occur after discontinuation of the birth-control pill or by irritation from an IUD. It could be a sign of a threatened miscarriage or an ectopic pregnancy.

Menorrhagia—Irregular Periods

Frequent and irregular bleeding can have a variety of causes: hormonal imbalance, abnormal ovulation, stress and nervousness, uterine trauma, polyps, fibroid tumors, or cervicitis. It can also be caused by inadequate hormone dosage in the birth-control pill or by irritation from an IUD. It could be a sign of a threatened miscarriage or an ectopic pregnancy. Abnormal bleeding should, however, always be evaluated since it can be a sign of cancer.

Bleeding Abnormalities in the Young Woman

The onset of menstruation (menarche) varies markedly from woman to woman. In the last decade, the onset seems to be arriving earlier. It is not abnormal to see a girl start menstruating at twelve years of age. It is not known if this is due to better nutrition or if it is entirely due to a woman's weight. During the first few years, menstrual periods may be rather irregular, light periods may be followed by very heavy ones, and menstrual periods may be absent entirely for a few months. This is due to inadequate ovulation and abnormal hormone levels. A young girl does not ovulate regularly or have regular menstrual periods until she becomes sexually mature. Such menstrual irregularities might continue for three or four years. This often causes uneasiness and nervousness, as well as fear of pregnancy if the young woman becomes sexually active. This nervousness can again influence the brain hormones, thus causing absence of bleeding. If this is the case, menstruation can usually be brought on by progesterone (Provera tablets). When menstruation starts after a prolonged absence, too much tissue has often built up

THE REPRODUCTIVE CYCLE 115

inside the uterus, resulting in heavy menstrual bleeding. This can usually be controlled with progesterone administration, which is often more effective than a D&C.

Dysfunctional Bleeding

Abnormal bleeding is usually not serious, but if it persists, it should be evaluated. It could be a sign of danger and could even result in anemia. If minimal bleeding occurs, you should not do anything about it for a month. If it persists, you must see a gynecologist.

Any malfunction in the delicate hormonal balance can cause abnormal bleeding. Menorrhagia is usually characterized by prolonged menstrual bleeding or spotting.

Many physicians treat this condition with a D&C. Women should be aware that a D&C does not often cure menorrhagia if the problem is a hormonal one. A hormonal cause must often be treated by estrogen and progesterone administered in a cycle regimen, or by progesterone administered for a few days to bring the body back to its regular cycle. Sometimes birth-control pills will also be effective.

Bleeding Due to Trauma

A young woman often experiences severe bleeding during the first intercourse. This is usually a result of the tearing of the hymen. Some women do not experience this, whereas others bleed during their first *several* times of intercourse, or until the hymen is completely open. Older women, who have more fragile vaginal tissue, often experience tearing of this vaginal tissue, especially if they have not had sex for a long time and have become too tight. This is particularly true if they did not have time to lubricate sufficiently. It is common to experience some bleeding during the first intercourse, after childbearing, or after different types of vaginal surgery. This is usually due to tearing or laceration of the scar tissue. Many women describe bleeding after intercourse, particularly if the man is well endowed. This could be a sign of cancer and should, of course, be evaluated, though it is more likely to be due to an infection of the cervix (cervicitis) or to a cervical polyp that has been irritated during the sexual activity. Women with IUDs might also experience some bleeding, particularly after strenuous intercourse. This is due to strong uterine contractions immediately after intercourse, which can cause part of the endometrium to shed.

If you develop severe bleeding after your first intercourse and it does not stop spontaneously, you should insert a tampon into the vagina and squeeze your legs together. If the bleeding is uncontrollable, you should go immediately to the nearest emergency room, since you may need a few stitches to control the bleeding. Do not be embarrassed about this; it happens quite frequently. The same advice applies if you have any form of bleeding after intercourse, no matter what your age.

Bleeding Associated with Pregnancy

Abnormal uterine bleeding can also be due to an abnormal pregnancy or threatened miscarriage in which the placenta has not implanted firmly in the uterine wall and has started to slough off. This bleeding is usually pinker and brighter than menstrual bleeding, and can often start painlessly. However, if a miscarriage is on the way, severe cramps follow, and a physician should be consulted immediately.

This type of bleeding also occurs as a result of an *ectopic* pregnancy (pregnancy outside the uterus, often in the fallopian tubes). If the egg is growing in a fallopian tube, the hormones which maintain the uterine lining in pregnancy are inadequate and bleeding occurs, though usually without pain at first. As the tubal involvement becomes more extensive, there will be severe lower abdominal pain. If this occurs, particularly in association with bleeding, a woman must see her physician immediately.

Polyps and Cervicitis

A cervical polyp can cause menorrhagia, especially if it is irritated by sexual intercourse. A polyp in the uterus can also cause abnormal bleeding. Either of these conditions can be treated with a D&C, with the polyp being scraped off. However, the removed polyps should always be sent to a pathology laboratory to make sure they are not cancerous.

Cervicitis, an inflammatory condition of the cervix, often causes bleeding or spotting. This is particularly true after a Pap smear or intercourse. This should be treated with either coagulation or freezing of the cervix.

Bleeding Associated with IUDs and Birth-Control Pills

An IUD is a foreign object in the uterus and can irritate the uterine wall and cause bleeding. This is quite common for the first few months, or until the uterus adjusts to the IUD, but if it persists, a gynecologist should be consulted. Bleeding due to an IUD is usually treated with either progesterone or birth-control pills. Progesterone decreases the cramps that contract the uterus against the IUD. Birth-control pills help relax the uterus in the same way. Antiprostaglandins, such as Motrin or Naproxen, also can be used to decrease this excess bleeding. This bleeding is also sometimes due to a low inflammatory reaction, in which case antibiotics should be added to the treatment.

Birth-control pills can also be responsible for abnormal bleeding. Usually, the first few months a woman takes the pill, particularly the minipill, the hormones in the pills are not strong enough to take over the woman's ovarian function and bleeding results. This is called *breakthrough bleeding* and is usually treated by doubling the dosage of the pill temporarily and, sometimes, doubling it again. This may be done for several months before the cycle comes under the pill's control (see Chapter 10 on Contraception).

Bleeding and Fibroid Tumors

If a fibroid tumor breaks through into the uterine cavity, it affects the endometrium (uterine lining) in the same way a polyp would, causing bleeding. This is the only time a fibroid tumor is potentially dangerous, because it can cause severe hemorrhage and necessitate transfusion. In this case, the tumors usually must be surgically removed by a myomectomy. A hysterectomy is not necessarily indicated. (See Chapter 13, Uterine Abnormalities.)

Postmenopausal Bleeding—A Warning

Nowadays, the menopause occurs later than in the past, probably because of better nutrition and living conditions. However, if a woman experiences menstrual bleeding after a cessation of at least six months, she should see a gynecologist immediately to have a D&C or a biopsy of the uterus. This bleeding could be a sign of cancer and early diagnosis leads to more successful treatment. Therefore any bleeding, slight or heavy, after change of life should be evaluated immediately. This is even more important if you are in estrogen-replacement therapy. Then you should have a biopsy from the endometrium every one or two years, and a D&C as soon as bleeding or spotting occurs, to rule out any premalignancies.

Bleeding as a Sign of Cancer

Of course, abnormal bleeding *can* be an indication of uterine or cervical cancer. If this bleeding occurs after menopause, you should see a gynecologist immediately, since older women are especially susceptible to genital cancer. Extra caution is necessary if you have high risk factors, such as obesity or high blood pressure, or if you have had no children. Abnormal bleeding is the first sign of such cancers, because the uterus tries to slough off the tumors. Cancer of the cervix causes bleeding in its advanced stage, but if a woman has her Pap smear regularly, cancer is usually detected before the cancer advances to stages in which it causes postcoital bleeding.

MENOPAUSE

Of all the mammals on earth, human females are the only ones to stop menstruating in midlife. The "change" usually occurs around age fifty, but variations are great. Genetic factors are important in determining when a woman will reach menopause; if your mother stopped bleeding in her forties, so, probably, will you.

Women are born with about half a million oocytes, ovarian cells which can theoretically grow into an egg. Every month after puberty, one of these oocytes forms into a Graafian follicle and ovulation occurs. These cells also produce the female hormone, estrogen. As the woman approaches middle age, the oocytes begin to degenerate and their estrogen production decreases. This process varies from woman to woman, and might be responsible for the great difference in menopausal symptoms between women. Many women have minimal symptoms because their *ovarian stroma* (supporting tissue) continue to produce estrogen after ovulation ceases. Testosterone also continues to be produced in the ovaries.

The average lifespan for an American woman is seventy-five years, so during the last third (twenty-five years) of her life, she will not ovulate and probably will not have menstrual bleeding.

WHAT HAPPENS DURING MENOPAUSE

The first sign that menopause is approaching is usually abnormal menstrual bleeding ranging from skipping just one period to intramenstrual spotting, to a sudden cessation of menstruation for several months or permanently. This pattern can persist for several years, depending on the individual's estrogen level. Irregular menstruation can, however, be a sign of several conditions and a woman who experiences those symptoms should see a gynecologist to have the bleeding abnormality evaluated and her estrogen level checked. This is particularly true for a middle-aged woman who experiences a resumption of vaginal bleeding after more than a six-month cessation of menstruation. She should be alerted to the fact that this could be an early sign of uterine cancer (see Postmenopausal Bleeding, p. 117).

Other symptoms of menopause include a change in skin tone or texture, an abnormal vaginal discharge or pain due to atrophic vaginitis (see Vaginitis after Menopause, p. 138), a decrease of breast size and firmness, back pain (which should alert women to the possible onset of osteoporosis, a decrease in bone substance and a lowering of the bone calcium content), and arthritic symptoms.

SEVERE MENOPAUSAL SYMPTOMS

Only 25 percent of American women suffer any significant menopausal symptoms other than cessation of ovulation and menstruation. The most severe and abrupt changes occur in women who have undergone surgically induced menopause via hysterectomy and oopherectomy (removal of the ovaries).

This 25 percent suffer two distinct types of symptoms. One type is due to vascular instability and is characterized by hot flashes and sweating, especially at night. The other type is primarily psychosomatic, and can manifest itself in a variety of ways. These latter symptoms are generally consistent with what a woman has been brought up to expect during menopause, and can include heart pain, hysteria, constipation, ulcers, and severe depression.

To the extent that they are physical, menopausal symptoms are probably due to low levels of estrogen and high levels of gonadotrophins, FSH and LH. These hormonal changes affect the brain, and it should be understood that although many symptoms may be psychosomatic, they are grounded in physiological imbalance.

Treatment of Menopausal Symptoms

The best treatment is often psychological counseling and understanding. Tranquilizers can help a woman over the tense period of adjustment, which can last from one to ten years.

The most severe symptoms are often seen in women with surgically induced menopause who have hysterectomies with removal of the ovaries. Many gynecologists insist that the ovaries are useless after menopause, but this is not altogether true. Despite the loss of their reproductive value, they probably still function to maintain a hormonal balance, and their absence is felt.

With or without estrogen treatment, women should understand that the change of life takes time—probably a few years—and that they will eventually adapt and have no further symptoms.

Good nutrition is essential to minimizing menopausal symptoms. Dietary supplementation of B vitamins and vitamin D, calcium, and iron can help protect against cardiovascular diseases, diabetes, osteoporosis, and obesity. Some physicians report that the use of 400 to 1600 international units of vitamin E daily cures hot flashes. It is important for women to watch their weight after menopause, as the risk of heart disease increases greatly at that age and obesity multiplies the risk geometrically. A proper dietary supplement of vitamins and minerals such as calcium and zinc will keep the bones strong and supply the energy that many women feel they lose at menopause. Protein is also important, though excessive animal fats should be avoided. Large amounts of water will flush the system and keep all the cells in balance.

Does Estrogen Replacement Cause Cancer?

Estrogen is thought to protect against *arteriosclerosis* and *cardiovascular diseases,* as well as arthritis and *osteoporosis* (a condition characterized by a loss of calcium in the bones, making them brittle and weak and easily broken). Despite this, many physicians are against estrogen treatment for menopause because of the risk of cancer. Estrogen is said to keep the skin and breasts looking young and firm and to keep the vagina soft. For these reasons, many women consider it a rejuvenating drug. Research, though, has revealed that some of the same results can be obtained with calcium pills and vitamins.

Still, if a woman wants estrogen treatment, she should be aware of the dangers. High doses of estrogen have been linked to both uterine and breast cancer. It is said to increase the chances of endometrial cancer sevenfold. However, endometrial cancer is relatively simple to treat when caught early, and many physicians feel the risk is worth taking. The first symptom of this type of cancer is bleeding. If a gynecologist is consulted immediately and he diagnoses endometrial cancer, the cure rate is almost 100 percent. It is thought this *cancer* is caused by an abnormal buildup of the uterine lining and *can be prevented by prescribing estrogen in three-week cycles, each cycle followed by progesterone treatment (the last week)* to prevent the endometrium from thickening very much. This, too, is a controversial treatment. Of course, a woman who has had a hysterectomy needn't worry about cancer of the uterus, but she does have to consider the danger of breast cancer.

Women with higher amounts of estrogen in their bodies have a greater tendency toward breast cancer. However, many physicians feel that women who take estrogen treatment offset the risk of death from breast cancer by visiting their gynecologist more often, thereby catching any tumor early enough to treat it effectively and prevent its spread.

Some scientists believe estrogen might actually have some preventive effect on the development of ovarian cancer. This is the worst type of female cancer, because there are no warning signs and by the time it is diagnosed, it is usually too late to cure. Some gynecologists, therefore, feel that even if estrogen might stimulate the development of uterine or breast cancer, it is worthwhile if it aids in the prevention of ovarian cancer. Nevertheless, if estrogen therapy is indicated, a woman should be started on the lowest dose. This dose can be carefully increased if the low initial dose proves ineffective. Probably the most widely prescribed estrogen replacement is Premarin, manufactured from the urine of pregnant mares. It is used by an estimated three million American women, and is the fifth most prescribed medication in America.

Unfortunately, there are no definite answers. Until there are, every woman should be informed of the possible risks and/or benefits of estrogen treatment by her physician in order to make an informed and appropriate decision.

Other Hormonal Treatments

Some women take progesterone to alleviate the symptoms of menopause. It has apparently been effective, but the side effects have not yet been fully explored.

Male hormones have been used therapeutically on menopausal women for many years. Certain women gain energy and maintain a positive calcium balance, making their bones stronger, when treated with testosterone. This hormone also has an aphrodisiac effect on many women. However, testosterone treatment may initiate hair growth on the arms, legs, and face. Again, the pros and cons must be weighed in each case.

Should a Woman Take Estrogen, the "Antiaging" Pill?

The change-of-life symptoms can be so severe that many women become extremely depressed. These women cannot control their own minds, and life becomes a misery for both the woman and her family. The change-of-life symptoms can range from mild headaches to symptoms of heart attacks, asthma attacks, and severe abdominal pain. A woman with severe symptoms often visits many physicians, who perform a series of unnecessary tests and X-rays without any further solution or treatment. Many of these women can benefit from love, care, and understanding, but some women do not feel better until they start estrogen treatment. After initiation of hormone replacement, one can often see a complete transformation of these women; from being tired, depressed, and miserable, they become happy, energetic, and in good spirits. For women who respond well to estrogen replacement, the treatment can only be recommended. If a woman does not take estrogen, her skin will get thinner and start to sag. Her vagina will get dry, she will lose her hair, and her bones will be affected with osteoporosis, a condition causing pain and, occasionally, a collapse of the vertebrae. A woman will then start to shrink in stature and experience increasing pain. Therefore, if a woman either has symptoms that warrant estrogen treatment or if she is well motivated and does not want aging to accelerate when she is at her best age, she could take the estrogen-replacement treatment. If the estrogen is taken in a three-week cycle, followed the last week with progesterone treatment, the chances of developing uterine cancer should be very slim. During hormone administration, it is now recommended to have a Pap smear and a biopsy from the uterus once a year to detect any early cancer sign. A woman should examine her breasts thoroughly every month and perhaps have a mammogram once every one or two years.

If a woman knows about the natural changes that take place in her body during menopause and the therapies available to modify or nullify the less acceptable of these changes, then "change of life" can be, in many ways, a change for the better, a time when she is free from the problems of contraception and wise in the ways of life.

chapter 6

VAGINITIS—THE MOST COMMON COMPLAINT

One out of every two women visiting a gynecologist's office is suffering from vaginitis. In the broadest sense, vaginitis is any type of vaginal infection. It is usually characterized by an abnormal vaginal discharge and symptoms such as vaginal pain, itching, irritation, painful intercourse, and painful urination.

Women always have some type of normal vaginal secretion. This secretion depends on a number of factors: age, time of the menstrual cycle, sexual stimulation, type of contraception, and mental state.

NORMAL VAGINAL SECRETION

A delicate balance of microorganisms, bacteria, and yeast coexist in the vagina. The *Döderlein* bacillus, one of the most important components of the vaginal flora, is responsible for the maintenance of the proper vaginal pH, which should be between 4.5 and 5.0. The normal vaginal milieu, which is slightly acidic, is produced via the fermentation of lactic acid from glycogen (sugar) by the *Döderlein* bacillus. When a woman receives antibiotic therapy for infection, the *Döderlein* bacillus can be killed. If this happens, the acidity of the vagina diminishes, providing an ideal environment for the growth of yeast. The yeast can multiply, creating a yeast infection.

The quantity and quality of normal vaginal secretions change throughout the menstrual cycle. Secretion is thick and sticky just after the end of menstrual bleeding and immediately prior to the next menstrual flow. Secretions are influenced by estrogen; when the estrogen level rises prior to ovulation, the vaginal secretion becomes clear, watery, and slippery. These are sometimes called the wet days.

After menopause, as a woman's estrogen level decreases, vaginal cells usually atrophy and the amount of normal vaginal secretion decreases. The vagina becomes dry and the protective vaginal flora disappear, leaving postmenopausal women more susceptible to vaginal infection. The same situation occurs in prepubescent girls, who also have no estrogen production and are susceptible to infection.

Sexual intercourse allows transmission of the microorganisms which cause vaginitis. As the use of the condom has decreased and the number of a woman's sexual partners has risen, the occurrence of vaginitis has sharply increased. During sexual intercourse, the friction produced by the penis on the walls of the vagina can cause the sloughing off of the cells of the vaginal surface, and thus permits microorganisms to be pushed into the vaginal mucosa and become a source of vaginal infection. The more frequent the intercourse and the more numerous the partners, the higher are the chances of vaginal infections.

An IUD sometimes causes uterine irritation and the formation of a clear, watery discharge secreted through the vagina. This is a normal side effect and should not be a source of concern. Birth-control pills, particularly those with low estrogen content, can decrease the amount of acidity, predisposing the user to monilia vaginitis. Pregnancy also alters vaginal secretion, making a woman more susceptible to vaginitis.

Tension, anxiety, and insufficient rest can cause a decrease in normal secretion, upsetting the balance and rendering the vagina more susceptible to infection. Extreme tension can tighten perineal muscles (the muscles around the vagina) to such an extent that normal vaginal secretions cannot drain. These secretions can become a source of irritation and even infection.

You can examine normal vaginal secretions by placing a finger within the vagina to obtain a small amount of secretion. You can then look at this secretion on a glass plate. If you know what normal secretion looks like, it will help you to spot abnormal secretions. You should examine your vulva with a mirror if you suspect vaginal secretions are abnormal in any way.

LEUKORRHEA

If vaginal secretion increases to an abnormal amount, loosely defined as any secretion truly bothersome, the condition is called *leukorrhea*. Leukorrhea is a white vaginal discharge containing white blood cells and excreted dead, or damaged vaginal cells. Leukorrhea can be caused by a vaginal infection or irritation by a foreign body, such as an IUD, a forgotten tampon, or even a vaginal tumor. When leukorrhea becomes a source of vaginal pain or irritation, a woman should see her gynecologist.

HOW TO PREVENT VAGINITIS

The vagina is the perfect environment for the growth of microorganisms. It is warm, dark, wet, and provides sufficient nourishment and oxygen. The normal vaginal flora offer some protection against vaginitis, and a woman should do everything she can to maintain the balance. She should stay in good physical condition, getting proper nourishment and sufficient rest. She should avoid stress and deal appropriately with tension.

A woman should learn voluntary control of her perineal muscles so that she can relax these muscles to permit the passage of vaginal secretions. Some women can gain voluntary control of the perineal muscle by simply being told they are there, but most women need further help. One method is to start and stop the flow of urine (see Kegel's exercise, Chapter 21). Another is to place a clean finger within the vagina, tensing and relaxing the muscles around it. Once a woman learns the feeling of tension and relaxation of the perineal muscles, she can relax these muscles two or three times a day. Some find it a pleasant feeling—a warmth in the perineal area when the muscles are relaxed.

While on antibiotic therapy, a woman should also receive antiyeast pills or suppositories to prevent disturbance of the vaginal milieu.

A woman should keep herself clean, washing the area of the vulva at least once a day. After urination or bowel movement, a woman should wipe from front to back—*never* from back to front—to prevent the passage of bacteria from the anus to the vulva.

She should make sure that her sexual partner is clean. A man should wash his penis once a day. Women could learn a useful trick from the professionals by carefully inspecting and milking the penis prior to intercourse. This is particularly appropriate with a new sexual partner. The use of a condom may not be a bad idea for the primary sexual encounter. If a couple engages in anal sex, the penis must be cleansed prior to vaginal intercourse.

Diabetes and obesity predispose a woman to vaginitis by causing changes in the vaginal milieu. Diabetics should avoid excessive sugar intake and obese women should lose weight.

A foreign body in the vagina can cause irritation. Therefore, a diaphragm should not be worn for longer than the required time. A forgotten tampon can also be a frequent source of vaginal infection.

Excessive douching can disturb the protective balance of the vagina and predispose a woman to vaginitis. If a woman wishes, she can douche safely approximately once a week with an appropriate solution (see Douching at the end of this chapter).

Pantyhose and Vaginitis

The constant wearing of pantyhose can increase a woman's chances of getting vaginitis. When pantyhose are worn, the temperature and moisture of the vagina are increased. The vagina becomes more susceptible to infection. This is a particular problem in the summer. Pantyhose also stimulate the growth of bacteria by preventing the circulation of air in the vulvar area. If a woman has

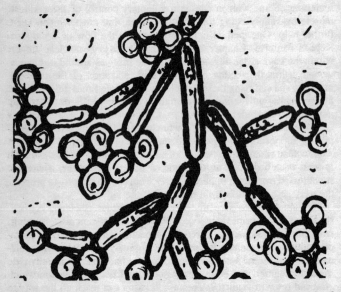

Fig. 6–1: A drawing of the microscopic view of a typical growth of monilia *(Candida albicans)*. The yeast microorganisms multiply by forming new "branches," and can thus spread very rapidly. *Candida albicans* grow better in a moist, warm environment with only a mild degree of acidity.

vaginitis or has had recurrent episodes of vaginitis, it is recommended that she refrain from wearing pantyhose, or wear pantyhose with a cotton crotch.

MONILIA OR YEAST INFECTION

Monilia (or *Candida albicans*), a fungus of the yeast family, is a normal resident of the oral cavity, the vagina, and the rectum. When the normal balance among the vaginal flora is disturbed, particularly when the vaginal acidity decreases, monilia starts an uncontrolled growth. The result is a monilia infection.

About half of all vaginitis is due to monilia or yeast infection. There has been an increase of monilia in recent years, thought to be the result of increased use of antibiotics and oral contraceptives and a decrease in the use of condoms and diaphragms. Antibiotics kill the *Döderlein* bacteria and the pH of the vagina becomes more conducive to yeast growth. Low-estrogen birth-control pills also alter vaginal acidity. Pregnancy, diabetes, and obesity all produce a hospitable vaginal environment for yeast.

Transmission of Yeast Infection

A monilia infection need not be transmitted. It can flare up spontaneously whenever the vaginal milieu is disturbed. However, a yeast infection can be transmitted through sexual intercourse. Yeast is viable for some time outside the body if moisture is available. A common site is moist towels. Infection often spreads this way in such places as college dormitories, where women sometimes share the same towels.

Symptoms of Monilia Infection

The symptoms of monilia vaginitis are discharge, itching, burning, and painful intercourse. The discharge is white and curdy, looking something like cottage cheese, and is easily discovered by self-examination. It has a yeasty odor. The vagina, which is usually pale pink, turns bright red. This redness often spreads to the vulva, which you can see with a mirror. The discoloration can reach all the way to the anus. It can cause swelling and become very painful. Sometimes the irritation becomes so severe that walking is difficult. Often there are whitish or grayish areas or spots either in the vagina or on the vulva.

It is possible to have monilia in the mouth. This is usually caused

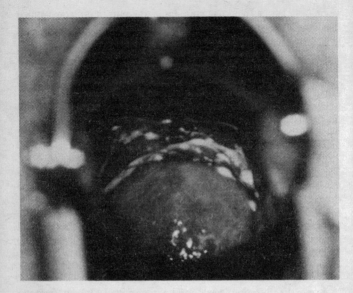

Fig. 6–2:   A physician's view of the cervix through a speculum. The cream cheeselike discharge on the cervix and on the top of the vagina is characteristic of a monilia vaginal infection. (Reproduced by permission of the Emko Company, St. Louis, Missouri.)

by antibiotic therapy, although sometimes also by oral sex. It looks like curdy white patches in the mouth, which bleed if scraped. Oral pain and fever can occur.

Diagnosis of Monilia

The diagnosis of monilia vaginitis can be made by the characteristic appearance and odor of the discharge, the presence of white or gray patches in the vagina, and the inflammation of the vulvar area. To substantiate this clinical diagnosis, the physician microscopically examines a wet smear of the vaginal discharge for the typical yeastlike organisms. A swab of the vaginal discharge can also be placed on a special culture medium, such as Nickerson's medium. The culture will grow within a few days, even at room temperature, if it contains *Candida albicans*.

Treatment of Monilia Vaginitis

Antiyeast suppositories and creams are the most common treatments for monilia infection. Nystatin suppositories (mycostatin) are the most commonly prescribed and are very effective. The usual dosage is two suppositories a day for fourteen days. The suppository melts, coating the vagina with medication which may leak from the vagina and stain underwear. Follow insertion of the suppository with a vaginal tampon, cut in half and placed in the lower part of the vagina, or use a minipad to protect your clothing.

Mycostatin can be taken orally, but high doses are needed for effective treatment of monilia infection. Oral mycostatin can be used to treat men who have monilia infections.

There are a number of other very effective antiyeast suppositories available. There is a new vaginal cream, Monistat, which appears effective and needs only a single application daily.

If the monilia infection causes swelling of the vulvar tissue and irritation, symptomatic relief may be provided by local application of a soothing medicated cream such as Mycolog. This cream may also be applied to the penis of a man who has a yeast infection.

These antiyeast suppositories and creams should be stored in the refrigerator, and it might be wise for a woman who is subject to recurrent monilia infections to keep medication on hand. When she identifies the initial symptoms of the monilia infection, she can then immediately initiate treatment before she becomes too uncomfortable.

If a monilia infection resists treatment with any of the antiyeast suppositories or creams, successful treatment may be achieved by the use of gentian violet, probably the most common treatment for monilia before the development of the antiyeast drugs. Gentian violet is a deep purple dye that can either be painted on the cervix, vagina, and vulva by the physician twice weekly for three weeks or can be applied by the woman in the form of a suppository with one application daily for three weeks. Although effective, this treatment is extremely messy.

In recurrent cases of monilia infection, it is important to restore the proper acidity of the vagina to inhibit the uncontrolled growth of yeast. This can be accomplished by vaginal administration of acetic and boric acid gel (Aci-jel), or by douching with a vinegar-and-water solution. Some physicians recommend douching with a one-percent potassium sorbate solution to inhibit yeast growth (this chemical is used to inhibit yeast growth in wine making). Still others suggest douching with an iodine solution like Betadine, an agent used for preoperative cleansing.

It would be a good idea for women to eat yogurt while taking antibiotics. In fact, yogurt is a useful addition to the diet of any woman who has or is predisposed to yeast infections. She must, of course, eat yogurt that contains *live* cultures; this counterbalances the yeast in the vagina. If a woman does not like yogurt, she could take oral acidophilus tablets instead. It has been suggested that plain yogurt (again, only yogurt with live cultures) could be applied like a vaginal cream for the treatment of a monilia infection. The effectiveness of this yogurt treatment has not been tested.

Oral monilia infection can be treated with an antifungal mouthwash. Mycostatin comes in the form of a mouthwash, and although its taste is anything but appealing, gargling two or three times a day until symptoms disappear cures an oral monilia infection.

TRICHOMONIASIS VAGINITIS

Trichomoniasis vaginitis is caused by a single-cell parasite called *Trichomonas vaginalis*. This organism lives only in the female vagina and the male urethra. The organism is usually transmitted by sexual intercourse. The *Trichomonas* organism can dwell within the reproductive tract without causing any symptoms. It is estimated that approximately 15 percent of men have trichomoniasis within the urethra. The organism can be detected by Pap smear in asymptomatic women.

Transmission of *Trichomonas*

Trichomoniasis is usually spread by sexual intercourse directly from an infected person to her or his partner. After transmission, the organisms can remain dormant in the body for extended periods of time. Alterations in the vaginal milieu can trigger the reproduction of this organism, with subsequent appearance of symptoms. Nonvenereal transmission of trichomoniasis is possible from contaminated toilets, towels, and instruments.

Symptoms

The vaginal discharge that accompanies a trichomoniasis infection is frothy and greenish yellow. The *Trichomonas* organism ferments the carbohydrates in the vagina, producing a gas which is the source of both the froth and the foul smell of the discharge. Trichomoniasis

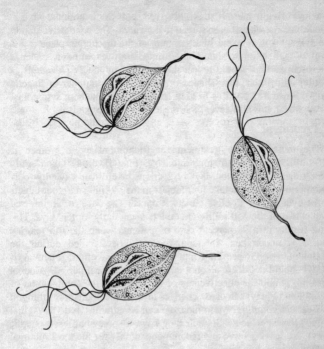

Fig. 6–3:   The form and the shape of *Trichomonas* organisms as they appear under the microscope. The trichomonads are identified by their characteristic form, also by their active twisting movement, caused by swinging movements of the four threadlike tails.

causes an irritation of the membranes of the vagina, producing severe itching. Since the membranes are irritated and sensitive, intercourse is painful, and so, sometimes, is urination. The inflammation can spread to the uterus, causing pelvic pain and a general feeling of malaise.

Diagnosis

The presence of the characteristic greenish, foul-smelling discharge leads a physician to suspect a trichomoniasis infection. A pelvic examination should confirm the diagnosis. If *Trichomonas* is present, the vagina is usually inflamed with a typical strawberry-red color, and there are often numerous small, deep red spots throughout the vagina. The inflammation can even spread to the vulva. The conclusive step in the diagnosis is to take a small amount of the discharge, place it in a drop of saline on a slide, and immediately examine it under a microscope. This should reveal the presence of the *Trichomonas*, a motile, unicellular, pear-shaped organism with a number of flagella (tails). Since it is possible to have trichomoniasis without symptoms, a Pap smear can also reveal the presence of the organism.

Treatment

The most effective treatment for trichomoniasis in women is 250-milligram tablets of metronidazole (Flagyl), either taken orally three times a day for ten days or 2 grams taken over a twenty-four-hour period. (You can take four tablets in the morning and four tablets in the evening, or all eight tablets at once.) The dose for an infected man is two of the 250-milligram tablets taken daily for ten days. This drug results in a 90-percent cure of patients when the full ten-day course is undertaken. Intercourse should be avoided during the treatment period to prevent contamination or reinfection. A person on Flagyl should not drink alcohol during the treatment period. Alcohol does not inhibit the effectiveness of the drug, but the combination of alcohol and Flagyl can cause changes in body metabolism resulting in nausea and vomiting. Metronidazole can be administered via vaginal suppositories, which, although they have a somewhat less systemic effect, are less effective and recommended only for the most minimal trichomoniasis infection.

It has been reported that fetal abnormalities have occurred in the offspring of pregnant laboratory animals given Flagyl. Therefore Flagyl is not recommended for women during the first three months of pregnancy, and if possible, should be avoided throughout pregnancy. A pregnant woman with a trichomoniasis infection is best treated with a nonmetronidazole suppository.

There have been reports that cancer developed when high doses of metronidazole were given to laboratory rodents over a period of time. There has been no evidence that metronidazole is carcinogenic in humans. Still, it is prudent to avoid overexposure to this potent drug. A woman should be sure to take the full course of metronidazole treatment to control the trichomonal infection completely and, most importantly, to avoid reinfection. She should also be sure that her sexual partner or partners are simultaneously treated. In this way, overexposure to metronidazole is avoided.

Warning!

Symptoms of vaginitis often elicit a diagnosis of trichomoniasis without proper identification of the infecting organism. Many women who have monilia infections are incorrectly treated for trichomoniasis and are given Flagyl, which can actually exacerbate the symptoms of monilia. If trichomoniasis cannot be clearly demonstrated, therapy for trichomoniasis should not be initiated.

HEMOPHILUS VAGINALIS VAGINITIS

Hemophilus vaginalis is a bacterial infection of the vagina now believed to be the third most common cause of vaginitis.

Transmission of Hemophilus Vaginalis

Hemophilus vaginalis is a Gram-negative bacteria that may be part of the normal vaginal flora. The uncontrolled reproduction of this bacteria, triggered perhaps by a change in the vaginal acidity, produces the infection. On the other hand, since the *Hemophilus* can occur in both women and men, the infection may be transmitted by sexual intercourse with an infected partner.

Symptoms of Hemophilus Vaginalis Vaginitis

In the earliest stage of the infection, a woman notices a scant vaginal discharge associated with mild burning and itching. As the infection spreads, the discharge becomes more profuse, either white or gray, and carries a foul smell. Vaginal itching and irritation increase, intercourse may become painful, and there may be a sensation of burning during urination.

Diagnosis of Hemophilus Vaginalis Vaginitis

A pelvic examination by a trained physician is required to diagnose hemophilus correctly. The symptoms of this infection are similar to the clinical symptoms of a trichomoniasis infection, often resulting in a misdiagnosis. The examination should reveal inflammation of the membranes of the vagina. Occasionally there will be small spots of hemorrhage. A sample of the discharge is examined under a microscope, where the absence of either *Candida albicans* or *Trichomonas* rules out these two organisms as being implicated in the infection. Hemophilus vaginalis is difficult to identify, but the presence of granular epithelial cells, called clue cells, and numerous white blood cells helps establish the diagnosis.

Treatment of Hemophilus Vaginalis Vaginitis

A mild hemophilus vaginalis infection can be successfully treated by intravaginal administration of triple-sulfa cream twice a day for two weeks. In more advanced cases, oral antibiotics are indicated. Ampicillin in doses of 500 milligrams, four times a day for five days, or tetracycline in doses of 250 milligrams four times a day for seven days, or other broad-spectrum antibiotics, is usually effective. When oral antibiotics are administered for treatment of a bacterial vaginitis, antiyeast suppositories should be given to prevent the overgrowth of yeast and a flare-up of monilia vaginitis. Intercourse should be avoided during the treatment period, and a woman's sexual partner or partners must be treated simultaneously to prevent reinfection.

NONSPECIFIC VAGINITIS

If the cause of vaginitis is not identifiable as trichomoniasis or monilia, it is often designated as nonspecific. This is usually a nonvenereal bacterial vaginitis with a gray, homogenous, foul-smelling discharge. It can be caused by poor hygiene in the vulvar area, which allows the growth of bacteria, which are then pushed by penile penetration into the vagina. Poor hygiene in the man has had the same effect.

Hemophilus vaginalis is still classified by many physicians as a nonspecific vaginitis, but the frequency of this rather specific infection merits its consideration as a separate entity.

E. coli bacteria are also found in some vaginitis discharge smears. These come from the rectum; they are normally in the intestines and are involved in the digestion process. *E. coli* can reach the vagina because of poor hygiene or mixing anal and vaginal intercourse. Women should be careful after defecation to clean themselves from front to back, not from back to front, to ensure that *E. coli* do not get into the vagina.

Mycoplasma is a microorganism associated with vaginitis; alone it causes no symptoms, but it has usually been found with bacteria. It can cause infertility.

When these bacteria infect a man, they grow inside the urethra and occasionally spread to the prostate. If either sex partner is diagnosed as having nonspecific infections, both should be treated.

A great number of bacteria can cause nonspecific vaginitis—too many to be listed here. The treatment for nonspecific vaginitis is the same as for hemophilus vaginalis vaginitis.

MIXED VAGINITIS

Vaginitis can have more than a single cause, and a woman may be infected with *Monilia, Trichomonas,* and *Hemophilus* bacteria all at the same time. Vaginitis must be carefully diagnosed, and a woman must be treated for *each* of the infecting organisms in order to achieve an effective cure.

CERVICITIS

Cervicitis is an inflammation of the tissues of the cervix, caused by a variety of infecting microorganisms. Cervicitis is classified as either acute or chronic.

In *acute cervicitis,* the inflammatory reaction is fresh and the symptoms are a purulent discharge and pelvic pain. Gonorrheal infection is one of the main causes of acute cervicitis, but it can be caused by any number of bacteria.

Chronic cervicitis is extremely common and may be present to some degree in ninety of every hundred women after childbirth. Chronic cervicitis can be very mild and the symptoms so minimal that a woman does not suspect anything. On the other hand, a woman may experience discharge, backache, and urinary problems. Chronic cervicitis is often associated with pregnancy or the use of birth-control pills with high estrogen levels. This is probably due to an increased blood supply to the cervix secondary to the increased hormone levels.

The cervix is extremely vulnerable to infection, since it is traumatized during childbirth and can even be mildly affected during sexual intercourse. Any infection within the vagina is easily passed to the cervix, where the infecting organism can be harbored. The tissue of the cervix can be so inflamed by the infection that *cervical erosion,* an open sore on the cervix, is formed. With cervical erosion, the outer, protective layer of cervical tissue has been destroyed and the cervix becomes even more vulnerable to infection. One of the symptoms of cervical erosion is a puslike vaginal discharge which, when cultured, often yields *E. coli* bacteria or any of the bacteria found in mixed vaginitis.

Chronic cervicitis can lead to cervical erosion. There may be a minimal, yellow discharge with early chronic cervicitis, but the amount of discharge increases appreciably when cervical erosion develops. As tissue destruction becomes more severe, cervical erosion may develop into a *cervical ulceration,* which can be a source of intermenstrual bleeding and spotting and bleeding after intercourse.

Diagnosis

The diagnosis of acute cervicitis is made after obtaining a smear of the cervical discharge during pelvic examination. The smear is cultured and the infecting organism identified. The cervix is red and swollen with a purulent discharge. In the diagnosis of chronic cervicitis, it is most important to differentiate this condition from cervical cancer, since some of the symptoms of cervical erosion are identical to the symptoms of a cervical malignancy. A Pap smear must be obtained; and any suspicious area should be biopsied during the pelvic examination. The biopsy can be obtained during a culposcopic examination or after the cervix has been stained with an iodine solution. A culture of the cervical discharge should be obtained to identify the infecting bacteria.

Treatment

Acute cervicitis is treated by administration of the appropriate antibiotics to eliminate the infecting organism.

Mild *chronic cervicitis* often spontaneously subsides, even without treatment, once the proper vaginal milieu is reestablished. This can be achieved postdelivery or when a woman stops use of birth-control pills. As with acute cervicitis, the infecting organism associated with chronic cervicitis must be eliminated by the administration of the proper antibiotic. If cervical erosion is present in a mild state, the physician may apply silver nitrate, which destroys the damaged cells and permits the growth of new, healthy cervical cells. When the cervical erosion is more advanced, electrocauterization or cryosurgery is performed to eliminate the damaged cells, making way for new, healthy tissue growth (see Chapter 16 on Operations).

Chronic inflammation of the cervix might predispose a woman to cervical cancer. Therefore, if symptoms of cervicitis appear, a woman should consult her physician.

CERVICAL POLYPS

Cervical polyps are small, fragile protrusions of tissue that grow from the inside of the cervix, sometimes protruding from the cervical opening into the vagina. Polyps usually grow when there has been a persistent cervicitis or other minor cervical abnormalities. The symptoms of cervical polyps are bleeding or spotting following intercourse or bowel movements, and some vaginal discharge. Since any abnormal vaginal bleeding is considered a potential sign of cervical cancer, a Pap smear must be obtained when the presence of polyps is suspected. Some cervical polyps can be removed by forceps in the physician's office. However, since the polyps usually have their origin within the cervix, they are more often removed during a D&C. A physician can then easily scrape the bases of the polyps to ensure that they do not grow back. Polyps are sent for pathological examination to rule out any malignancy.

VAGINAL DISCHARGE IN CHILDREN

A vaginal mucous discharge is not uncommon in girls around the time of menarche, the beginning of menstruation. This discharge signals the onset of estrogen production by the ovaries during the maturation process. Both trichomonas and monilia infections are seen in children. Mothers and elder sisters can spread these infections through towels and contaminated clothing, as can girls in boarding schools. Early sexual experimentation must also be considered, and any persistent vaginal discharge should be examined for gonorrhea. Cancer can also cause vaginal discharge. Although vaginal cancer is very rare in children, there have been cases of clear-cell carcinoma reported in the young daughters of women who received the antimiscarriage drug known as DES during pregnancy.

The combination of discharge, odor, and scant bleeding often means a foreign object in the child's vagina. Children have a tendency to satisfy their natural curiosity by exploring their bodies. Little girls may actually stick some small object into the vagina, which may catch inside the hymen, causing irritation, discharge, and odor. Physicians have extracted a wide variety of objects from girls' vaginas, such as hairpins, pencils, apple cores, and small toys.

When diagnosing a vaginal discharge in a child, the physician should probably perform a rectal examination rather than chance breaking the hymen with a vaginal examination. However, the findings may indicate the need for a vaginal examination, either to confirm the diagnosis of an infection or to remove a foreign body. The treatment of vaginitis in a child must be determined by the child's physician on an individual basis.

Intestinal parasites such as pinworms can also cause vaginal discharge in children, and there are oral medications for the adequate treatment of these conditions.

VAGINITIS AFTER MENOPAUSE

The vaginal milieu is enormously dependent upon hormonal influences. As the level of estrogen in the blood drops drastically during and following menopause, the cells of the vagina change. The vaginal tissue becomes atrophic, the mucosa loses its normal pink color and becomes gray, and the vagina is more easily traumatized, with slower healing due to decreased blood supply. These atrophic changes in the vagina later spread to the tissue of the vulva, and the skin becomes thin and loose. These changes can be accompanied by symptoms such as itching and burning. These symptoms vary enormously from one woman to another.

The atrophic changes which occur following menopause significantly alter the normal vaginal milieu and render the vagina very susceptible to infecting organisms such as yeast, *Trichomonas,* and even gonorrhea.

Treatment

The best treatment for simple *atrophic vaginitis* is local application of estrogen cream. This results in a thickening of the vaginal mucosa, an increase in blood supply to the vaginal tissue, and may help in the restoration of the vaginal milieu. The usual course of therapy involves daily applications of the vaginal cream until the symptoms have subsided. It is then advised that estrogen cream be applied at least once or twice weekly to prevent recurrence of symptoms. There is some systemic absorption of the vaginally applied estrogen; therefore, this treatment cannot be used by women for whom estrogen is contraindicated. If a woman is receiving estrogen-replacement treatment for menopausal symptoms, there is very little chance she will develop atrophic vaginitis.

If a woman contracts a secondary infection such as yeast, trichomoniasis, or gonorrhea with atrophic vaginitis, it should be treated by the usually prescribed medications.

VAGINAL DISCHARGE DUE TO FOREIGN BODIES

One of the most foul-smelling discharges results from a retained tampon. Quite often a woman uses two tampons during heavy bleeding, then removes only one of them. After a while, she notices an odor, and has a discharge that no amount of douching stops. When she finally goes to a gynecologist, the tampon is simply removed, and the symptoms immediately abate.

This same type of discharge can be caused by anything that becomes lodged in the vagina. It is surprising how many things gynecologists find in the vagina. Masturbatory objects are extremely common, and quite embarrassing to the patient. Small vibrators and bottles are frequently found.

Women with prolapsed uteri are often given pessaries, which act like crutches to hold the uterus in place. These, too, are foreign bodies, and can cause irritation and discharge. Retained and forgotten diaphragms do the same thing.

Some women use their vaginas as secure hiding places for money and gems, then either forget their valuables or can't get them out. This used to be a more common practice than it is today, but gynecologists in high-crime areas still extract a sizable booty from vaginal banks.

PSYCHOSOMATIC VAGINITIS

As with many other illnesses or disorders, the origin of vaginitis can be psychosomatic. This does not mean the vaginitis should be ignored or that it is not real; psychologically caused vaginitis is physically identical to any other type of vaginitis.

This type of vaginitis often has a sexual basis. Itching of the vulva or vagina may occur in women who are lonely, sexually frustrated, guilty about certain sexual practices, or overly fearful of venereal disease. Any of these can be especially acute when the woman engages in casual sex with a new partner.

When a woman has intercourse after a long abstinence and then experiences a discharge, it can be very upsetting. She can easily persuade herself that she has VD when her discharge actually stems from emotional stress. Unfortunately, the fear of VD only increases the symptoms.

The same thing can occur when a woman has an abnormal discharge and suspects cancer—the anxiety can easily affect hormonal balance and produce more discharge. On the other hand, some women ignore a discharge, afraid they might have cancer. The reasoning is that what they don't know can't hurt them. Of course, this is dangerous, even if there is no cancer, because any untreated infection can develop into serious physical problems.

Tension is a common cause of vaginitis. Stress causes more steroids to be produced by the adrenal glands, which decrease the body's formation of antibodies (immunoglobins). Thus, stress can make the body especially susceptible to infection by weakening its natural defense system.

The only way to treat tension-produced vaginitis is to learn to relax. Relaxation is not a luxury for the idle rich alone; it is a vital function of good health. It doesn't matter whether you are involved in organized relaxation—yoga, transcendental meditation, hypnosis, biofeedback, psychoanalysis—or whether you just sit back and enjoy music with a glass of wine. Relaxation is good for you and should be done regularly, every day.

One recommended method of relaxation is sex. Orgasm is a normal release of built-up tension, and it can relieve the entire body of anxiety. A healthy life most definitely includes a healthy sex life.

URINARY INFECTIONS

Because a woman's urethra is so much shorter than a man's, she is much more susceptible to urinary infections. These can be caused during intercourse by the penis pushing dirt and bacteria from the vagina into the urethra, or they can occur when a woman cleans herself after bowel movement from back to front rather than front to back, spreading rectal bacteria into the urethra.

Urinary infection is usually an infection in the bladder or kidneys. If it is left untreated, permanent damage may occur. Usually, symptoms are burning during urination, pressure on the bladder, fever, and backache.

If a severe urinary infection is suspected, tests should be performed to determine the source. Urine should be obtained for culture. Kidney X-ray and cystoscopy (examination of the bladder by introducing a scope through the urethra) may be performed. A thorough examination is especially important in children with recurrent infections.

When the clinical symptoms present the characteristic portrait of a urinary tract infection (UTI) with burning during urination, bladder pressure and pain, and low back pain, treatment is usually initiated immediately with one of the sulfa drugs such as Gantrisin. However, once the urine culture returns, treatment may be altered. If the infecting organism is more susceptible to a different antibiotic, it will be prescribed. While on antibiotic therapy for UTI, a woman must drink at least six to eight ounces of fluid every hour during her waking hours. She might also drink cranberry juice and take vitamin C to render the urine more acidic and less hospitable to the growth of bacteria.

If a woman suffers from recurrent urinary tract infections, she should have a careful evaluation by a qualified urologist to determine if these recurrent infections are the result of any urinary tract abnormality or kidney damage.

HONEYMOON CYSTITIS

A common bladder condition is called *honeymoon cystitis;* it is usually the result of very frequent intercourse, hence the name. The symptoms of this condition are bladder cramps, burning during urination, and blood in the urine. Honeymoon cystitis need not be the result of a bladder infection; it may be caused by an inflammation of the wall of the bladder. Excessive stimulation of the cervix during sexual intercourse can lead to a low-grade cervicitis, and the inflammation can spread via the lymphatic pathways to part of the bladder wall, resulting in honeymoon cystitis. Honeymoon cystitis may also be caused by an infection, with bacteria pushed up the urethra into the bladder during sexual intercourse. Adequate personal hygiene on the part of a woman and her partner may help prevent bacterial honeymoon cystitis.

Treatment of Honeymoon Cystitis

If it is suspected that honeymoon cystitis is not of bacterial origin, the first step in the treatment is to abstain from sexual intercourse. A woman should drink large amounts of water and increase her intake of cranberry juice and vitamin C. If the bladder pain is severe, pain killers such as Darvon and aspirin may be prescribed. If a urine culture reveals that the cystitis is of bacterial origin, appropriate antibiotic therapy is initiated.

BARTHOLIN'S GLAND INFECTION

There are two small glands inside the opening of the vagina, midway between the anus and the lower edge of the opening of the vulva. These are the Bartholin's glands, and their principal role is to secrete mucus to lubricate the vagina and facilitate penetration of the penis.

An infection or inflammation in the vulval area can cause swelling and irritation of any of the genital glands. The little ducts of the Bartholin's glands can become so inflamed that they will swell shut, trapping the mucous secretions. The trapped secretions cause the glands to swell into lumps the size of small eggs (Bartholin's gland cysts). This swelling is usually not painful, but often frightens a woman. If the Bartholin's gland becomes infected with a virulent organism, it leads to an abscess (Bartholin's gland abscess). This condition can be so painful that the woman is unable to walk. Abscess of the Bartholin's gland is most often caused by gonorrheal infection, but any kind of bacteria can be responsible.

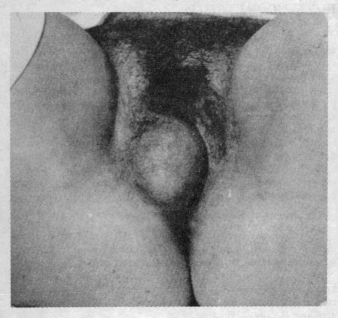

Fig. 6–4: A view of the vulva area. The woman's legs are resting in the stirrups. The large egg-shaped mass seen in the lower aspect of the right *labia majora* is an abscess of the Bartholin gland. (Reproduced by permission of Edmund R. Novak, M.D., from *Textbook of Gynecology*, 9th edition, The Williams and Wilkins Company, Baltimore, Maryland.)

Treatment

Bartholin's gland cysts and inflammation of the duct can heal spontaneously and, as the swelling of the duct subsides, the trapped secretions drain and the gland usually returns to normal size. This initial inflammation of the duct may be treated with oral antibiotics in combination with local application of an antibiotic-antiyeast cream. Sitz baths may also be advised. In some women, the gland may remain somewhat enlarged over a period of years, but this enlargement is not painful and requires no medical treatment. If reinflammation of the duct occurs, drainage of the cyst is impaired and the cyst will swell. If this reenlargement is asymptomatic, sitz baths may be the only treatment required, but if there are symptoms of pain, antibiotics should be taken. Women with Bartholin's gland cysts should be particularly attentive to their personal hygiene to avoid infection.

When the Bartholin's gland becomes abscessed, the pain usually becomes so severe that hospitalization is necessary. Cultures are obtained to determine the infecting organism and intravenous therapy with the appropriate antibiotic is initiated. Sitz baths are given to help reduce and ease the pain and swelling and aid the drainage of the gland.

In cases of very severe infection, a surgical procedure is required to drain the gland; this procedure is called *marsupialization*. A portion of the cyst wall is removed, the purulent material is drained, and the incision is sutured in such a fashion that the gland drains directly into the vagina, bypassing the ducts. Antibiotic treatment and sitz baths are continued postoperatively until complete healing has occurred. This procedure should have no sequel.

DOUCHING

Women have probably been douching, or instilling various fluids in the vagina, as long as they have been cleansing other parts of their bodies. In the past, douching was thought to have therapeutic effects, from the control of pelvic infections to the prevention of conception. The types of douches are widely varied and women have to the present day used everything from wine and garlic (as reported in the Ebers Papyrus of 1450 B.C.) to the perfumed and even flavored solutions available in today's pharmacies. In the past, one of the most common reasons for douching was contraception; recipes for the prevention of pregnancy were handed down from mother to daughter rather like a prized recipe for apple pie. Today, douching is used almost solely for cleanliness.

About fifty percent of American women douche at least occasionally. Most of them douche when they notice excessive or bad-smelling discharge. If this discharge is the result of an infection, douching will probably not help. On the other hand, it will probably do no harm, and although it does not treat the infection, it can clean out excess vaginal secretions.

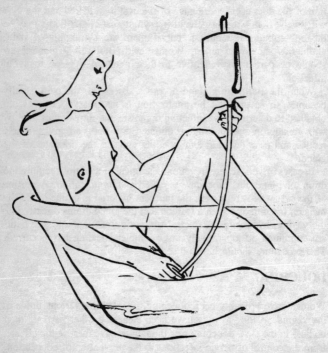

Fig. 6–5: Douching should be done in the bathtub. The douche tip is within the vagina and the labia are held by one hand to keep the fluid in the vagina. In this drawing, the douche apparatus is slightly higher than it should be, no more than 2 feet above the hips.

Is Douching Recommended?

Douching is not necessary to cleanse the vagina, since the normal, healthy vagina cleans itself. If a vaginal discharge is present, douching usually increases, rather than decreases, the amount of vaginal secretions. Too-frequent douching can alter the vaginal milieu and render the vagina more susceptible to infections. Douching tips and the douching solutions are seldom sterile and can even be a source of infection.

However, in general, douching is a benign procedure. If a woman feels it is personally necessary, she may douche perhaps once a week with little problem. On the other hand, the *perineal area* should be carefully washed every day as an essential part of personal hygiene. The Europeans have a good system in the bidet, which washes the external perineal area to prevent infection from spreading into the vagina.

How to Douche

If a woman wishes to douche, she should douche lying down in the bath tub rather than sitting on the toilet. The douche bag should be filled with one to two quarts of douching solution and placed no more than two feet above the level of the hips. The tip is inserted gently into the vagina as far as it will go, and the labia are pressed against the tip with one hand to keep the tip in place and to keep the douching solution from leaking out. The woman uses her free hand to release some of the solution from the douche bag and allows it to flow into the vagina until she feels a sense of fullness in the lower abdomen. She then stops the flow and holds the labia shut for fifteen to twenty seconds, during which time she tries contracting the muscles of the vagina to circulate the solution. The labia are then opened and the solution drains from the vagina. This procedure is repeated until all the douche solution has been used.

Douche Apparatus

There are three important don'ts when it comes to douching apparatus:

1. Don't use anyone else's douche apparatus—it is the perfect way to spread infection from one woman to another.
2. Don't douche with an apparatus that has been used at any time for an enema—bacteria from the rectum can live inside the tubing and easily be spread to the vagina.

3. Don't use a positive-pressure, bulb-type apparatus—if the pressure is too high, the douching solution, and possibly infection, can be forced into the uterus and even into the abdominal cavity.

A douche apparatus should be carefully cleaned and dried following each use, and should be placed where it will be as free from contamination as possible. A disposable douche bag is highly recommended, since their tips are sterile.

Douching Solutions

An enormous variety of commercially produced douching solutions is available, but probably one of the best, most benign solutions is one quart of ordinary tap water containing one tablespoon of plain white vinegar. If a woman wishes to use a commercially available preparation, she should carefully follow the instructions concerning the preparation of the solution to avoid damage to the vaginal tissue resulting from too strong a solution. An iodine solution, such as diluted Betadine, can be used as an effective cleansing douche and may alleviate the symptoms of herpes Type II infection. The FDA is expected to propose that commercially produced solutions carry an insert stating that their only proven therapeutic effect is that of cleansing.

Douching and Pregnancy

Douching is not recommended during pregnancy, since it is feared that if the douching solution enters the uterus it can harm the fetus and perhaps cause miscarriage. There is the possibility that some of the chemicals in the douching solution might enter the general circulation, pass the placenta, and even cause fetal abnormalities. Some douching solutions contain phenylmercuric acetate (PMA), and it has been shown that mercury can be damaging to a developing fetus.

TOXIC SHOCK SYNDROME

A widely publicized and serious new disease, *toxic shock syndrome* (TSS), was first described by Dr. James Todd in a paper published in the prestigious medical journal *Lancet* in 1978. Very rapidly over the ensuing months, reports of incidents of TSS surfaced, and as these cases were analyzed, a disturbing picture began to emerge. During the period from 1970 through 1980, 941 cases of TSS were confirmed in the United States. Ninety-nine percent of the TSS victims were women, and 98 percent of these women experienced onset of the disease during the menstrual period. As the disease was intensively studied, another significant fact emerged: Almost 100 percent of the menstruating women with TSS had used tampons; the occurrence of TSS appeared to be linked to tampon use during menstruation.

What Is Toxic Shock Syndrome?

The causes and true nature of toxic shock syndrome remain a mystery, although the disease has been the object of intensive scientific investigation. The disease is identified and characterized by its symptoms. These symptoms usually begin within five days of menstruation, most frequently on day 3 or 4 after the start of bleeding. Initially, an abrupt onset of high fever, 102 degrees or higher, is accompanied by vomiting and watery diarrhea. Other possible symptoms include sore throat, headache, and muscle pain. Within forty-eight hours, the condition of the TSS victim can deteriorate into hypotensive shock, a drop in systolic blood pressure to below 90 millimeters of mercury (mmHg) (normal systolic blood pressure would be 110 to 120 mmHg). A diffuse, sunburnlike rash appears over the body, mainly on the palms of the hands and soles of the feet. As the disease progresses, the skin on the hands and feet peel and the tongue and the mucous membranes become deep red in color ("strawberry tongue"). The victim can approach total collapse and requires large amounts of liquids to avoid dehydration. TSS runs its course in seven to ten days. A fatality rate as high as 8.4 percent has been reported for TSS, but in the presence of intensive surveillance of the disease, the fatality rate has dropped to 2.6 percent.

How Many Women Get TSS?

Toxic shock syndrome is a frightening and serious disease, but fortunately, a very rare one. The estimated incidence among all menstruating women is 6.2 cases of TSS per 100,000 women per year. Tampon use increases the chance to 8.8 cases of TSS per 100,000 women per year. The chance of developing TSS decreases as a woman's age increases. A woman over thirty runs a risk of developing TSS that is only about one-third that of her under-thirty counterpart. If, however, a woman has experienced an episode of TSS, her chances of developing TSS again are much higher than the general population's. In a study Dr. Jeffery Davis and his coinvestigators at the Bureau of Prevention, Wisconsin Division of Health found that ten of thirty-five patients (just over 28 percent) with previous history of TSS experienced recurrence of the disease, usually within one to two months of the first episode.

What Causes TSS?

It may be easier to say what does *not* cause TSS than to identify the real cause. TSS is not caused by being a woman, by being under thirty, by menstruating, or by using tampons, though these factors do appear to render a person more susceptible to TSS. Intensive investigations seem to point to a certain bacterium, *Staphylococcus aureus*. *Staph aureus* has been isolated from the vagina of 73 to 100 percent of women with TSS. *Staph aureus* is found in approximately 10 percent of women during menstruation. When bacteria such as *Staph aureus* multiply uncontrolled, a toxin is produced by the bacteria. In TSS, the toxin of *Staph aureus* passes into the circulation and causes the characteristic symptoms. The role of menstruation and tampons in this chain of events is not yet clear. The tampons themselves are not contaminated; this was vigorously tested. It is theorized, however, that the blood-soaked tampon could act as a sort of "culture medium," an enhanced environment for bacterial growth.

It is interesting to note that the peak of reported cases of TSS occurred in August 1980. The disease received much publicity during that summer, and women were well alerted to its possible threat. The Rely tampon, which had been involved in a number of TSS cases, was voluntarily withdrawn from the market. Over the next few months, the number of reported cases dropped by two-thirds. Tampon use also dropped from 70 to 55 percent, but even this significant decrease was not enough to explain the encouraging drop in the number of TSS cases.

Who Gets TSS?

The startling appearance of this serious new disease spurred epidemiologic investigation that attempted to isolate those factors that made one woman more likely than another to succumb to TSS. Menstruation and tampon use were soon isolated, but millions of women use tampons during their period, and investigators searched for other isolating characteristics. Women with TSS were matched with control groups; aspect after aspect and difference after difference were carefully examined. It had been suggested that frequency of sexual intercourse, intercourse during menstruation, or the number of sexual partners could be contributing factors, but careful scientific studies negated these possibilities.

The use and form of contraception were studied, and it was shown that, in fact, contraceptives seem to have a protective effect. In one study, only 31 percent of women with TSS used contraception, and only 4 percent used oral contraceptives. This is in vivid contrast to the use of some form of contraception by approximately 70 percent of all women nationwide, the pill being the most widely used. It is theorized that the protective effect of birth-control pills, if indeed there is a protective effect, comes from their ability to reduce the amount of menstrual bleeding, and/or the hormone changes they induce. This theory gains some support from the fact that the incidence of TSS is lower in older women, who, like women on the pill, frequently have a decrease in menstrual flow.

Neither the use of feminine hygiene sprays nor frequency of douching were shown to have any significant effect on the incidence of TSS.

The use of tampons *was* linked to TSS, and it was thought that tampon insertion might produce some laceration in the vaginal wall that could render women more susceptible to infection. This has proved not to be the case. Another suggestion was that the syndrome was linked to how frequently the tampon was changed, but again this was shown to have no influence on TSS statistics. One factor that *was* shown to have a significant effect on TSS incidence among tampon users was how continuously the tampon was used. Women who used tampons continuously throughout menstruation were shown to be more at risk than women who used tampons intermittently, perhaps wearing tampons during the day and sanitary napkins at night.

How Is TSS Treated?

TSS is a bacterially caused syndrome and can be treated with antibiotics. *It is a very serious disease and must not be treated by self-medication at home.* Once the syndrome has been identified, the patient will be hospitalized and antibiotic therapy will be initiated. The bacteria will be cultured to determine which antibiotic can be used most effectively. In many cases, *beta-lactamase*-resistant, anti-staphylococcal antibiotics have been used successfully. In addition, the patient will be treated symptomatically with intravenous fluids; and if shock should occur, intensive antishock measures will be instituted. Early detection is, of course, vital, for the earlier that treatment can be initiated the greater the chance of avoiding or minimizing the serious, and possibly fatal, effects of TSS.

How to Avoid TSS

The chances of contracting TSS are very small. Only 6 of 100,000 menstruating women will suffer from TSS in one year, and even this minimal chance seems to be lessening as the number of reported cases drops. A woman, however, can almost entirely eliminate even this minimal chance by not using tampons. The informed woman will wish to balance the benefits and convenience of tampon use against the very slight risk of this disease. This risk can be significantly reduced by simply using tampons intermittently over the menstrual period. On the other hand, women who have experienced a single incidence of TSS run a high risk of recurrence and should not use tampons at any time during menstruation.

The most important therapeutic measure that a woman can take in relation to TSS is to learn its early warning signals. If, during menstruation, a woman develops sudden high fever, 102 degrees or higher; vomiting; and diarrhea; she should immediately remove her tampon, if she is wearing one. She must immediately go to a doctor or emergency room, not the next day, not even the next hour, but immediately. She must inform the doctor of the possibility of TSS. This is no time to test your physician's diagnostic capabilities by playing guessing games. Early detection and early treatment are vitally important.

chapter 7

VENEREAL DISEASE

WHAT IS VD?

Basically, venereal disease (VD) is an infection contracted and transmitted primarily through sexual intercourse. The organisms which produce the various types of VD are extraordinarily fragile and cannot survive for any length of time outside the body. Air, light, lack of moisture, and even minor variations in temperature will destroy *most* VD organisms.

VD cannot be contracted from inanimate objects such as toilet seats, bed linen, or clothes, despite the stories you may have heard. It is transmitted directly from one partner to another in the act of sexual intercourse. These organisms invade the body where tissues provide a favorable environment (dark, moist, and warm), and are susceptible to the organism. These tissues are the mucous membranes of female and male genitalia, the mouth, the eyes, and the anus. VD in a pregnant woman can infect her unborn child.

Most VD is either a *bacterial* or a *viral* infection. Syphilis is caused by a microscopic, unicellular, spiral bacteria called *Treponema pallidum*. Gonorrhea is a bacterial infection caused by the bacteria *Neisseria gonorrhoea*. Other venereal diseases are discussed later in this chapter: *chancroid, lymphogranuloma venereum, granuloma inguinale*, and *herpes simplex* virus. All but the last are relatively rare, but herpes is a major problem as it becomes widespread because there is no known cure.

Venereal disease may be detected by the appearance of certain symptoms after intercourse with an infected individual. The symptoms vary, and the interval, or incubation period, between the time of exposure and the onset of the active disease may extend from two days to as long as six months, depending on the type of infection. The early signs of venereal infection are usually obvious in the male, although they may be ignored, tolerated, rationalized, or perhaps even unrecognized due to ignorance of the disease. In the woman, however, manifestations of venereal infection in the genital tract are often neither felt nor seen and cause no distress. Unknowingly, she becomes a *carrier of the disease,* completely unaware of the infection spreading inside her that she, in turn, may transmit to others.

You Can Have VD Without Knowing It

In women, both syphilis and gonorrhea can be asymptomatic (without symptoms). Gonorrhea can be asymptomatic eighty percent of the time, but a syphilis sore can also go unnoticed, since these sores are not painful and often disappear spontaneously. For this reason, women should be checked frequently for VD if they engage in sexual activity with many partners. If you do not know where to obtain information regarding VD symptoms and treatment, call the National VD Hot Line (Operation Venus) at the following toll-free numbers, 9:00 A.M. to 9:00 P.M. 7 days a week:

(800) 523-1885 (National)
(800) 462-4966 (For Pennsylvania)

VD on the Rise

With the discovery of penicillin, it appeared that venereal disease had finally been conquered. The past decade, however, has seen a dramatic resurgence in venereal disease. Today, the number of cases reported far surpasses the number reported before the advent of antibiotic treatment. Venereal disease is now considered an epidemic and reportedly strikes one person every two minutes in this country.

The term venereal disease (VD) refers to both syphilis and gonorrhea. These two diseases are, however, different; syphilis can, in its final stage, cause death, whereas gonorrhea is rarely fatal but can cause permanent sterility in both women and men. The required premarital blood test, VDRL (Venereal Disease Research Laboratory), detects only syphilis. Gonorrhea can be detected only by a culture obtained from the infected area.

Both syphilis and gonorrhea (GC) are on the rise, but there are about twenty-five cases of GC reported for each case of syphilis. The reported incidence of VD is higher in men than in women, particularly among male homosexuals.

HISTORY OF VD

At the end of the fifteenth century, the first documented epidemic of syphilis ravaged western Europe, spreading rapidly from the southern countries to their northern neighbors. The Europeans had not acquired immunity and the initial stages of the disease were far more severe and deadly than what is seen today. People fearfully recalled the Black Death, which had decimated the population of Europe 150 years earlier.

When syphilis was first reported, it was not known by that name but labeled differently in each country, usually by a form of political epithet. In France it was *le mal de Naples* or the Neapolitan disease; the Italians reciprocated by calling it the French pox. Depending on an Englishman's political preference, he suffered from either the French or Spanish disease. The Turks indicted all of western Europe by calling it the disease of the Christians.

By 1530, it appeared that the epidemic was over, and an Italian physician and philosopher, Hieronymus Fracastorius, left descriptions about the disease in the form of a poem, "Syphilis, Sive Morbi Gallici." In this poem the author invented the myth of Syphilis, a shepherd in the land of Opyhre who cursed Apollo, the Sun, and led his people from the worship of Apollo to that of their king, Alcithous. Reacting to this blasphemy, Apollo

was vexed in spirit, and shot forth harsh rays of angry light . . .
Forthwith a pestilence unknown before sprung up on the unhallowed earth.

The shepherd was the first victim of the new disease; his name was Syphilis.

The poem achieved such widespread popularity that the name of the unfortunate mythical shepherd, Syphilis, later on became the name of the disease.

There are two theories on the origin of syphilis: *the Columbian* and *the pre-Columbian*. *The Columbian theory* holds that syphilis is the gift of the New World to the Old. While there is no evidence that syphilis existed in Europe prior to the voyage of Columbus, ancient skeletons bearing the marks of syphilis infection have been discovered in the Americas. In 1492, Columbus explored the island of Hispaniola. Syphilis was present among the native population; the crew of Columbus acquired the infection through intercourse with native women and carried it back to Europe. A physician, Ruy Diaz de Isla, wrote in later years that he had treated Columbus's men for syphilis when they landed in Barcelona in 1493. More members of the crew were infected after the second voyage in 1494, and the contagion spread rapidly to groups of Spanish mercenaries.

These soldiers were sent to help King Alphonso II, a Spaniard who held the throne of Naples and was being threatened by King Charles VIII of France. As King Charles besieged Naples with an army of fifty-thousand men gathered from all the countries of Europe, the city was being infected with syphilis from the troops of Alphonso. Naples surrendered to King Charles on February 22, 1495, and it is generally accepted that the fall of Naples marks the beginning of the first epidemic of syphilis in Europe.

King Charles was eventually defeated and his army was disbanded in November, 1495. The troops returned to their respective countries carrying with them the contagion. Cases of syphilis were reported in France, Germany, Switzerland, Holland, England, and Greece in 1496. The pestilence reached Scotland by 1497 and Hungary and Russia by 1499.

The *pre-Columbian theory* recognizes the role played by the siege of Naples and the armies of Charles in the spread of syphilis but holds that the disease was present in Europe prior to the voyage of Columbus, though it went unrecognized or was confused with other diseases such as leprosy. It was the great flux of armies and people precipitated by Charles's invasion and the subsequent retreat from Naples that probably initiated the epidemic.

Syphilis has not readily yielded the secrets of its nature. In many parts of Europe, it was originally thought that syphilis was spread by any form of contact with an infected individual. Cardinal Wolsey was accused of infecting Henry VIII with syphilis by whispering in his ear. In other areas, the transmission of syphilis through sexual intercourse was acknowledged quite early.

The ultimate recognition of the venereal aspects of syphilis both promoted a clearer understanding of the disease and led to further confusion. In the sixteenth century, the history of syphilis was intertwined with that of a far more ancient condition, gonorrhea. For centuries following the first syphilis epidemic in Europe, GC and syphilis were regarded as variations of the same ailment. This fallacy was perpetuated by the tragic self-experimentation of John Hunter in the eighteenth century. He thought that gonorrhea and syphilis were two different diseases, and he deliberately inoculated himself with pus from a gonorrheal patient. Unfortunately for both Hunter and science, the gonorrheal patient also had syphilis, and the pus with which he infected his own body was contaminated with syphilitic organisms. In his report of the experiment, Hunter objectively described how he developed gonorrhea and then syphilis, erroneously convinced that they were indeed the same disease. Hunter eventually died of syphilis and so great was his reputation that evidence opposing his theories was disregarded for the next half-century. Finally, in 1838, Philippe Ricord, after studying the results of 2,500 human inoculations, published a report which irrefutably established the distinctions between syphilis and gonorrhea and identified them as separate diseases.

SYPHILIS

Transmission of Syphilis

Syphilis is known in the vernacular as lues, pox, syph, or bad blood.

The nature of the infecting organism, the *Treponema pallidum*, dictates the mode of syphilis transmission. *T. pallidum* is an anaerobic microbe; that is, it cannot survive or be transmitted through the air. Syphilis is spread by direct contact; the *T. pallidum* must be transmitted from the infectious syphilitic lesion of a carrier to the susceptible body surface of her or his partner. The most infectious syphilitic lesions, those swarming with *treponomes*, are located in the area of the genitals. The most susceptible body tissues, those which provide the proper environment for treponemal survival, are the membranes which line the reproductive tract. Sexual intercourse provides the opportunity for contact between infectious genital lesions and susceptible genital tissue and is the most efficient means for the transmission of syphilis. Nine out of ten cases of acquired syphilis are contracted through sexual intercourse.

Syphilis can be spread without sexual intercourse. Infectious syphilitic lesions can appear in the throat, and the lining of the oral cavity also offers the proper conditions of susceptibility—warmth and moisture—required for treponemal survival. In these cases, the infection may be passed by kissing. It is doubtful that the *T. pallidum* can pass directly through the skin into the body, but the slightest break in the skin, even a cut or abrasion of microscopic size, permits treponemal invasion. Thus, contact between broken skin surface and an infectious syphilitic lesion allows passage of the infection.

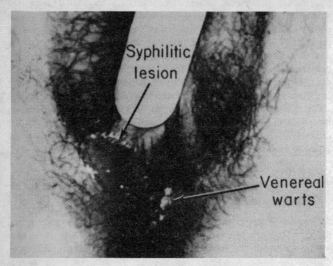

Fig. 7–1: A primary syphilitic lesion on the right labia of a woman, with the characteristic sharp edge of the chancre. This woman also has venereal warts on the perineum, the area between the vagina and anus. The presence of venereal warts should lead a physician to check for venereal diseases such as syphilis or gonorrhea. (Reproduced from *Syphilis: A Synopsis*, by permission of the Dept. of Health, Education & Welfare; Public Health Service; Center for Disease Control; Atlanta, Georgia.)

Finally, a pregnant woman infected with syphilis can transmit the disease to her unborn child. During the first five months after conception, the fetus is protected by the developing placenta, which blocks passage of the treponomes. After the fifth month, this barrier weakens and syphilitic organisms can invade the body of the infant and cause congenital malformations, miscarriage, or infant death.

Primary Syphilis

When syphilis first invades the body, some of the treponomes spread through the lymphatic system. Most of them, however, remain at the point of infection. The organisms alter the tissue surrounding this point, producing a *chancre*—a painless, hard, open sore—which occurs between three to four weeks after exposure. This is the characteristic sign of primary syphilis.

Chancres can appear singly or in groups. They look like small craters, ranging from an eighth of an inch to an inch in diameter. The raised edges are firm, but the surface is shiny red, raw, and sometimes crusted. When chancres occur in the genital area, they are usually painless. They generally develop in men on the shaft of the penis, but sometimes they develop invisibly beneath the foreskin or within the urethra. In women, genital chancres are often hidden within the vulva, on the walls of the vagina, or on the neck of the cervix. Chancres of the anus are becoming increasingly common as a result of homosexual intercourse. Extragenital chancres—on the lips, tongue, tonsils, or lining of the mouth—are frequently painful. These can also develop elsewhere on the body where syphilis has invaded a break in the skin, occurring most frequently on the nipples and fingers. Lymph glands near chancres often become infected and swell, aiding in diagnosis.

The chancre, or *primary syphilitic lesion,* appears to heal spontaneously one to five weeks after its appearance. This does not mean the syphilis has gone away. Instead, it signals a passage from primary to secondary syphilis.

Secondary Syphilis

In this stage of the disease, the effects of the spread of the infection throughout the body are first seen. Although transmitted locally, usually through the mucosa of the genitalia, syphilis is a *systemic* disease. In the secondary stage, its effect on the organs of the body becomes more evident. This stage usually occurs about two and a half months after initial exposure to the disease. In approximately one fourth of the cases, the signs of secondary syphilis appear before the chancre has healed, while in some cases these symptoms may be delayed for up to six months. The symptoms include fever, general malaise, and loss of appetite. Some may experience headaches, pain in the joints and long bones (which seems to worsen at night), sore throat, and swollen lymph glands.

There is also a skin eruption in the secondary stage. First, a rash called *macular syphilide* appears in small, round, rosy spots on the upper torso and arms. This rash may be so light that the discoloration of the skin cannot be seen under artificial light. It may disappear after a few days, or it might develop into a more common and prominent rash called *papular syphilide*. This rash is characterized by dull red,

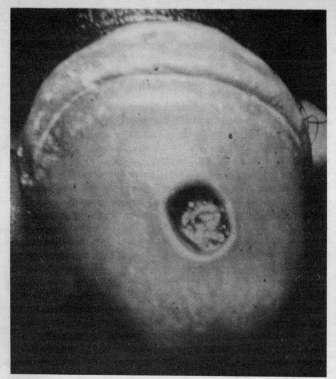

ABOVE
Fig. 7–2: A primary syphilitic lesion on the glans of the penis, with the characteristic smooth and sharp edge of the chancre. This type of sore heals very slowly but is not painful. (Reproduced from *Syphilis: A Synopsis,* by permission of the Dept. of Health, Education & Welfare; Public Health Service; Center for Disease Control; Atlanta, Georgia.)
RIGHT, TOP
Fig. 7–3: A primary syphilitic lesion on the shaft of the penis. This type of sore can be mistaken for venereal herpes lesion. Any abnormal sore in the genital area that does not heal easily should be immediately evaluated. Herpes lesions are, however, painful. (Reproduced by permission of Robert Boyers, M.D., from *Hospital Medicine,* July, 1972.)
RIGHT, BOTTOM
Fig. 7–4: A primary syphilitic lesion on the upper lip. This is a characteristic chancre with sharp edges. Oral syphilitic chancres are frequently painful. (Reproduced by permission of Robert Boyers, M.D., from *Hospital Medicine,* July, 1972.)

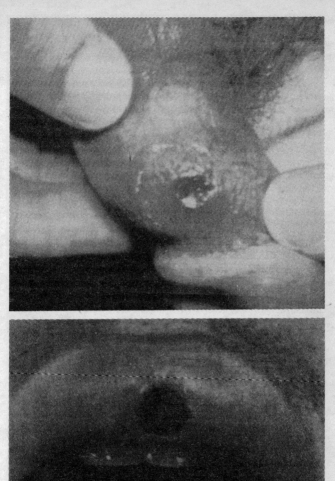
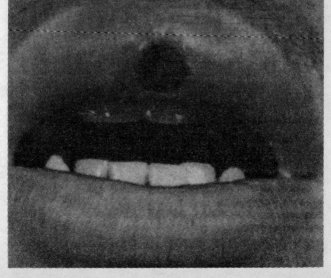

slightly raised spots from an eighth of an inch to half an inch in diameter, appearing all over the body, on the arms, legs, palms, soles, and face.

The treponomes may attack the hair follicles (*follicular syphilides*), causing the hair to fall out in patches, looking moth-eaten. Hair loss may also occur at the outer edges of the eyebrows.

Papular, or raised, lesions, may occur where skin surfaces meet in warm, moist areas—between the buttocks, or the inner surfaces of the upper thighs. These can become large, fleshy masses with broad bases and flat tops (*condylomata lata*). Initially dull red, they become grayish white. As the dead surface skin is shed, the lesion may ooze fluid swarming with infectious treponomes. A very rare form of secondary syphilis, malignant syphilis, a condition reminiscent of the first syphilis epidemic of the fifteenth century, is characterized by deep, ulcerating lesions which, if left untreated, can lead to death.

Mucous patches, or lesions of the mucous membranes, are also common in secondary syphilis, occurring in the throat and mouth or on the tonsils. These are round, grayish white lesions with dull red areolas. They can cause sore throat and, sometimes, deepening of the voice. Mucous patches resembling chancres can also appear on the genitals. Whether in the oral cavity or on the genitals, these lesions are extremely infectious.

Even if untreated, the symptoms of secondary syphilis disappear after two to six weeks, although the skin rashes may reappear. Syphilis then enters the latent stage.

Latent Syphilis

This stage is basically a symptomless period in which the only indication of the disease is a positive serological test (VDRL). During this phase, the disease cannot be transmitted except by a pregnant woman to her fetus. In one third of the cases, the disease disappears entirely. There is a spontaneous cure. In another third of the cases, the syphilis will never progress past the latent stage and no further manifestations of the disease occur, even though the blood tests remain positive. In the final third of the cases, the latent syphilis takes its time invading the various organs of the body. This can take up to forty years, or it may take only a year. Then the late, or *tertiary*, stage begins.

Late or Tertiary Syphilis

Twenty-five percent of all victims of *tertiary syphilis* die of the disease. One of the symptoms is *gummas*, relatively benign skin lesions appearing anywhere on the body. Gummas on the skin are disfiguring, but not deadly. If they occur on the spinal cord or in the brain, gummas can cause blindness, insanity, paralysis, or death. The *T. pallidum* shows a preference for cardiac tissue, and eight of every ten syphilis deaths result from cardiac problems. Syphilis can weaken the aorta, causing a huge *aneurysm* (a ballooning in the wall of the artery) which may burst and cause death. Likewise, the aortic valve may be attacked, causing the blood to back up into the heart instead of being pumped into the body, resulting in cardiac insufficiency. By this stage, damage is irreversible, and treatment can only slow down deterioration or perhaps stem it.

Congenital Syphilis

Congenital syphilis is a misnomer, since it is not an inherited genetic defect but rather an infection that is transmitted from mother to fetus. Since the placental barrier prevents the transmission of syphilis to the baby during the first five months after conception, congenital syphilis is a preventable disease. Early detection and treatment of syphilis in the mother completely protects the fetus, while an undetected syphilitic infection in a mother can result in death or permanent damage to the infant. The more recent the syphilitic infection in the mother, the greater the chance that she will miscarry or deliver a stillborn infant. If the mother has had the disease for an extended period of time, there is less chance that she will pass it to her child, but if passage of the infection does occur, it is more difficult to detect without the proper serological tests.

The manifestations of congenital syphilis are varied, since syphilis is a systemic disease and can attack any organ system. The effects of syphilitic infection on the developing organs of the fetus can be particularly devastating, and death *in utero* is commonly seen in cases of congenital syphilis. During the seventeenth century, congenital syphilis was probably the major cause of fetal mortality. If a child with congenital syphilis survives, it may suffer anything from skin lesions to blindness and deafness. Congenital syphilis detected before the age of two years is often characterized by a bloody nasal discharge called the snuffles. In some children, the signs of syphilis do not appear until after the age of two, but the destructive disease processes have been occurring since birth and these children often bear "stigmata" of congenital syphilis. These are often bone malformations, such as notched teeth, perforated palate, and disfigurement of the nasal bone called saddle nose. Congenital neurosyphilis is one of the most serious forms and may lead to paralysis and mental retardation.

Diagnosis of Syphilis

The symptoms of syphilis vary, and the incubation period (the length of time between the infecting intercourse and the onset of symptoms) may extend from ten days to as long as three months. The early signs of syphilis are usually obvious in men, although they may be ignored or tolerated. Conversely, a woman can be a carrier of syphilis but not be able to see or feel anything abnormal.

Serological blood tests are the most valuable tools in the diagnosis of syphilis. During certain stages of syphilis, for example, they are the only way to detect the presence of the disease. These blood tests fall into two categories: *specific* and *nonspecific*. The nonspecific tests (the famous Wassermann test, now largely replaced by the more accurate VDRL, or Venereal Disease Research Lab), are useful for general screening and searching for antibodies produced by the body to fight this invading organism. Such tests are required in most states before issuance of a marriage license.

Specific tests are required when the nonspecific test results are positive but no further clinical evidence is available to pinpoint the disease. This frequently occurs with syphilis, in which certain stages exhibit no symptoms. Tests like the TPI *(Treponema pallidum* immobilization) and the FTA—ABS (Fluorescent Treponemal Antibody—Absorbed) can detect the specific antibodies the body develops to fight syphilis.

The serological tests not only indicate the presence of syphilis, but also serve as guides to treatment. When serology reverses from positive to negative, VD has been cured.

When there is a fresh lesion, syphilis can also be diagnosed by scraping the surface of the lesion and examining this material with a specific microscope (dark field microscope). Only venereal-disease specialists have access to this diagnostic technique.

Treatment of Syphilis

Fifteenth-century physicians discovered ancient Arabic writings that prescribed an ointment containing mercury to cure scabies. Since syphilis produced similar skin ulcerations, this treatment was applied to VD for the next four hundred years. Patients were anointed, swathed in heavy clothing, and confined in hot, vapor-filled rooms for up to thirty days to sweat out the disease. Many were given overdoses of poisonous mercury by unknowing physicians. The patients salivated continuously, their lips and mouths became covered with sores, their gums swelled, and their teeth fell out. Many chose to die of syphilis rather than undergo this rigorous treatment.

Today, penicillin is the most effective antibiotic in the treatment of syphilis. The *T. pallidum* is particularly sensitive to this drug. The amount of penicillin depends on the stage of syphilis, but the usual dosage in primary and secondary syphilis is 2.4 million units of benzathine penicillin G given intramuscularly at one time and repeated seven days later. Early, active syphilis responds very rapidly to this therapy, but the more advanced stages of syphilis require higher doses. The treatment, however, varies individually and should only be administered by specialists in venereal disease who check the response to treatment. If the response is not satisfactory, a higher dose of penicillin will be administered. If the treatment is initiated prior to a positive serology in primary syphilis, the serology remains negative, since the infecting organism is destroyed before it can effect major tissue changes. If the serology is already positive, the effectiveness of the treatment can be judged by a serology reversal and by the disappearance of symptoms. It is prudent to advise patients to refrain from further intercourse for one week after the relief of the clinical symptoms and reversal in serology. In patients sensitive to penicillin, other antibiotics are employed, such as erythromycin and tetracycline. In late syphilis and congenital syphilis, the effectiveness of antibiotic treatment is not as great; the syphilis may be cured but the destructive effects of the disease cannot be reversed. Syphilis is such a dangerous disease that it should only be treated by specialists familiar with the latest developments in diagnosis and treatment of this condition.

GONORRHEA

History of Gonorrhea

Gonorrhea, the most common form of venereal disease, is perhaps also the most ancient. It is referred to several times in the Bible and is described in the writings of most ancient civilizations. Gonorrhea is recognized as a purulent, or pus-filled, discharge arising from the reproductive organs.

The name *gonorrhea* is derived from the Greek, meaning a "flow of seed," and was first applied by Galen in 300 A.D. The venereal origin of gonorrhea was recognized during the Middle Ages by Guillaume de Salicet, a physician who believed that the disease was contracted by sexual exposure to unclean women and manifested itself by a urethral or penile discharge several days later. Cleansing of the penis with water was one of the first suggested means of prophylaxis. There are no medical references to syphilis prior to the fifteenth century, and most of the writings on venereal disease concerned gonorrhea. It was only after the first syphilis epidemic, in 1497, that confusion developed between the two diseases, gonorrhea and syphilis. Paracelsus, in the sixteenth century, thought that gonorrhea was merely the initial manifestation of a syphilitic infection. The tragic self-experimentation of John Hunter in 1767 prolonged the fallacy that syphilis and gonorrhea were the same disease. Finally, in 1838, Philippe Ricord differentiated between syphilis and gonorrhea and noted the different ways they affect the human body and the development of the varying symptoms and signs.

In 1879, Neisser identified the bacterial organism that causes gonorrhea, earning himself the dubious honor of having the microorganism named after him *(Neisseria gonorrhoea)*.

Symptoms of Gonorrhea

Gonorrhea is recognized two to eight days following intercourse by a milky discharge from the vagina and female urethra or urinary tract or from a man's penis. The disease usually infects any glands in the genital area, including the sweat glands. Gonorrhea does not infect the skin, so no sores erupt; it is a disease of the mucous membrane or internal surfaces. It can also occur in the rectum in instances of anal intercourse, and in the throat, in cases of oral intercourse.

At the same time as the discharge first appears, a man will experience a sudden increase in frequency and urgency of urination, accompanied by some pain. Women will usually experience this to a lesser extent. Frequently, after several days of acute symptoms, even if no therapy is provided, a woman may enter the latent or chronic phase of the disease. Although she has no symptoms, she can still infect a male sex partner. She then becomes a continuous *carrier*.

Advanced Stage of Gonorrhea

In women, a spreading infection through the uterus and tubes causes tubal infections which can result in tubal damage and sterility. Gonococcal infection of the tubes must be treated as soon as possible or the damage is irreversible.

If an infected male is not treated, the urethra (the tube between the bladder and the tip of the penis) may become chronically infected, resulting in inability to void. A *urethral stricture,* or narrowing of the opening, may occur and infection of the ducts leading to the testicles produces *epididymidis* (infection in the first portion of the sperm duct), *cystitis,* and *infected prostate*. Gonorrhea frequently causes sterility.

There are systemic complications of untreated gonorrhea in both women and men and in children born of an infected mother. These include a generalized infection with high fever called *septicemia,* which can cause heart disease and death. Infection of the joints can lead to rheumatism and arthritis.

Gonorrhea in a pregnant woman can cause the infant's eyes to become infected during its journey through the gonococcal vagina during birth, leading to blindness. This is prevented by anointing the eyelids at birth with silver nitrate or antibiotic salve applied to the eyes of the newborn immediately after birth. This is now a requirement of the sanitary code.

How to Prevent Gonorrhea

The most reliable prophylaxis against gonorrhea is the use of a condom, a rubber sheath over the penis, which protects both male and female. The diaphragm and contraceptive foam also offer some protection against gonorrhea. It was recently reported that the incidence of gonorrhea in women using these methods was five times less common than in women using IUDs and pills. Cleansing of the genital areas with soap and an antiseptic solution immediately after intercourse, as well as urinating immediately after sex, offers other theoretical, but not confirmed, methods of protection. The prophylactic use of penicillin before exposure has many drawbacks, including development of individual immunity to penicillin and the production of a gonorrhea organism which becomes insensitive to the antibiotic. The prophylactic use of penicillin is particularly bad when a single individual is reinfected with gonorrhea. The more often the drug is used, the less are its chances of being successful. Successful prophylactic treatment with tetracycline in 500-milligram doses four times daily and vibramycin in 100-milligram doses twice daily for three to five days following suspected exposure have also been described. With any prophylactic drug, continuous use is not recommended because it can mask the infection.

In order to prevent the spread of gonorrhea, it is very important, once a case is recognized, to find all contacts of the individual over a period of several weeks. They should be brought in for specific testing for the organism. If there is some doubt about the contact, treatment with injectible penicillin should be instituted within a ten-day period. The only way to control the gonorrhea epidemic is by being honest about the disease and making sure all contacts are treated before they contaminate others.

The Incidence of Gonorrhea

The reported incidence of GC has increased by 15 percent per year in the past decade. The incidence of the infection in men is three times greater than in women. Gonorrhea in the male is usually a symptomatic disease, with clear symptoms of the infection. Since 80 percent of the women with gonorrhea are asymptomatic, a great number of women are, therefore, unknowing carriers of gonorrhea.

A great number of venereal diseases are not reported to the authorities, but it is estimated that there are approximately two to three million new cases of gonorrhea in the United States every year, and more than one hundred million new cases worldwide.

The chance of being infected is high, particularly if a person has many sex partners. Any suspicious discharge should be immediately evaluated by a physician to rule out VD.

Diagnosis of Gonorrhea

Gonorrhea can be diagnosed either by microscopic examination of the discharge or by culturing of the organism.

For many years, the most frequently used diagnostic technique was the microscopic detection of the *gonococci* bacteria. The obtained smear was treated with a series of complex chemical dyes (Gram stain) to reveal the presence of the bacteria. This rather involved procedure was lengthy and did not offer great accuracy in diagnosis. This technique was only correct in 30 to 40 percent of the cases and, therefore, is rarely used today.

Gonorrhea is almost entirely diagnosed through the culture technique. The gonorrhea bacteria is extremely fragile and can only survive in an atmosphere that contains very little oxygen. Immediately after being obtained, gonorrhea cultures are placed in a special transport medium, Trans-grow; the culture is taken as soon as possible to a special laboratory, where it is placed on a selective medium called Thayer-Martin (T-M) medium. The T-M is a growth medium which provides nutrition to the multiplying bacteria. The specimen in the T-M medium is placed in an incubator, where the cells multiply over a period of one to two days. After this time, the characteristic growth pattern of the gonorrhea can be diagnosed by specialists.

Unfortunately there is no quick, foolproof method that can diagnose gonorrhea within a few hours, and there is no simple blood test for the detection of this condition. When gonorrhea cultures are obtained, they must be sent to the specialized laboratories immediately, and if a culture is taken in a private physician's office or in a small clinic, it must be immediately transported for accurate diagnosis.

If a single smear is obtained from the cervix, it will detect gonorrhea in 90 to 93 percent of infected women. To improve the chances of detecting the condition, three cultures are obtained, one each from the cervix, from the urethra and from the anal canal.

Research is being performed to provide simple and inexpensive methods of gonorrhea screening. In one such program now in operation throughout the country, women come to a special clinic during the second or third day of their menstrual cycles. They are asked to use a vaginal tampon for at least fifteen minutes, and then the tampon is employed as the source of a smear for a gonorrhea culture. This simple technique eliminates the need for a pelvic examination by a trained physician, but is still only being carried out on a limited basis in a few institutions.

Treatment of Gonorrhea

For centuries, the most common treatment for gonorrhea was weekly injections of sandalwood oil, forced up the penis or into the upper vagina and female urethra.

Today, if caught in the primary stages, most VD is easily cured with antibiotics. Since this treatment was begun in the 1940s, however, the dosage has increased tremendously as various strains of VD have built up immunity to penicillin and other drugs. In the late 1950s and early 1960s, penicillin dosage was gradually increased from 600,000 units to 4,800,000 units. No one strain has developed immunity to *all* antibiotics, so gonorrhea can be treated.

The suggested treatment today is a one-time injection of penicillin. The recommended dose for women is 4.8 million units of procaine penicillin G divided into two doses and injected intramuscularly into each buttock. The dose for men is 2.4 million units of procaine penicillin G. If a person is allergic to penicillin, other antibiotics are effective. Procaine penicillin is more potent than regular penicillin because it is more self-sustaining. Oral tetracycline treatment has been widely used and provides an acceptable alternative. The recommended dose is an initial intake of 1.5 grams of tetracycline followed by 500 milligrams orally four times daily for four days. Vibramycin in the dose of 100 milligrams twice daily for five days is also recommended. Kanamycin and erythromycin, as well as other antibiotics, have also proven effective. The most important factor for a successful cure, however, is early treatment.

Because of the increasing number of antibiotic-resistant strains of gonorrhea, it is not safe to assume that a particular course of antibiotics has been 100 percent effective. The effectiveness of the treatment must be checked. Once an antibiotic has been given, the patient should return to the doctor seven days after the end of the treatment. A second culture will be performed at this time to make sure that the infection has been completely eliminated. If not, a different type of antibiotic can be administered.

GENITAL HERPES INFECTION

Infection with genital herpes virus or the herpes simplex virus Type 2, HSV-2, is considered a venereal disease since, in the majority of cases, it is transmitted by sexual intercourse. The infection is characterized by the appearance of painful blisters or sores in the area of the body below the waist, usually confined to the genitalia. The herpes 2 virus is closely related to the herpes simplex virus Type 1, which causes cold sores or fever blisters, usually in the area of the mouth, but they can occur in any area above the waist. The two viruses, Type 1 and Type 2, are closely related; they are generally confined to their respective areas of the body. A cold sore on the mouth, however, in 30 to 40 percent of people can be the source of genital infection during oral sex, and vice versa.

There is an increased interest in genital herpes, both in the lay press and in the medical community. There are a number of reasons for this attention, such as the reported association of herpes Type 2 virus with cervical cancer, reports in medical literature that genital herpes can be transmitted from an infected mother to the child at birth, and reports of the almost epidemic spread of this condition.

In the United States alone, it is estimated that 300,000 people are infected with this disease every year. The estimated number of people exposed to herpes Type 2 virus, determined by a specific blood test, is much higher. This blood test determines the presence of antibodies to the herpes Type 2 virus. Many more people have positive results than ever complain of the symptoms of a genital herpes infection. It is known that if a person experiences recurrent fever blisters around the mouth, her or his body produces antibodies of the herpes Type 1 virus, which appear effective in combating the herpes Type 2 virus, also. Thus, a person can be infected with the herpes Type 2 virus, but experience only minimal and transient symptoms that will not require medical attention. On the other hand, if a person has never had cold sores and is infected with herpes Type 2 virus, the infection is usually quite severe and there is a high incidence of recurrence of the symptoms until this individual has built up his or her own antibodies to the virus.

How Genital Herpes Is Transmitted

Genital herpes can be transmitted during sexual intercourse with a partner in the active phase of the disease, usually immediately after the genital blister has broken and the virus lies free on the surface of the mucosa. The virus can also be spread when there are open herpes sores.

The symptoms of infection can occur as soon as four days after exposure, or the virus can invade the cells of the genital mucosa and lie dormant for varying periods of time. What stimulates the virus from a dormant to an active phase is not clear, but it is known that a variety of stressful situations triggers the growth of the virus. In women, the cause of the stress situation can be the onset of the menstrual period, or perhaps being run down from too much work and too little sleep. Periods of emotional stress also appear to trigger viral growth. Stressful situations inhibit the immune response of the body and its natural ability to hold the growth of the virus in check, and thus the virus moves from a dormant to an active form.

Symptoms of Genital Herpes Infection

The virus in the active stages starts to multiply unchecked, inside the cells in which they have remained during the dormant state, causing the inflamed enlargement of one cell and then a number of cells. This causes the appearance of a blister or series of blisters. The first symptom may be itching and minor irritation in the genital area. The blisters may not appear on the vulva, in the vagina, or on the cervix until the infection has spread extensively in women. In men, the sores or blisters usually appear on the shaft of the penis, under the foreskin, on the glans or within the urethra. The blisters begin to enlarge, irritating nerve endings and causing pain. These soon rupture, becoming shallow, very painful ulcers, which interconnect and become extremely painful sores. These sores develop a secondary infection and then take up to six weeks to heal. During this period, the sores or lesions are extremely painful and are often mistaken by the sufferer for the primary chancre of syphilis. One point can be borne in mind to make the distinction between these two conditions—the chancre of syphilis in the genital area is usually not painful.

The first time a person has a genital herpes infection, the symptoms can be rather severe. High fever, general malaise, enlarged lymph glands, painful or difficult urination, and severe pelvic pain usually occur. These symptoms are often mistaken in women for pelvic inflammatory disease. They can, in various degrees of severity, last from a few days to a few weeks.

After the primary infection, the virus returns to its dormant state; it has not been destroyed, it is merely dormant. If a person has not had a previous herpes infection, this dormant state is usually transient and the symptoms of herpes genital infection may recur at any time from a few days to a year later. In some individuals, there may be up to ten recurrences of the symptoms. It should be emphasized that these recurrences are not caused by reinfection but by the transition of the virus from the dormant to the active state. Fortunately, the recurrent episodes of the disease are usually less severe than the primary infection, since antibodies are developed naturally. In the recurrent episodes, the lesions again appear, the lymph glands swell up, and urination becomes painful. Urinary-tract infections occur when the virus spreads to the urethra. When the body develops sufficient antibodies, the recurrent episodes of genital herpes cease.

Incidence of Genital Herpes Infection

Herpes virus Type 2 infection is very rarely reported in persons before they become sexually active. HSV-2 appears to be prevalent among teenagers and young adults. The mean age for people with a primary infection is about eighteen years and the mean age for recurrence is twenty-five years. There have been extensive studies to screen HSV-2 antibodies in the blood, and it has been found that the incidence of this virus is three to four times higher among lower socioeconomic groups, where it has been found in up to 30 percent of sexually active individuals. In some segments of the lower socio-economic population, amongst those who have a high rate of sexual activity, the incidences of herpes Type 2 antibodies have even approached 60 percent.

Genital Herpes Infection and Pregnancy

Herpes 2 erupts more frequently in pregnant women, possibly because the body's immune system is weakened during pregnancy. This has caused considerable concern, since the virus can be passed on to the infant during delivery through the vagina or even directly through the bloodstream, causing possible brain damage, meningitis, or death. Many physicians advocate Caesarean section delivery for women who have an acute HSV-2 infection within a few weeks of delivery to minimize the threat to the child.

Genital Herpes Infection and Cervical Cancer

Women with cervical cancer have been found to have HSV-2 antibodies in the blood more often than women without cervical cancer. This may be coincidental, since both cervical cancer and genital herpes infection are associated with an early and active sex life. There is no evidence that the herpes virus causes cancer, but studies indicate that women with HSV-2 antibodies have two to four times the chance of developing cervical cancer than women without these antibodies. There is no proof that if a woman has a genital herpes infection, she is necessarily a candidate for cervical cancer. She should, however, follow the prudent course by having a Pap smear performed every six months. Symptoms of the cancer would be detected while it is in a treatable stage.

How Can Genital Herpes Infection Be Prevented?

As with any venereally transmitted disease, the best prevention is avoidance of sexual intercourse with anyone in the active phase of a genital herpes infection. If there is any suspicion that a person's sexual partner has a genital herpes infection, the use of a condom may prevent the spread of the infection. Spermicides, such as contraceptive jellies and foam, in conjunction with a diaphragm may offer some protection, but the infection could still be transmitted. Any indication of a blister or sore in the genital area must raise the suspicion of genital herpes infection, and intercourse should be avoided.

Treatment of Genital Herpes Virus

At the present time, there is no cure for a genital herpes infection, but it can be treated symptomatically by a trained physician and complications avoided. A physician can prescribe antibiotics to prevent secondary infection, pain relievers, or a combination cream, such as Mycolog (cortisone and antiyeast) to reduce swelling and pain. An increased intake of vitamin A may be helpful, since this vitamin has been proven to stimulate the body's immune system. A person should also try to relax, giving the body a better chance to fight the infection.

There are several experimental treatments being used around the country today, and though none of them has been proven successful, the signs are encouraging. Studies have shown that 90 percent of patients treated with daily douches of a Providone-iodine solution (Betadine) showed symptoms of relief within one to three hours, with relief lasting up to three days. Interest has also been centered on photodynamic therapy, where proflavine, or "neutral red dye," has been painted on the external lesions, then exposed to fluorescent or ultraviolet light. This seems to dry up the lesion and speed healing, giving symptomatic relief and curing the lesions within seven days. The recurrence rate also seems to decrease, although studies show that the virus itself survives the exposure to the light and dye. Vaccination of BCG, a drug used to fight tuberculosis (made of tuberculosis bacteria), also seems to reduce recurrence, since it stimulates a person's immune mechanism. Recently, two therapies have shown promise in providing relief of the symptoms of herpes and preventing recurrent attacks. These new therapies are injections of adenosine 5'-monophosphate (AMP) and topical administrations of an ointment with 0.19 percent 2-deoxy-D-glucose. Intensive research into this widespread condition will hopefully yield an effective treatment in the near future.

RARE TYPES OF VD

Chancroid

Chancroid is a rare form of VD that derives its name from the resemblance between its symptoms and those of syphilis. However, the two diseases are distinct. Chancroid is caused by the *Ducrey* bacillus and is easily treated with sulfa drugs over a period of one to two weeks. If untreated, the lymph glands in the groin become infected and enlarged, sometimes requiring incision and drainage.

Granuloma Inguinale

Another rare disease, *granuloma inguinale*, is characterized by large areas of swollen, red, meaty skin around the genitals. The disease is diagnosed by the discovery of an organism, called Donovan bodies, in tissue scrapings from the infected area. This disease is much more common in tropical areas than it is in the United States. The treatment is tetracycline, given four times a day for ten to fifteen days.

Lymphogranuloma Venereum

This is another tropical disease, characterized by small, transient skin ulcers occurring seven to twelve days after sexual intercourse.

After the primary lesion, there is a tremendous enlargement of the lymph nodes in the groin, which blocks lymphatic drainage. In women, there is swelling of the labia, and in men, swelling of the scrotum and penis. Sulfa drugs or a broad spectrum of antibiotics are effective in treating *lymphogranuloma venereum*. If it goes untreated, sores of the rectum occur, followed after several months by a narrowing of the rectum, which requires corrective surgery.

PELVIC INFLAMMATORY DISEASE (PID)

Pelvic inflammatory disease (PID) is the term given for any extensive infection in the organs of the pelvic area. Vaginal or uterine infections can spread up into the fallopian tubes, causing an infection in the tubes, or *salpingitis*. The infection occasionally spreads into the abdomen and to the ovaries, causing a pelvic inflammatory disease. PID can lead to an abscess in the fallopian tubes or ovaries, or can spread to the peritoneum, causing peritonitis. This is an extremely serious condition that can lead to death if left untreated.

PID is often caused by a gonorrheal infection. The symptoms of gonorrhea often go untreated in a woman, who sometimes mistakes the gonorrheal discharge for minor vaginitis. Studies have shown that some 5 percent of women have undiagnosed gonorrhea that has spread dangerously far into the fallopian tubes, threatening sterility. It is essential for a woman, for this very reason, to consult a gynecologist whenever she notices an abnormal discharge.

PID can also be of nonvenereal origin due to other bacteria, including streptococcus, staphylococcus, or coli (from the rectum). Many of the anaerobic bacteria, which grow without oxygen, have also been found to cause PID. This type of nonvenereal infection is often found after childbearing or abortion, when bacteria have spread into the uterine cavity and continue into the fallopian tubes. If it is treated correctly with hospitalization and antibiotics, this infection rarely causes sterility. X-ray examination could, however, be conducted several weeks after treatment to ensure that the tubes are open.

With gonorrheal infection, the disease often spreads all the way through the tubes without causing any significant symptoms. The ends of the tubes swell shut, stopping the infection from spreading any further; the tubes then close their ends. This closure is often permanent and causes sterility, since the egg and the sperm cannot meet. Even though it is possible to open the tubes through plastic surgery, the chance of subsequent pregnancy is slim.

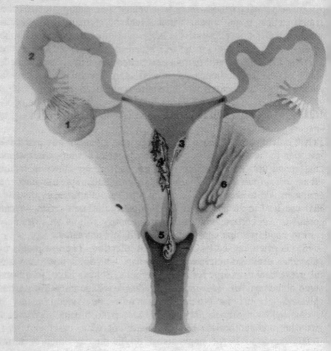

Fig. 7–5:   Areas subject to pelvic infection:

(1) Infection in the ovary is called *oophoritis;*

(2) infection in the fallopian tube is called *salpingitis,* and can distend the fallopian tubes, causing adhesions between the fimbriated end of the tube and ovary;

(3) infection of the endometrium within the uterine cavity, called *endometritis;*

(4) infection of placental tissue which has been retained in the uterus after delivery or after miscarriage;

(5) infection of the cervix is called *cervicitis* and could result in a sore or ulceration of the cervix. Cervicitis is usually accompanied by a discharge from the cervical os; and

(6) infection can spread outside the uterus, resulting in advanced pelvic inflammatory disease.

(Courtesy of Eli Lilly and Company, Indianapolis, Indiana.)

An unclean abortion, or intercourse a few days after abortion (allowing the penis to push bacteria into the uterus), can also cause PID. Sterility rarely results if prompt and proper treatment is carried out.

If the fallopian tube or the ovary becomes heavily infected, an abscess can form. The tube may be distended and damaged through the formation of extensive pelvic adhesions, so that the woman becomes sterile. A severe infection of this type is most properly treated with hospitalization, rigorous antibiotic therapy, and, on occasion, surgery (to drain the deeply infected abscess). In rare cases, a hysterectomy is indicated, but this procedure should be performed only as a last resort. It is a sad comment that many unnecessary hysterectomies are performed. A woman who refuses a hysterectomy, is adequately treated with antibiotics, and undergoes plastic surgery to reopen the fallopian tubes has at least a chance of conceiving. If a hysterectomy is suggested because of this condition, another physician should be consulted for a second opinion.

PID leading to tubal or ovarian abscesses occurs in women of any age. Often, when abscesses occur in postmenopausal women, the diagnosis is missed since the symptoms are ascribed to postmenopausal irregularities. Any irregularity at this age should be investigated with blood tests and cultures for VD. Women of any age can contract VD.

Women with IUDs are more susceptible to PID, particularly women fitted with early IUD models that have tails with many *filiforms*, several fibers acting as wicks for bacteria. It is now known that bacteria can climb up these tails into the fallopian tubes causing salpingitis. This often occurs on one side only, so if a woman has an IUD and pain on one side, it may be salpingitis, and she should be treated immediately with high doses of antibiotics. The later-model IUDs do not permit the entrance of bacteria, but tubal infection can still occur.

Peritonitis

The most advanced stage of PID is peritonitis, in which the fallopian tubes, both ovaries and the surrounding tissue, and the peritoneum (the thin, watery membrane covering the abdominal lining and the organs) are totally infected. This is probably the most painful condition a woman can have, and if untreated, it leads to death. The cure involves hospitalization, intravenous treatment with high doses of antibiotics, and several days of fasting to keep normal bowel functions from spreading the infection to other organs.

Pelvic Tuberculosis

Pelvic tuberculosis is very rare, but it can also cause PID. There are two types of tuberculosis: primary and secondary. Primary tuberculosis is probably transmitted through sexual contact. If a man has tuberculosis in his urinary tract, he can spread it to a woman's vagina. From there, it develops through the cervix, the uterus, the fallopian tubes, and often reaches into the abdominal cavity to cause peritonitis. This is rare, but it is probably the only way tuberculosis spreads as a primary infection of the fallopian tubes. Years ago, when tuberculosis was spread by unpasteurized milk, it often reached the peritoneum through the intestines. This, of course, is no longer a problem, except in the most isolated instances.

A secondary tuberculosis infection in the pelvic area is spread through the bloodstream from a primary infection in the lungs.

The diagnosis of this disease is usually made after the physician has detected an infection and takes cultures. It is sometimes noticed during surgery, when masses are found and sent for pathological examination. This type of tuberculosis is usually successfully treated with antituberculosis medicines, but should be treated by a specialist in this type of disease. Tuberculosis in the fallopian tubes usually causes sterility.

OTHER SEXUALLY TRANSMITTED CONDITIONS

There are several sexually transmitted conditions that are not considered real venereal diseases. They are, however, spread during sex acts and infect both women and men. These diseases do not have the same damaging consequences as VD.

Venereal Warts

Venereal warts *(Condylomata acuminata)* are caused by sexually transmitted viruses. Some women are not susceptible to venereal warts, while others catch them from only brief exposure. Women with monilia seem to have a higher incidence of contracting them, probably because the pH changes make the vagina more receptive.

Once a woman has venereal warts, it is common for the virus to drain out of the vagina down toward the anus. This causes spread of the warts, which look like small lumps, located anywhere from the vagina to the opening of the anus. If you find such lumps, contact your gynecologist immediately. Venereal warts are easy to treat in early stages, but if left untreated, they can overgrow the vagina to the

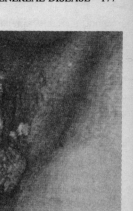

Fig. 7–6: An extreme case of venereal warts, or *condylomata accumulata*. The warts have grown on the vulva all the way down to the anus. These warts can occasionally become so large that they obstruct the entire vagina. (Reproduced with permission by Edmund R. Novak, M.D.; *Textbook of Gynecology*, 9th edition. The Williams and Wilkins Company, Baltimore, Maryland.)

point of closing it up, becoming football-sized lumps in severe cases. During pregnancy, this could necessitate a Caesarean section.

Though they are usually sexually transmitted, there are cases of apparent spontaneous eruption of venereal warts. The exact transmission in these cases is unknown. Normal warts on hands, feet, and so forth usually indicate a susceptibility to venereal warts. Warts on hands and fingers are not, however, caused by the same virus and cannot, therefore, spread to the female or male genitals by touching. Venereal warts on a man are usually located on the mucosa underneath the foreskin or on the glans. A woman who discovers venereal warts should immediately examine her sex partner. He might have only a tiny wart, but it is enough to transfer the virus. He should also be treated when you are undergoing treatment. If he is not treated, the warts will be transferred back, and you will be reinfected time after time.

Treatment of Venereal Warts

When external warts are seen, a speculum examination of the vagina and cervix is required to determine the extent of wart growth. Most venereal warts are treated with a medication called podophyllin, which burns the warts away. This is used for both women and men. This should be administered, only by a physician, directly to the head of the warts. It should never be applied to the skin because it causes painful burning and irritation. After application, the patient must remain on the examining table for a few minutes until the podophyllin dries. Then, after four hours, she should wash the area to remove the remaining podophyllin. To achieve a permanent cure, the milieu of the vagina should also be changed. Venereal warts are often associated with yeast infections. Treatment should, therefore, include antiyeast suppositories or cream.

If the podophyllin is unsuccessful in completely removing the warts even after several applications, your physician may have to coagulate or burn the warts. This is painful, and local anesthesia is used. If the warts are too extensive, this should be done under general anesthesia. If the warts are extremely developed, surgery may be required to cut them out. A vaccine can be developed from excised warts, but this is rarely done. Venereal warts during pregnancy usually disappear after delivery.

Sexually Transmitted Hepatitis B

Recent British studies have shown that 50 to 60 percent of hepatitis B cases not attributed to needles occur in homosexual men. American studies have found ten times as much hepatitis B antigen (a substance which induces the formation of antibodies) in the blood of homosexual men as in heterosexual men. The virus is also known to be present in saliva and semen and can be transmitted even by kissing and oral sex. Because of these findings, hepatitis B is thought to be, at least sometimes, sexually transmitted both in homosexuals and heterosexuals. Vaccines are presently being developed to prevent this disease.

Nongonorrheal or Nonspecific Urethritis

Discharge due to a nongonorrheal or nonspecific urethritis (infection in the urethra) is often identical to gonorrhea symptoms and is often misdiagnosed in both sexes. On closer examination, this infection can be identified as *Chlamydia trachomatis*. If a person has a discharge resembling gonorrhea and a test for that disease is negative, it could signal one of the lesser-known venereal diseases. Many laboratories do not have sufficiently sophisticated equipment to diagnose a *Chlamydia trachomatis* infection, yet an accurate diagnosis is important to ensure proper treatment—the discharge could also be due to trichomonas or other nongonorrheal infections. *Chlamydia trachomatis*, however, is the most common cause of nonspecific urethritis in both women and men. If you have no access to an adequately equipped lab, but gonorrhea has been definitely ruled out, treatment can be initiated against the Chlamydia infection with a fairly high rate of success.

The treatment is consistent with that of many other causes of nonspecific urethritis. A broad-spectrum antibiotic, like tetracycline, should be administered in a dose of 500 milligrams given four times daily to both sexual partners for seven to ten days.

Chlamydia infection is also common in pregnant women, and should be checked for since it can be transmitted to a child during delivery. It is now considered the most common cause of eye infection in newborn infants.

Crab Lice

Crab lice are tiny creatures which can be transmitted through sexual intercourse. They cause intense itching and, on close examination, can be seen at the base of hair shafts. Scratching often leads to secondary infection, with pus-filled areas in the genital region.

Crab lice survive only in pubic hair, in eyebrows, or in armpit hair. The crabs do not survive on the skin unless there is an extremely thick mat of body hair; they never survive on the scalp or on hairless skin. Though intercourse is generally the common method of transferral, crabs can be caught from infested bed linen.

If you begin itching in the pubic region, examine yourself under strong light. If you have crabs, you should be able to see them. There may also be eggs, like little lumps, at the base of hairs. These are

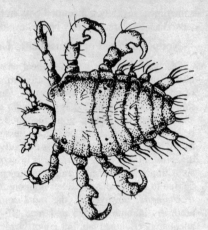

Fig. 7-7: A crab louse (*Phthirus pubis*). (Reproduced with permission of Beck J. Walter, M.D., and Barrett Connor, M.D.; from *Medical Parasitology,* St. Louis, 1971, The C.V. Mosby Company.)

black and visible, and can be removed with your fingernails. But be thorough; it takes only one egg to begin a new infestation. The first sign might often be small black spots or bloodstains on the underwear.

You can buy over-the-counter insecticide washes to treat crabs, but they may not be sufficient. The best medication is Kwell lotion or shampoo, available by doctor's prescription only. Use it liberally throughout the infected area, then wash carefully the following morning. Scrape up all the eggs with your nails and send all clothing and bed linen for cleaning. You may have to repeat the Kwell treatment several times until the crabs finally disappear. Your sexual partner should immediately be informed and treated.

There is no need to shave if you are infected with crabs. This will not help get rid of the lice or eggs.

Scabies

Scabies is a microscopic insect, *Sarcoptes scabiei,* that burrows into the skin, causing severe itching. The insects are seldom seen because they lie under the skin, but they spread rapidly from person to person, even without sexual contact. If one person in a house has scabies, everyone must be treated for it, including children.

The itch gets worse at night, usually attacking the palms, between the fingers, beside the scrotum, the breasts, the genitals, the beltline,

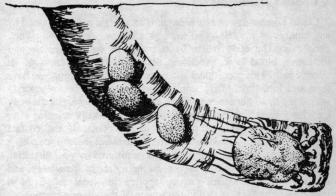

Fig. 7–8:   The scabies mite *(Sarcoptes scabiei)* tunnels under the surface of the skin and deposits its eggs. The upper line is the skin surface and the depth to which this parasite can infect the skin can be seen. The scabies are very small and the mite itself is usually not seen, but the infestation is detected by symptoms of itching and, occasionally, minute breaks in the skin. The openings of the mites' tunnels can be seen on very close inspection, particularly between the fingers and the toes. (Reproduced with permission of Beck J. Walter, M.D., and Barrett Connor, M.D., from *Medical Parasitology,* St. Louis, 1971, The C.V. Mosby Company.)

and the armpits. Scabies can be found anywhere except the face. The tunnels, though theoretically visible to the eye, are usually obscured by marks, irritation, and infection from scratching. If you have full-body itching, see your doctor. Kwell lotion will effectively treat the condition, working on the scabies overnight. All linen and clothing must be carefully washed the next day.

CONDITIONS OFTEN MISTAKEN FOR VD

Several conditions are often mistakenly thought to be cases of venereal disease, not so much by physicians as by patients who feel they are wise enough to diagnose their own ailments and prescribe their own cures. They may indeed have seen identical sores before and experienced identical symptoms, but that does not mean the cause of the symptoms is the same. This is especially common with skin diseases.

Contact Dermatitis

Contact dermatitis, or *skin eczema*, is an allergic reaction caused by any number of irritants—hair tints, skin creams, detergents, plants, chemicals. The body reacts by releasing its own chemicals and increasing blood flow, producing the characteristic redness of an allergic rash. This condition is often the result of something you have used for a long time. Many people assume that it must be a reaction to something new, since they have had no problems before. But the body may have been developing antibodies that are finally released after months or even years of exposure to a product. If the contact continues, the rash will worsen. Bacteria can infect the area, causing a secondary reaction. An antihistamine administered by your physician may help if you are unable to pinpoint the source of the allergy, and external cortisone cream can be applied for local relief. Most important, however, is to find the source of the allergic reaction.

Heat Rash

In hot, moist weather, the sweat ducts can become plugged, balloon up, and form red blisters. This heat rash usually occurs in folds of skin or in areas covered by tight clothing. It often occurs beneath breasts in women or under the scrotum in men. Women who wear pantyhose often develop it in the pubic area. The primary treatment is to discard restricting clothing in order to let the skin breathe. Keep the skin as dry as possible; powder and heat lamps can help. Cortisone cream helps clear up the rash at first; then proper skin care is required.

Nonvenereal Warts

Nonvenereal warts are caused by susceptibility to wart virus, possibly a hereditary trait. The warts on people's hands and feet are contagious only if a person is susceptible to warts. They are not the same as venereal warts and *cannot* spread to the genitals. Treatment is either special salve or cauterization.

Acne

Acne is a common skin disorder, most often seen during adolescence, on the face and shoulders. It is brought on by a hormonal imbalance. As oil is secreted from the skin and combines with the normal dirt and bacteria lying on the surface, the glands that cover the surface of the body become infected, causing pimples. Good skin care and cleanliness help to an extent, but often it is a matter of waiting for the body to grow into a normal hormone balance. Junk foods should be avoided, especially oily snacks like french fries, potato chips, or chocolate. For sugar, eat fruit instead of candy, and get plenty of vitamin B complex, even if it means taking daily vitamins. Drinking, smoking, and exhaustion all contribute to this skin problem. The skin is a mirror of your body's internal condition, the abuse of your body often manifests itself by breaking out on the skin. Lack of estrogen can cause acne, and women who develop this condition while taking low-estrogen birth-control pills might need a vitamin supplement strong in B complex to prevent breakout. If this does not help, they should change to a pill with higher estrogen content.

More severe cases are treated with tetracycline to prevent secondary infections. Drying therapy with alcohol or other astringent medications, or even heat treatments, is often prescribed. Exposure to the sun also helps. X-ray or radiation therapy used to be prescribed, but this is now considered dangerous because of the threat of cancer.

Boils

Boils are red, hot, swollen areas similar to large pimples. When a hair follicle is plugged and doesn't drain, it becomes a perfect medium for bacterial growth. White blood cells rush to the area to fight the infection and create pus. The blood brings nutrients to the trouble spot, causing redness. The skin stretches from the influx of all these fluids and the nerves stretch, causing pain. Scratching spreads the infection, creating multiple boils.

To treat boils, remove any tight clothing. This stops dirt from being rubbed into the infected area. Then soak a washcloth in hot water and place it directly on the boil to increase pressure and bring the pus out. A heating pad can also be used for this. Antibiotics help prevent further spread of the infection. The boil should drain after application of moist heat, and antibiotics for a few days should keep it from returning.

Ringworm

Ringworm is a fungus, often carried by cats and other animals, that causes itching and small, scaly, gray patches on the skin, sometimes forming a gray ring. It is easily treated with medication, prescribed by a dermatologist, which is applied directly to the irritated areas. If there is a cat in the household, it should be taken to a veterinarian to be treated or the infection will spread all over again.

Fever Blisters—Herpes Simplex Virus Type 1 Infection

Herpes simplex Type 1 causes fever blisters or cold sores, usually in the mouth and nasal cavity, but sometimes elsewhere above the waist. This is a nonvenereal virus, but is spread through direct contact —kissing, touching, and so forth. When the blister breaks, it is highly infectious. Like herpes simplex Type 2, Type 1 can hibernate in the cells, then erupt unexpectedly through the thinner skin surfaces—the gums, the lips, the tongue, the roof of the mouth. When the cold sore finally bursts, it takes a long time to heal and is quite painful. A secondary infection can develop if the area is not kept clean. The body usually heals the sore within seven to ten days and the virus goes back into the cells until it is ready to erupt again.

The virus usually comes to life when a person is in a weakened state —tired, run down, ill, under stress, or about to menstruate. This virus does not grow in the genital area. If you have a herpes lesion on your lips, you *cannot* transmit it to the genitals through oral contact. Although there is no known cure, researchers are looking into promising areas.

PREVENTION OF VD

The best prevention of VD, short of abstinence, is a condom (a rubber sheath over the penis). This protects both the male and the female, providing, incidentally, good and safe birth control if used correctly. Cleaning the genitals with soap and an antiseptic solution following intercourse offers theoretical, but not confirmed, protection. The prophylactic use of penicillin or other antibiotics is not recommended, since the body builds up a sensitivity to the drug necessitating increasingly larger doses until the antibiotic eventually becomes ineffective or subsequently results in an allergic reaction.

Once VD has been identified, it is essential to control its spread by informing everyone with whom the individual has had sexual relations during the previous weeks (this period depends on the type and stage of the disease). Each of these people should be examined and, if necessary, treated. All of these individuals should then contact all of *their* sexual partners, *ad infinitum*, until all possible spread has been checked.

chapter 8

A BRIEF HISTORY OF CONTRACEPTION

Before examining the techniques of modern birth control, it is important to stress that birth control is *not* a twentieth-century discovery. Contraception has been a continuing concern of humanity since the most primitive times. Techniques for birth control were described in the earliest forms of writing, and while most of them were ineffectual, some did provide protection from pregnancy.

Most modern birth-control methods have historical roots, and a review of society's struggle with this age-old dilemma can help us to understand the problems inherent to contraception.

Some of the history is both amusing and horrifying. Above all, it offers insight into society's concept of the position of women and the role of sex.

PESSARIES

A pessary is an object or substance placed in the vagina for contraceptive purposes. Pessaries were used by the ancient Egyptians, and the formula for a pessary described in the Petri Papyrus, dated 1850 B.C., called for a mixture of crocodile dung and honey to be placed in the vagina before intercourse. Interestingly, this mixture not only acted as a barrier to the sperm, but had some broad spermicidal effects. If a convenient crocodile wasn't available, elephant dung could be used.

Elephant dung and honey was used as a contraceptive pessary throughout India and Africa. In fact, this honey and dung compound appeared up to the eleventh century, when it was specifically mentioned by Constantinus Africanus in his Islamic book of surgery.

By the sixth century A.D., pessaries were a widely used contraceptive method; almost every ancient medical book prescribed their use and suggested varying formulas.

In Persia during the tenth century, a pessary was invented which not only acted as a barrier, but acted as a chemical spermicide as well. This pessary mixed rock salt and an oily material. Today, ordinary table salt is still recognized as an effective spermicide.

In his memoirs, Casanova describes the use of a gold ball—18 millimeters in diameter—which was inserted into his partner's vagina prior to intercourse. Unfortunately he did not comment on the actual effectiveness or reasoning of this elegant technique.

The onset of the industrial age in the nineteenth century saw the practice of family planning become an increasingly important social and political issue. Walter Rendell, a London chemist operating his own pharmacy in the 1880s, felt the rising concern. As he listened to his customers' stories of poverty and deprivation, it became apparent to him that an effective birth-control method was urgently needed. After much work and experimentation, he developed a pessary containing quinine, which he distributed freely to his customers with instructions on its proper use.

The results of this new pessary exceeded his expectations. Requests were logged so rapidly that the pessary was marketed commercially in 1886. By the turn of the century, the product was a best seller throughout the world. In fact, until the twentieth century, quinine was the only recognized spermicide which could be used with complete safety.

Today, quinine has been replaced by nonirritating substances in stronger spermicides like foam or antispermicide jelly, which are sold separately or in conjunction with diaphragms. Still, Rendell's discovery was a landmark in the history of birth control—it was the crowning peak of pessaries even as it ushered in a new age of birth-control products.

SPONGES, DIAPHRAGMS, AND CERVICAL CAPS

Diaphragms and pessaries originated from the same idea—to create a barrier to keep semen from entering the uterus. While pessaries were used to block the semen, other early methods were used to absorb it. The earliest reference to such absorption devices was made in the Ebers Papyrus, around 1500 B.C. The papyrus described a tampon made of lint and soaked with acacia and honey to be placed in the vagina before intercourse. Ancient Talmudists considered the sponge an effective contraceptive device—a method which has persisted almost unchanged for a thousand years. Even as recently as ten years ago, one could still buy sponges for contraceptive purposes in Paris.

Early physicians suggested a round or cuplike device placed in the vagina to block the sperm. In the first century, Dioscorides prescribed vaginal insertion of a swordlike leaf filled with honey. By the sixth century, Aetius of Amida created a barrier in a natural shape. He suggested cutting a pomegranate, removing the seeds and pulp, and inserting the hollow end into the vagina before intercourse. This was probably the first real diaphragm.

In 1883, Dr. Frederick Wilde, a German physician, described a rubber cap as a blocking contraceptive, but it was Dr. Mensinga of Germany who popularized the method. The function of this cap was to block, or close, the cervical canal to semen. This method spread from Germany to Holland, then to England, where it became known as the Dutch cap.

Once the popularity of the cap-type contraceptive was established, doctors realized that it was necessary to completely seal any gap in its fit against the cervix to prevent sperm from entering.

DOUCHING AND FUMIGATING

Douching and fumigating (in this context, sending fumes or gases into the vagina) were long believed to be effective contraceptive methods. Douching appeared very early in Egyptian literature. Inscriptions have been found giving details of the solutions. Drawings and instructions for douching, plus an actual douching instrument, have also been uncovered.

After coitus, the woman was advised to douche with such ingredients as wine and garlic with fennel. These solutions were administered through instruments made from horns of animals or bills of birds. The most common was the bill of the ibis, which was used as a conductive tube to pour liquid into the vagina.

In the early 1880s, Charles Knowlton, in his book *The Fruit of Philosophy,* offered various recipes for contraceptive douching solutions, such as mixing alum with the juice extracted from hemlock plants or green tea.

Today there are various spermicides available, but these are inserted into the vagina immediately prior to intercourse, not after. Douching is advocated simply as a hygienic, not a contraceptive, method.

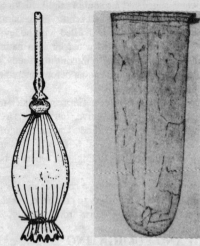

LEFT
Fig. 8-1:   A douche bag from the thirteenth century. The bag was constructed of sow bladder and the nozzle of wood. (Reproduced by permission from: *Contraception through the Ages* by B. Finch and H. Greene, published by Peter Owen, London.)

RIGHT
Fig. 8-2:   A condom from the eighteenth century. This condom was made from the cecum of sheep. (Reproduced by permission from: *Contraception through the Ages* by B. Finch and H. Greene, published by Peter Owen, London.)

The condom, or sheath, was not developed to prevent conception, but to prevent the spread of venereal disease. Even before the connection between intercourse and conception was recognized, people were concerned with disease passed between women and men during coitus.

The earliest known condom was depicted in paintings on cave walls of Cambarelles dating from prehistoric times. One of the drawings showed a man and a woman engaged in the sexual act, the man seeming to have his penis covered with some sort of coat.

In ancient and imperial Rome, the guts and bladders of animals were used to cover the penis. The animal cebum had a fineness, an elastic quality, and a tensile strength which made it an excellent sheath.

Dr. Falloppio, an Italian authority on syphilis, described in his book, *De Morbo Gallico*, first published in 1564, a linen sheath to fit on the glans to help prevent infection. His definitive instructions on the use of this sheath apply even today.

When the connection between intercourse and pregnancy was established, the dual-purpose sheath came into focus, and what is known as the condom was gradually perfected.

Curiously, one of the first manufacturers of condoms was a woman, Mrs. Phillips, who operated a small warehouse in London in the latter part of the eighteenth century. She advertised her wares, made from dried gut of sheep, by circulars and handbills. Gradually the condom was refined and redesigned using rubber and, finally, synthetic rubber.

COITUS INTERRUPTUS

Once it was established that male semen was, indeed, a fertilizing agent, society dealt with means of preventing the semen from reaching the egg. The simplest and least expensive method was simply to withdraw the penis before ejaculation. This was the most widely adopted method in early history, known as the practice of *coitus interruptus*. It has retained its popularity for over two thousand years, and it is only with the dissemination of more effective methods that coitus interruptus has become one of the lesser-used methods of birth control.

STERILIZATION AS A MEANS OF CONTRACEPTION

One of the more efficient ways to prevent conception has been sterilization of men and/or women.

Men

It was probably in China that the practice of castration had its earliest history. The Chinese studied animals to discover the role of testicles and ovaries in conception. They castrated dogs, cocks, and bulls with remarkable success. They also castrated men. In early Chinese medical history, castration was originally adopted as a means

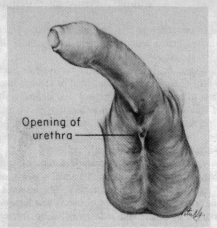

Opening of
urethra

ABOVE

Fig. 8–3: Subincision, or *koopli*. This was a form of male surgical contraception used by Australian tribes. A man in a tribe who had this operation could be easily recognized, since he would have to stand with his legs far apart to urinate.

BELOW

Fig. 8–4: Male *infundibulation* consists of attaching a ring or clasp to the penis. This procedure was performed by the Romans, but only on uncircumcised males, since the ring was placed through the foreskin. The purpose of the ring was to prevent the insertion of the penis into the vagina. The ring was usually larger than the one shown in this drawing and could be considered a type of chastity belt for men, since it prevented intercourse.

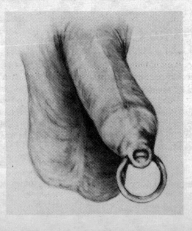

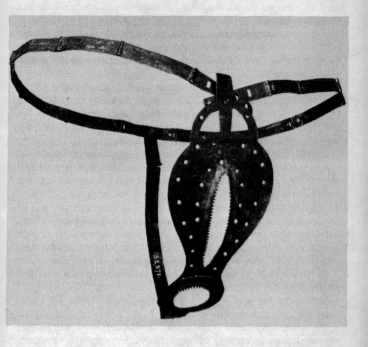

Fig. 8–5: The chastity belt was a frequently used apparatus, apparently introduced in France at the time of the Crusades, circa 1180. The belt consisted of two main parts—a band of flexible metal and a perforated plate (or a pair of hinged plates). The band was worn around the hips. The underportion passed just above the buttocks, with the second part of the apparatus attached by a joint to a band in the front. The second piece (constructed of metal, bone, or ivory) was convex so it could press firmly against the mons Veneris. It extended downward, completely enclosing the vulva. A dentured or plain perforation permitted the natural functions but was too small to admit even the tip of the penis. (Reproduced by permission of Nordiske museet, Stockholm, Sweden.)

of punishment for certain grave offenders. About 1200 B.C., it was used on servants or attendants of the emperor and his family in the Chou Dynasty.

Other civilizations, including the Assyrians and Babylonians, castrated slaves and made them guardians of the home. These slaves became known as eunuchs, men rendered incapable of the act of sexual intercourse.

Another surgical sterilization means used by aboriginal tribes in Australia was called *Koolpi,* or subincision. Basically, it was a ritual operation in which a slit was cut along the urethra close to the testicles. At the time of ejaculation, the semen would not go into the vagina, but would, rather, spill through the slit.

The Romans are credited with a semisurgical procedure which was a highly effective contraceptive. Called *infundibulation,* it consisted of attaching a ring, or clasp, to the penis. During this procedure, the foreskin was pulled forward over the glans of the penis until it formed a complete cover. Two threads were then drawn through the edge of the foreskin. Each day the threads were moved backward and forward until two clear holes were formed. A ring was then placed through these holes, making it impossible to have intercourse. Infundibulation was one of the only reversible surgical methods of early times.

In the twentieth century, the X-ray was discovered as a means of sterilization for both men and women, but the harmful effects of radiation and the possibility of it causing cancer in later life ended most research in this area.

Vasectomy (the surgical removal of the *vas deferens*), has become the most popular method of sterilization. Developed in the early 1900s, the procedure has been refined over the years and is now considered a very viable birth-control alternative.

Women

The problem of fertility in women has been researched during all of human history.

Hippocrates, in the fourth century B.C., was one of the first to notice that fat women appeared to bear fewer children than lean women. It followed that fatness was encouraged in women wishing to remain sterile. Curiously, modern medicine has reached the same conclusion. If a woman is too fat, she does not experience normal ovulation and is, therefore, less fertile.

The most drastic measure to ensure female sterilization was removal of the ovaries, known as female castration. In ancient Egypt, kings castrated the young women of their harems. It was thought that if women were castrated at a young age, female sex characteristics would not develop and their youth would be preserved.

There were, of course, many other ideas and concoctions and devices, some far-fetched and some fairly sound, used through history to prevent conception. When these failed, more extreme measures, like abortion and infanticide (the slaughter of babies), were instigated. These, of course, were not contraceptive techniques; rather, they were early exercises in population control.

Most of the old methods, though, never really freed women from the worry and concern of unwanted pregnancies. It has only been in the twentieth century that women have been able to approach contraception with any sense of self-dignity, safety, and reliability.

chapter 9

MODERN METHODS OF CONTRACEPTION

Birth control has become increasingly important in an era of dramatically increasing population and changing personal life-styles. Attitudes of greater sexual freedom have been accompanied by growing knowledge of contraceptive methods. Nearly everyone has the ability, and certainly the right, to use their own bodies as they desire. To exercise that right, you must understand how your body functions. Full control of your sexual life means being able to take advantage of the various methods of birth control. The more you know, the greater your personal choices.

In this chapter, the current methods, trends, and notions about birth control are discussed. Some of these methods are effective, advanced, and changing every day, while others are misunderstood, outdated, or just plain ineffective. Several methods are especially well suited to couples planning families and can help in the spacing of children. Couples who have completed their families may find other, more acceptable methods for preventing further pregnancies. People who have infrequent or unexpected sexual relations might find some of the more traditional methods better suited to their needs. Virtually everyone should be able to find contraceptive techniques compatible with his or her thoughts on family planning, not to mention particular sexual desires. This chapter will give you a thorough understanding of the various forms of contraception, as well as of their safety and effectiveness.

Many people have been justifiably concerned with the reported side effects of various contraceptives. Oral contraceptives and intrauterine devices (IUDs) have been criticized for producing harmful side effects, or even fatalities. Many contend that not enough is known about the full effects of such powerful or potentially dangerous methods. Medicine should never be taken for granted; an educated concern about what we do to our bodies is beneficial. The side effects and the changes that contraceptives produce in the body, as well as the risks involved in their use, are discussed here to give you a basis for making your own informed decision.

Control of your body and sexual freedom without the worry of unwanted pregnancy are advances made in the last twenty years. To take full advantage of these, you must know your choices, and what you do not know *can* hurt you!

VAGINAL SPERMICIDES: FOAM, CREAM, AND JELLY

Vaginal spermicides, called a *barrier method* of contraception, have been around a long time. The ancient Egyptians were said to place mixtures of honey, vegetable gum, sodium carbonate, and crocodile dung into the vagina to prevent pregnancy. Aristotle reported using a combination of frankincense, oil of cedar, and olive oil for the same purpose. In the Middle Ages, people were fond of rock salt and alum. Walter Rendell, the founding father of modern spermicides, introduced a suppository of cocoa butter and quinine sulfate to England in 1885. Rendell's, probably the first commercial spermicide, is still available today.

Modern spermicides are made of two basic components: a spermicidal (sperm killing) chemical and a harmless, bulky base. This base is heavy enough to block the cervix, so that even if some sperm are not killed by the chemical, they cannot enter the cervical canal.

Spermicides are available in a number of different forms. There are spermicidal foams, creams, jellies, foaming tablets, and suppositories. Foaming tablets and suppositories are not widely available since they do not work as well as the other methods. Foams are the *most* effective spermicide—they spread quickly and evenly coat the cervix. Creams and jellies are more likely to fail because they do not spread as easily, nor as evenly, throughout the cervix. Emko and Delfen are two of the most popular spermicidal foams, and their names have nearly become synonymous with contraception. Many foams are now available in factory-filled, premeasured doses for easy use.

The Pros and Cons of Spermicides

Spermicides offer several advantages. They are relatively benign to the body and can be purchased in almost any drugstore or pharmacy without a prescription. Almost everyone finds a spermicide quite simple to use, and it can easily be combined with other birth-control methods for added protection. There is no device involved, which may prevent the artificial or physically unsatisfactory feeling that condoms sometimes cause.

On the other hand, a spermicide must be used *immediately* before intercourse, which some people feel interrupts the spontaneity of lovemaking. It also must be inserted before *each and every* intercourse. Some women do not like having to touch their genitals in order to insert the spermicide high up in the vagina. Other users report a mild burning or similar vaginal irritation after application, but this may be relieved by changing to another, perhaps less irritating, brand. Then, of course, there is the complaint of messiness due to the dripping or leaking of the spermicide from the vagina, which is simply unaesthetic. Some men object strongly to the taste of the foam or spermicide.

How to Use Foam, Cream, and Jelly

The first step in the use of a spermicide is to fill the applicator with the preparation. A prefilled applicator, such as Emko's brand Because, can also be used. Creams and jellies usually have applicators that screw onto the top of the tube for easier handling. Next, the woman lies down and gently inserts the applicator as far up into the vagina as it will go. The applicator is then pulled back about a half an inch, the plunger depressed or the tube squeezed to deposit the spermicide near the cervix, allowing the preparation to coat it evenly. Creams and jellies do not spread as easily as foam, so the careful positioning of the applicator is more important with these preparations.

Spermicides should be applied no more than a half-hour before intercourse. If more than an hour passes, there must be a second application. There should be an interval between application of the spermicide and intercourse. Two to three minutes should pass to allow creams and jelly preparations to coat the cervix. Waiting is not necessary if foam is used. After the vaginal spermicide has been applied, a woman must remain on her back to prevent leakage prior to intercourse. After intercourse, she should wait at least six hours before douching. Douching too early dilutes the spermicide, weakening its ability to kill any sperm still left in the vaginal tract.

The spermicide kills sperm by coating the surface and preventing the passage of oxygen into the cell. There is evidence that spermicides may inhibit the growth of VD and herpes organisms spread during intercourse, but they are by no means totally effective as protection against VD. Women who use spermicides, however, have a lower

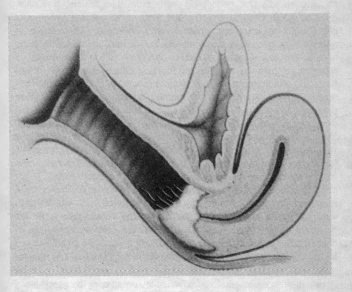

Fig. 9–1: Once a spermicidal foam has been injected, it coats the upper part of the vagina, covering the cervix and preventing the entrance of sperm, which can be seen immediately underneath the foam. (Courtesy of the Ortho Pharmaceutical Corporation, Raritan, New Jersey.)

incidence of VD than women who use nonbarrier forms of contraception or no contraception.

ENCARE OVALS AND OTHER FOAMING TABLETS

Foaming tablets and suppositories contain a spermicide that melts and spreads through the vaginal vault at body temperature. Most American pharmaceutical manufacturers have been reluctant to introduce this type of contraceptive to the United States since they felt its effectiveness was significantly below that of contraceptive foam or jelly. The foam and jelly immediately coat the upper vaginal region, forming an effective barrier of spermicide. The tablets, however, must be given time to dissolve and there is no óptimal spermicide effect until at least ten minutes after insertion. This delay in effectiveness from the time of administration until the tablet has time to coat the vagina may be one of the reasons for the number of reported pregnancies by users of foaming tablets. Encare Oval and Semicid, which recently have been introduced into the American market, are characteristic of the foaming tablets. It appears that more pregnancies occurred than were initially anticipated from the European experience when Encare Oval was introduced in the United States. This higher rate may be due to the improper use of the suppository. A clinical study sponsored by the manufacturers of Encare Oval demonstrated that the optimal spermicidal activity was from ten minutes to one hour following administration. Many physicians believe that the contraceptive effectiveness of Encare Oval remains to be demonstrated by closely controlled U.S. studies and, until such data are available, the foams and creams are to be the preferred spermicides. These tablets, however, offer the advantage of being available "over-the-counter" and easy to use. The disadvantages include delay between insertion and effectiveness. Also, the inserter used with vaginal creams and foams permits application of these agents high in the vaginal vault. When a woman uses the suppository she must make a conscious effort to place the tablet high in the vagina. A number of women fail to do this, reducing the effectiveness of the spermicide. Finally, there have been reports of an unpleasant burning sensation experienced by either or both sexual partners accompanying the use of the Encare Oval.

When Should Spermicides Be Used?

Spermicides are more effective when used in combination with condoms, and are acceptable for women who experience infrequent or unexpected sexual relations. They provide some contraceptive protection, as well as convenient lubrication, during coitus. They may be used when nursing children, during the first month on the minipill until the pill becomes effective, or during the time shortly after an IUD insertion for added protection. A spermicide can also be beneficial if more than one pill of an oral contraceptive series is forgotten. Some of the prefilled foams such as Because are ideal in these instances. They are prepacked in a relatively small applicator not much larger than a tampon and are, therefore, very portable.

How Effective Are Spermicides?

They can be very effective, but they often are not. Actually, the pregnancy rate for the foam spermicide is about thirty per one hundred women years. In other words, for every hundred women using spermicide for one year, thirty will get pregnant. The high failure rate results largely from not using the preparation with every intercourse or from not inserting an additional application before a second intercourse. The effectiveness is also higher for women who use the missionary position, since spermicides tend to leak in any other position, thus not covering the cervix completely. It is the user of the method, rather than the method itself, that causes failure. Proper use of a good-quality foam has produced reported pregnancy rates of five pregnancies per hundred women yearly. Because of their high failure rate, however, spermicidal preparations should not be relied on by women who must not get pregnant. These women should choose another more effective means of birth control. Creams and jellies are even less effective than foams.

The use of spermicidal preparations has declined in recent years with the advent of the pill and IUDs. It is estimated that between two to four million women use these products in the United States.

Side Effects

The worst side effect of spermicides for the user is probably a mild vaginal irritation, which can vary from one woman to another. If this happens, change brands. The preparations do not cause cancer.

Warning on Spermicides

The incidence of late miscarriage and severe birth defects in infants has been found to be twice as high in women who have used spermicides at or near the time of conception. It is thought that the spermicide may damage the sperm or the egg prior to conception or may directly attack the embryo. The use of spermicides should be suspended either for at least two months prior to a planned pregnancy or as soon as a woman learns that she is pregnant. She might, in such a case, choose to have the pregnancy interrupted.

COLLAGEN SPONGE—A FUTURE BARRIER CONTRACEPTIVE?

Dr. Milos Chvapil of the University of Arizona Medical Center has developed an intravaginal collagen sponge made of bovine skin which is being tested as a new barrier contraceptive. The sponge is placed in the vagina and absorbs the sperm. The natural acidity of the sponge will actively kill sperm for up to one month. It was originally thought that since the sponge was an active spermicide for one month it could be left undisturbed in the vagina for that period of time. However, as sperm were deposited on the sponge during periods of sexual activity the problem of malodor arose, and it was determined that the sponge should be removed and rinsed with a vinegar solution periodically. This is only during periods of sexual activity; if a woman is not sexually active the sponge may be left in place. At the present time only patient acceptability of the sponge has been tested on women with tubal ligation or intrauterine contraceptive devices. The contraceptive effectiveness is now being evaluated in a group of women using no other form of birth control. The availability of this sponge is presently limited to the research group at the university where it has been developed.

THE DIAPHRAGM

A diaphragm is a soft, latex rubber dome stretched around a steel spring. Although it acts as a mechanical barrier, preventing sperm from entering the cervical canal, its major contraceptive function is as a container holding a spermicidal jelly against the opening of the cervix. The dome of the diaphragm covers the cervix; in the front it fits snugly behind the pubis bone, and in the back into the posterior fornix, a small pocket behind the cervix. A spermicidal cream or jelly *must* be used with a diaphragm to kill sperm which pass the rim of the diaphragm. The diaphragm acts *primarily* as a container for the spermicide and *secondarily* as a physical barrier to sperm.

How to Be Fitted for a Diaphragm

Each woman must be individually fitted for a diaphragm, either by a doctor or by trained paramedical personnel. With diaphragms, there is no such thing as one size fits all. The doctor first performs a pelvic examination to determine the distance between the pubic bone and the back of the vagina. The doctor then inserts, in sequence, a series of diaphragm rings; these are diaphragm springs covered with latex, with the center domes missing. The doctor determines which size diaphragm most correctly suits each woman. Diaphragms range in diameter from 55 to 95 millimeters (approximately 2⅛ to 3¾ inches). The majority of women are fitted with a diaphragm of 70 to 80 millimeters in diameter (2¾ to 3⅓ inches). The type of diaphragm employed depends on the contour and size of the vagina as well as on the position of the uterus and adjacent organs. Some women with anatomical disorders (such as poor vaginal muscle tone, lacerations of the vaginal wall from birth trauma, or a complete uterine prolapse) are not able to use a diaphragm.

To function effectively, a diaphragm must fit properly. If it is too small, it can slip out during coitus; too large a diaphragm may buckle and will be both uncomfortable and ineffective. As a general rule, it is best to use the largest diaphragm that fits properly without the user being aware of its presence.

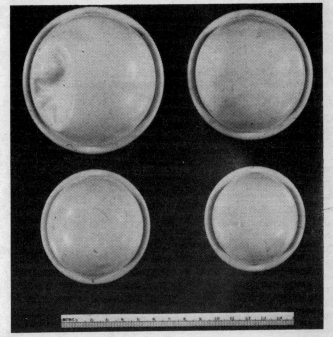

Fig. 9–2: Four different sizes of the Ortho-All-Flex diaphragms, clockwise from upper left: 90, 80, 65 and 70. The number of a diaphragm indicates its diameter in mm.

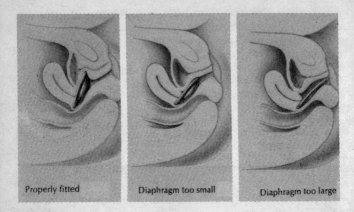

Properly fitted   Diaphragm too small   Diaphragm too large

Fig. 9–3: The diaphragm on the extreme left is properly fitted; the one in the center is too small; the diaphragm on the right is too large. When a diaphragm is not properly fitted, it will not provide proper contraceptive protection and can even interfere with intercourse. (Courtesy of Ortho Pharmaceutical Corporation, Raritan, New Jersey.)

A diaphragm must be refitted after childbirth, miscarriage, any surgical operation, or a weight change in excess of ten pounds, and routinely every two or three years. The fit of a diaphragm can be affected by the emotions—if a woman is nervous at the time of the examination, her vaginal muscles can tense, making proper fitting difficult. A virgin, with hymen intact, can be fitted for a diaphragm. She should be refitted shortly after she becomes sexually active, since vaginal muscles stretch with intercourse. If you choose to be fitted for a diaphragm, the doctor will ask you to examine yourself so that you recognize the position of the diaphragm in relation to the cervix and pubic bone. You should be able to feel that the cervix is completely covered by the dome of the diaphragm. If it is properly positioned, you can press one side of the diaphragm without tilting the device. It is most important that you know how to insert the diaphragm properly and are able to check its position for a correct fit. Do not leave the doctor's office until you understand this and have tried to insert and remove the diaphragm a few times with a nurse's supervision.

Insertion and Removal of the Diaphragm

Before inserting the device, smear about a teaspoon of spermicidal cream or jelly on each side of the diaphragm dome (the instructions suggest placement of jelly only on the inside of the dome, but since you often do not know how the diaphragm lies inside the vagina, it is safer to apply the jelly on both sides of the dome). Also, smear the cream with your fingertip around the rim of the device to kill any sperm that may slip past. To prevent the introduction of bacteria, you should wash your hands prior to insertion. Read the personal instruction booklet enclosed with the new diaphragm carefully.

The device is most easily inserted if you are crouching, squatting, lying down, or standing with one foot raised on a chair or toilet seat. Insert the diaphragm by squeezing it into a long, narrow shape with one hand, while the other hand holds the vaginal lips open. You slide the device up the vagina until the far rim passes the cervix. Then gently push the front rim up under the pubic bone, checking to see that the cervix is covered. If a woman has short fingers or dislikes handling herself, a plastic or metal inserter may be used. The diaphragm should now be far back in the vagina so neither partner is aware of it during coitus. A diaphragm is held in place by the spring tension of the rim, by vaginal muscle tone, and by the pubic bone. You remove it by hooking your index finger behind the forward rim and gently pulling downward. Be careful not to puncture it with your finger or nail.

A diaphragm should not be inserted more than *two* hours before intercourse. If coitus is delayed for more than two hours, you need to re-cover the diaphragm with spermicide or to apply a spermicidal foam. Likewise, reapply the cream or jelly before each successive intercourse. *Do not* remove the diaphragm to reapply the spermicide; simply insert some cream or jelly into the vagina. The diaphragm can be left in place overnight, but insert additional jelly before morning intercourse. You may bathe, walk around, or urinate with a diaphragm in place, but check its position after each bowel movement. Leave the diaphragm in place for at least *six hours* after the last intercourse to make certain the sperm in the vaginal tract have been killed. Douching is not necessary, but for that, too, you must wait at least six hours after intercourse or you will rinse away all the spermicide.

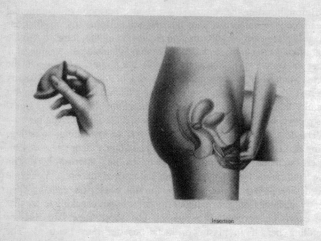

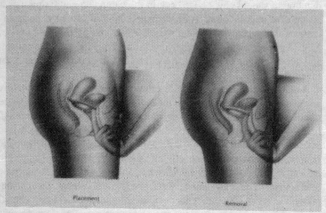

Fig. 9–4: The sequence of insertion and removal of the diaphragm. The diaphragm *must* fit snugly behind the pubis bone in front. (Courtesy of Ortho Pharmaceutical Corporation, Raritan, New Jersey.)

Care of the Diaphragm

To clean the diaphragm after removal, wash it with a mild soap and water, dry it, and then put it in its container. Unscented soaps and powders are best, for they will not corrode the rubber. Never use Vaseline or any petroleum products on your diaphragm. Regularly check the diaphragm for holes, cracks, or leaks, especially near the rim. Hold it up to the light, or fill it with water to see if there is any leakage.

Types of Diaphragms

There are four basic types of diaphragms. The most popular, the Ortho-All-Flex, has a spring ring that is flexible and easily adjusts to the vaginal contour. The Koromex has a stronger spring that does not bend much, which gives a better fit with weaker vaginal muscles. Other varieties curve or bend to provide a better fit for women with poor muscle tone or other individual disorders.

The Diaphragm in Historical Perspective

Women have used many things to block the cervical entrance during coitus. Casanova recommended squeezing the juice from half a lemon and placing the lemon shell in the vagina. The lemon shell acted as a barrier, while the citric acid was a spermicide. Dr. C. Hasse, using the name Mensinga, popularized the first modern diaphragm in Germany and Holland in the 1880s. It spread to England, where it was called a Dutch cap, and helped move Victorian women to responsibility for their own contraception. The material and construction of modern diaphragms has improved, but the basic concept goes directly back to Mensinga.

The Pros and Cons of Diaphragm Use

The diaphragm is an attractive form of contraception primarily because it affords protection from unwanted pregnancy without causing physiological or systemic changes in the body, and secondarily because, if used properly, it is a very effective form of birth control. The use of the diaphragm is under the control of the woman and has to be used only when needed. This technique appeals to women who have infrequent intercourse and also to women who have established relationships with intercourse on a routine basis. It is a very acceptable method for spacing children, since the spermicide jelly will not harm the fetus if pregnancy should occur. Since the use of a diaphragm causes no physiological changes in the body, it is also safe to use during breast feeding. Some women find that the cream or jelly used in conjunction with the diaphragm is helpful in providing extra lubrication during intercourse. It is interesting that a number of women employing other methods of birth control such as oral contraceptives or IUDs use a diaphragm when having intercourse during menstruation to contain the menstrual flow.

The major problem with a diaphragm is that it requires a high degree of motivation to make it work. It must be used with a spermicide for each and every intercourse, and this can deprive a relationship of a certain amount of spontaneity. In short, if your diaphragm is at home and you're not, you had better not. The use of a diaphragm requires that a woman handle her genitals; some women find this a problem. Other women have difficulty learning the proper method of insertion, which is all-important to the effectiveness of the diaphragm. Another objection is that the spermicide can be messy and expensive and some sex partners find the taste sour.

Use and Effectiveness

Before the pill and IUDs became popular, the diaphragm was used by about 30 percent of American couples practicing birth control. Today its popularity has fallen behind the pill and IUDs, probably because of the ease and effectiveness of the newer methods. Recently, however, there have been a great number of women who have resumed the use of diaphragms, mainly because of the adverse publicity the pill and IUDs have received. It is, therefore, difficult to estimate the exact number of women who are using diaphragms today. Many women are pleased with the switch from the oral contraceptive and IUDs to the diaphragm, but others have found the diaphragm too inconvenient and have subsequently gone back to newer and more acceptable types of pills and IUDs.

Successful use depends largely on a woman's motivation. There are failure rates of anywhere from six to twenty-nine pregnancies per year per hundred women using the device. If the instructions are carefully followed, however, rates as low as four pregnancies per hundred women a year have been reported, certainly well within the limits of acceptability. Younger women have higher failure rates, perhaps due to their inexperience in using the device. The method may fail for several reasons: improper use, improper fit, slippage during coitus, or a leak in the diaphragm. Diaphragms slip more frequently in woman-dominant positions, as the female organs hang slightly

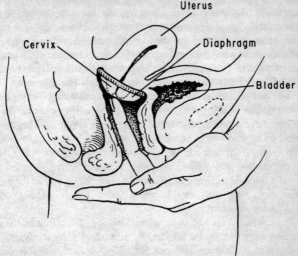

Fig. 9–5: How a woman should check for proper placement of a diaphragm. The cervix must be completely covered with the diaphragm dome, as shown in this illustration.

downward. They can also be dislodged by repeated penile thrusts. The vaginal walls expand during sexual orgasm, and the diaphragm can slip out of position. Such failure is the exception rather than the rule, but you should be aware of it. Although the pill and the IUD are highly effective, the diaphragm, which causes no side effects, can be equally safe if properly fitted and intelligently used.

THE CERVICAL CAP

The cervical cap, which is gaining popularity in this country, is, like the diaphragm, a barrier form of contraception. It is a small, cuplike device of either soft rubber or rigid plastic. Unlike the diaphragm, which blocks the entire upper portion of the vaginal canal, the cervical cap blocks only the cervix. Compared to a diaphragm, it is smaller in diameter, deeper, and most important, it is held in place by suction rather than by spring tension. The cap, like a diaphragm, must be fitted by a doctor.

To use the soft-rubber cap, fill it about a third full of jelly spermicide. Squatting or reclining, grasp the cap, dome down, separate the vaginal lips, and push it up the vagina as far as it goes. Then press the rim around the cervix until the dome covers the cervical opening and the cervix can be felt under the dome. The cap is then on tightly. You remove it by breaking the suction. It can be used without spermicide, but this decreases the cap's effectiveness.

The rigid-plastic cap uses no spermicide. It can be applied for a full month. When inserted after menstruation it remains on the cervix for the entire cycle, and is removed at the next menstruation. This device —and its regimen— has become less popular due to relative contraceptive *ineffectiveness*. On the other hand, the soft cervical cap, used in combination with jelly spermicide, is quite effective. It is inserted by the woman herself and can be left in place for up to two days. Not surprisingly, the soft cap is much more widely used than its rigid-plastic counterpart.

The cervical cap has been around a long time. It was used in England even before the diaphragm, and offers several advantages. Because it is held on with suction, it is unlikely to slip during intercourse. It can also be used by women with abnormalities or poor muscle tone who cannot use a diaphragm. And because the cap covers only the cervix, you will not need constant refitting as your vaginal muscles change. It is, however, difficult to insert. As it must be placed deeply within the vaginal canal, many women cannot learn the technique of proper insertion.

There are several varieties of cervical caps to fit women with differing anatomical features or problems. Several studies on the effectiveness of the cervical cap are still in progress in the United States, but at this time the cap is thought to be at least as effective a contraceptive as the diaphragm.

The cooperative venture of a gynecologist, Dr. Uwe Freese, and a dentist, Dr. Robert A. Goepp, has led to the creation of a permanent cervical cap. The cap is made of a soft, plasticlike material molded to fit the cervix of each woman. It is fitted by a physician and left in place indefinitely. The cap has a one-way valve that permits menstrual blood to flow out but does not permit sperm to pass into the uterus. The contraceptive effectiveness and patient acceptability of this cap are still being tested; it is not generally available.

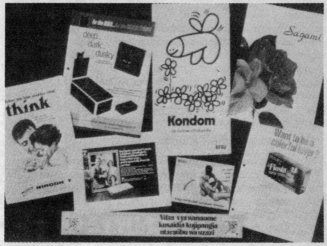

Fig. 9–6: Examples of condom advertisements from different parts of the world. These promotion techniques are used by various family-planning agencies as well as by the condom manufacturers to encourage the use of condoms. (Courtesy of I. Dalsimer, P. Piotrow, and J. Dumm; *Condoms: An Old Method Meets a New Social Need. Population Reports,* Series H, #1. Washington, D.C., George Washington University Medical Center, Population Information Program—1973.)

THE CONDOM

The condom, also called a rubber, a prophylactic, and a safe, is a sheath the man wears on his penis during intercourse. This much-celebrated device is still widely used, and when handled properly, is an effective mechanical barrier for contraception.

Most condoms today are made of a strong, thin, latex rubber. Condoms made of animal membrane, usually sheep intestines, are also available. Looking much like a skinny balloon, the condom is slightly thicker near the open end and has a ring around the opening to keep it on the penis. It is possible to get condoms with reservoir ends to contain the sperm, lubricated to facilitate intercourse, transparent for the latest in the see-through look, or in different colors to match whatever turns you on.

Most condoms come dry and powdered, but, as stated above, lubricated condoms are readily available. The sheep membrane condoms, while considerably more expensive, are said to conduct heat better and to provide more sensation than the latex variety. With proper care, membrane condoms can be reused several times. Condoms may be obtained in virtually any drugstore or pharmacy. The cheaper brands sold in washrooms or gas stations are generally of inferior quality and should be avoided. Tip condoms, or condom caps, which cover only the tip, or glans, of the penis can easily slip off and should *not* be used.

The History of the Condom

The condom has a long history. The name itself may come from the Latin *condus*, meaning a receptacle, or may even date back to the Persian word *kendu* or *kondu*, which refers to long vessels made from animal intestines and used to store grain. Possibly it refers to the unfortunately named Dr. Condom, who supplied England's Charles II with methods to prevent illegitimate children.

In its early days, the condom was probably used primarily to prevent venereal disease, and only secondarily for contraception. Since the days of Casanova, however, it has been associated with secret rendezvous and illicit sex. Its reputation has been tarnished further by being standard equipment issued by many armies, and by American labeling requirements stating it is "for the prevention of disease." For years, the condom has remained one of the most popular methods of birth control in England, Sweden, and Japan. Its unsavory reputation is not worldwide.

How to Use the Condom

Some couples actually incorporate unrolling the condom into their regular foreplay. Whatever your routine, unroll the condom a half-inch and place it on the man's penis, squeezing this half-inch reservoir to keep out the air. This allows the sperm to collect after ejaculation without leaking from the top of the condom. If the man is not circumcised, he should have his foreskin rolled down before using the condom. Roll the condom down the length of the penis, being careful not to tear it with rings or fingernails. It should cover the penis, with a half-inch hanging limply at the end. When inserting the penis, be careful not to catch the reservoir on the outside of the vagina, or to insert it too quickly—you may tear it.

Trying to force the condom into a dry vagina is very uncomfortable. Unless you have a lubricated condom, you will probably want some artificial lubrication, like a sterile jelly, a spermicidal foam or cream, or even saliva. Never use Vaseline or any petroleum jelly or oil, as this quickly *destroys the latex rubber*. For complete protection from unexpected or premature ejaculation, the condom should be worn throughout intercourse.

After ejaculation and loss of erection, the man should hold the condom tight against the base of his penis to avoid leakage. When he wishes to withdraw from the vagina, the condom is held on the penis at the base. If it slips off during coitus, remove it from the vagina immediately, holding the open end closed. To remove it from the penis after withdrawal, stretch the open end and pull down. Quickly inspect it for holes or leakage. If there is a leak, the woman should immediately use spermicidal foam. There is also a high-estrogen "morning after" pill to prevent pregnancy, which is taken for five days following intercourse (see information on "morning after" pill). While this can be used in cases of certain condom failure, this pill has very unpleasant side effects.

A good-quality condom can be used several times. After removal from the penis, drop it in a glass of water. As soon as is convenient, wash it in warm, soapy water, dry it, and powder it with cornstarch to preserve the latex. Skin condoms can be cleaned in a solution of mild household boric acid and water. Inspect all condoms for leaks before reusing them. Condoms should not be kept in a wallet or pocket for any length of time, as heat causes the latex to deteriorate.

The Pros and Cons of Condoms

There are a number of advantages to using condoms; they are inexpensive, completely harmless, compact and disposable, readily available, easy to use, fairly effective, and may inhibit the transmission of venereal disease in people who are very active sexually (there are no studies to support this assumption at the present time). If the man is willing, it is an excellent method for infrequent or unexpected sex. Couples involved in a continuous relationship will probably find that other methods (such as the pill, an IUD, or a diaphragm) are more suitable and more effective as a long-term contraceptive.

The condom is, of course, used by the man alone, although it can be combined with spermicidal foam. Many women, however, are reluctant to trust their protection solely to the man, wondering if he is reliable in the heat of passion. Many men say they dislike a condom because it is a mechanical device which disrupts spontaneity and dulls pleasure. This latter claim is rather dubious, for modern condoms are extremely thin. Nonetheless, some people dislike their artificiality, which is psychologically understandable.

How Effective Is It?

The condom is recognized as an effective method of contraception, and nearly a billion condoms are sold yearly in the United States and Canada. It can be used successfully by itself, but is more effective when used with a spermicidal foam or cream. Studies have shown this method is about as effective as the diaphragm and jelly technique of contraception. The failure rate has been measured at anywhere from five to twenty-five pregnancies per hundred women per year.

This method depends largely on motivation and on how strongly you wish to prevent conception. Failure is due mainly to not using the condom consistently for every intercourse. Not using the condom "just this once" can be a big mistake, as no contraceptive works well when it's still in the drawer.

Automated machinery produces high-quality condoms which are electronically tested at the factory, so the old "pinhole" problems of the 1940s have been virtually eliminated. Thus, condom failures can be attributed to human mistakes rather than the latex. The shelf life of a condom is about two years, after which time the latex or lubrication has deteriorated, making the condom undependable for use.

THE RHYTHM METHOD

The rhythm method means programed abstinence from sexual intercourse during those days of her cycle that a woman is most likely to become pregnant. It is based on the simple principle that egg and sperm must be in the same place at the same time for conception to occur. The rhythm method is so named because there is a rhythm to the periodic abstinence, and it is still the only method of birth control, short of complete abstinence, officially approved by the Catholic Church.

The Theory behind Rhythm

A woman can only become pregnant if she has intercourse during a fertile period of her menstrual cycle. This fertile period consists of those days immediately prior to and immediately following ovulation (the release of the egg from the ovary). Intercourse prior to ovulation must be avoided since the sperm can live in the female reproductive

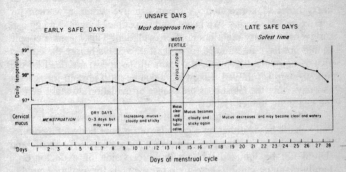

Fig. 9–7: The Rhythm Method. When using the rhythm method, it is most important to avoid intercourse around the time of ovulation. The chance of conception is much higher with intercourse prior to ovulation than after ovulation, because the sperm can survive for several days prior to ovulation in the female reproductive tract.

tract for up to seventy-two hours, and intercourse after ovulation must be avoided since the egg can live for up to forty-eight hours. If a live sperm meets a live egg, there is a very good chance for conception.

Since it is almost impossible to determine the *exact* time of ovulation, the principle of rhythm is simple in theory but difficult in practice. In general, a woman ovulates fourteen days *before* the start of the menstrual period, but not necessarily fourteen days *after* the onset of her menstrual period. Only for the rare woman with a consistent twenty-eight-day cycle is there a good chance that she ovulates exactly mid-cycle at day 14 (counting from the first day of menstrual bleeding). Very few women have twenty-eight-day cycles month after month, and even the most regular women usually have cycles that vary between twenty-seven and thirty-one days. It is with this variation that the problems of rhythm arise. If a woman cannot determine when she ovulates, she cannot determine her fertile period. The estimation of ovulation is all-important to the success of the rhythm method.

Predicting Ovulation—Safe and Unsafe Days

Ovulation occurs in mid-cycle, making this the most likely time of conception. Conversely, the beginning and end of a cycle are the least likely times of conception. A sperm can live within a woman for approximately seventy-two hours, and sometimes longer. An egg can survive up to forty-eight hours after ovulation. This means a couple should not have intercourse for at least three days before the earliest chance of ovulation, to make certain all the sperm are dead by the time the egg is released. Likewise, a couple must abstain for at least two days after the latest possible chance of ovulation, to make certain the egg is no longer viable.

The two most widely used methods for predicting ovulation involve daily charts based either on a calendar or on your body temperature. These methods are complex, involve a large chance for error, and should not be initiated without the supervision of a doctor or a family-planning clinic. There are other methods for ovulation prediction: One involves the estimation of the consistency and amount of cervical mucus, and another is based on the determination of the acidity of the vagina.

The Calendar Method

Often called the Ogino-Knaus method, this method assumes that ovulation occurs at some point during a five-day period approximately twelve to sixteen days before the onset of the next menstruation. Therefore, intercourse must be avoided for three days before this five-day span and for two days following it. For example, if a woman has a completely regular twenty-eight-day menstrual cycle, the length of abstinence during her fertile period will be ten days.

Most women, however, do not have menstrual cycles with textbook regularity. To determine what her individual cycle will be, a woman must keep a calendar record of her cycles for eight months. To determine her cycle variation, she counts the first day of her menstrual flow as day 1. She records on a calendar chart the length of each cycle for eight consecutive months. From the ninth month, she is theoretically able to determine her unsafe period. She subtracts nineteen from the length of her shortest cycle to determine her first unsafe day (ovulation may be a maximum of sixteen days before menstruation plus the three days the sperm can survive). If a woman's shortest cycle was twenty-six days her first unsafe day is seven days after the *onset* of menstrual bleeding ($26 - 19 = 7$ days). To determine her last unsafe day, a woman subtracts ten from the length of her longest cycle (ovulation can occur a minimum of twelve days before menstruation, minus two days for the life of the ovum). If a woman's longest cycle was thirty-one days, her last unsafe day is twenty-one days after the onset of menstrual bleeding (31 − 10 = 21). There should be no intercourse from the first to the last unsafe day; thus a woman with a cycle varying between twenty-six and thirty-one days must avoid intercourse from day 7 to day 21 of her cycle. For a woman with cycle variation of this degree, the only safe days for intercourse would be the first six days after the onset of menstruation and the last seven days before the beginning of menstruation.

Basal Body Temperature Method

A more accurate procedure for determining the time of ovulation is based on measurement of subtle changes in the normal, or "basal," body temperature. Called the Basal Body Temperature (BBT) method, it resulted from the discovery that immediately prior to ovulation body temperature drops slightly, rising rather sharply directly after ovulation. This change in body temperature (only 0.15° − 0.3° Centigrade [or 0.5° − 1.00° Fahrenheit]), can give a reasonable estimation of the time of ovulation. The temperature remains elevated for about two weeks if ovulation has occurred. This temperature increase is due to progesterone production by the corpus luteum (these physiological changes are thoroughly described in Chapter 5, The Reproductive Cycle).

If a woman wishes to use the BBT method, she must take and record her temperature every morning as soon as she awakens. This procedure must be performed faithfully before the woman even gets out of bed. The obvious drawback with this technique is that it does not predict when ovulation will occur; it only gives an indication of when ovulation *has* occurred. The safest period for intercourse with the BBT method would be three days, a full seventy-two hours, after the temperature elevation, since by that time ovulation would have occurred and the ovum would have disintegrated. The most unsafe period, as estimated by the BBT method, is the preovulatory time, particularly from five to seven days prior to the expected time of ovulation. Since the BBT method does not attempt to predict ovulation, in order to be completely safe, a woman should avoid intercourse during the entire first half of the menstrual cycle, from the time she bleeds until the seventy-two hours after the rise in Basal Body Temperature.

Because of the prolonged abstinence required in the BBT method and factors such as illness that impair its accuracy, women often combine the BBT with the calendar method to shorten the abstinence period. In this combined approach, the first unsafe day is taken from the shortest cycle on your calendar chart, and the last unsafe day is the third day after the rise in the BBT.

Mucus Method

It has been observed that the time of ovulation can be estimated by changes in the quality and quantity of the cervical mucus. During the period of time immediately following the end of menstrual bleeding, there is very little cervical mucus. These are known as the dry days. As ovulation approaches, there is an increase in the production of mucus, and it becomes cloudy and sticky. At the time of ovulation, the mucus is clear and highly lubricative. During the immediate postovulatory period, it again becomes cloudy and sticky. During the late safe period, more than seventy-two hours postovulation, the amount of mucus decreases, and it may become clear and watery until the time of menstrual flow. With this technique, the post menstruation dry days and the late postovulatory period of decreasing, clear, watery mucus may be considered safe days for intercourse.

The acidity of the vaginal mucus also changes throughout the menstrual cycle. The mucus is slightly acidic throughout the majority of the menstrual cycle, but it changes to a slightly alkaline factor around the time of ovulation. These changes can be determined with the use of litmus (pH) paper to estimate the time of ovulation. With this method, the safe period begins three days after ovulation has occurred.

Cervical Method

The cervix changes over the menstrual cycle. Through self-examination, a woman can monitor these changes, which will help her determine the time of ovulation. Immediately after menstruation, the cervix is closed and points backward. At ovulation, the cervix moves forward, the cervical canal opens to about 3 millimeters, and the cervical mucus is clear and watery. After ovulation, the cervix again tilts backward and the mucus dries up (see Fig. 12–2 in Chapter 12).

Natural Family Planning

The *natural family planning* technique involves utilizing all the bodily signs of basal body temperature, cervical mucus, and cervical changes to determine the time of ovulation. A couple wishing to employ this form of contraception can undergo training in the technique at the Human Life Center; for more information, contact the Couple to Couple League, Central Office, P.O. Box 11084, Cincinnati, Ohio 45211.

Effectiveness of the Rhythm Method

The reported effectiveness of the rhythm method varies tremendously from study to study and from country to country. The lowest incidence of unplanned pregnancy, ranging from 0.3 to 6.6 pregnancies per 100 woman years, was observed with the BBT method when intercourse was restricted to the postovulatory period only. When there was intercourse in both the pre- and postovulatory phases of the period, the failure rate was high, ranging from 0.7 in a West German study to 19.5 pregnancies per 100 woman years in a United States study. The failure rate with the calendar method alone was quite high, ranging from 14.4 in the United States to 47 pregnancies per 100 woman years in Colombia. The cervical mucus method also has a high failure rate.

The Pros and Cons of Rhythm

The major and perhaps only advantage of the rhythm method is that there are no devices or medication involved. However, the rhythm method requires an extremely high degree of motivation, since it requires abstinence for a minimum of ten days a month. Furthermore, it has one of the highest failure rates of any of the widely used birth-control methods. This is why this method is facetiously called Vatican roulette. The rhythm method should not be used by women who must not become pregnant, and cannot be used by women with irregular cycles.

The use of the rhythm method has declined dramatically in the last few years, because of the trouble and effort in predicting ovulation and the development of newer and more effective contraceptive methods. In 1955, approximately 22 percent of American couples practicing birth control used rhythm; the current level is about 6 percent.

Increased psychosexual stress is associated with the rhythm method. Lack of spontaneity and so-called programed sex can put pressure on a relationship. There is also strong evidence that the fertilization of an overaged ovum has been linked to fetal abnormalities. What this means is that the rhythm method fractionally increases the chances for fertilization of aged ova during the late, supposedly safe days. This creates a greater incidence of spontaneous abortion and abnormal children due to chromosomal abnormalities. There is a greater danger of this in older women or those with a history of habitual abortion or miscarriage.

COITUS INTERRUPTUS

Coitus interruptus is a variation on birth control's equivalent of Russian roulette. If you don't get pregnant, you are just plain lucky. This ineffective method allows unprotected intercourse to continue until the male is about to reach orgasm. He withdraws his penis from the vagina as he feels ejaculation coming. In biblical times, Onan threw his semen out to fertilize the land, and forever gave his name to coitus interruptus as the "sin of Onan," or onanism. A male must withdraw completely and ejaculate away from the vagina. Sperm cells move on their own. Sperm deposited anywhere between the labia majora (the external vaginal lips) can move all the way through the vagina to the uterus and fertilize the egg. The hymen need not be broken for conception to occur.

The Pros and Cons of Coitus Interruptus

The primary advantage of coitus interruptus is that it is always available. Since it does not require use of any type of medication or device, it is also physically harmless.

The great disadvantage of coitus interruptus is that it is a most ineffective method of birth control and results in a high pregnancy rate. The exact failure rate of coitus interruptus is not known, since there have been no recent studies of this technique. Some couples use coitus interruptus as a means of sexual foreplay and achieve orgasm either by oral or anal sex or by mutual masturbation.

One of the reasons for the high failure rate is that as orgasm approaches, both men and women find that complete voluntary control of the muscles becomes difficult. A man in the excitory phase just prior to orgasm may forget to withdraw, or he may suddenly decide he does not want to. Also, only about 50 percent of men ejaculate in one single burst; others expel semen sporadically or in a slow stream. Many men do not know exactly when they should withdraw, since there may have been a small ejaculation of semen prior to actual orgasm. Even a small ejaculation can contain millions of sperm, each one capable of fertilizing an ovum.

Some men can maintain an erection for five to twenty minutes, while others ejaculate within two to five minutes of intercourse. Men who ejaculate more quickly have greater difficulty with control and withdrawing. Younger men ejaculate more sperm, and thus have a greater chance of fertilization. They also have less physical control and more difficulty pulling out at just the right moment. All this makes successful coitus interruptus particularly difficult for younger men. If there is a second coitus, sperm left in the urethra (the tube of the penis) from the first intercourse can easily enter the vagina prior to the second orgasm.

Coitus interruptus also presents some psychological problems. Some women find it difficult to trust completely their sexual partners to withdraw in time. The man must be aware of when he will ejaculate, and must then be willing to withdraw. A woman may find that withdrawal interrupts her attempts to reach orgasm and causes her frustration. Both men and women may fear that ejaculation will occur before withdrawal. This subconscious fear of unwanted pregnancy does nothing to help the pleasure of the moment.

THE INTRAUTERINE DEVICE

An intrauterine device, or IUD, is a small object placed in the uterus to prevent conception. Intrauterine types of devices have been used in one form or another for centuries.

There are three basic types, or generations, of modern IUDs: The first generation was a *closed circular ring*, first developed by Gräfenberg in the 1920s and modified by Ota. The second generation is *open devices* of various shapes, such as the popular Lippes Loop or Saf-T-Coil, and devices such as the Dalkon Shield, which is a single, closed plane. It should be noted that because of their serious side effects, the closed ring devices are not recommended for use. The Dalkon Shield is used in special cases, but requires extra supervision. The third generation devices are either devices of improved design, such as the Ypsilon or Antigon-F, medicated IUDs such as the Copper-T or -7, or progesterone-impregnated devices such as the Progestasert.

Most modern devices are made of plastic, a body-friendly substance. All devices made exclusively of stainless steel have been removed from the market. The malleability of plastic is a great advantage, as it can be bent and threaded into a narrow "introducer," which inserts it into the uterus with a minimum of pain. Metallic salts are usually molded inside the plastic so the position of the IUD can be checked with X-ray. Many IUDs also have little tails made of nylon to facilitate their removal. The tail, extending from the cervix (the mouth of the womb), can be felt by the woman or seen by the doctor to be certain the device is still in the proper position.

History of IUDs

IUDs in one form or another have been used for a variety of purposes over the past twenty-five hundred years. Hippocrates reportedly used a hollow tube to insert medication or pessaries into the uterus. Translations vary as to whether this was for contraception or some other purpose. For centuries, nomads placed stones in the uteri of their female camels prior to a long caravan trip across the desert. This prevented these animals from becoming pregnant on the trip. It was many years before the contraceptive potential of a foreign object in the human uterus was widely recognized.

In the late nineteenth and early twentieth centuries, devices made of wood, glass, ivory, silver, gold, pewter, ebony, and other materials were inserted into the cervical canal. Some of these were inserted into the uterus, with the bottom of the devices extending into the cervix. The lower portion acted as a ladder, enabling bacteria and infection to climb from the cervix into the uterus. These devices may have prevented conception, but they generally functioned as uterine supports or were attempts to correct irregular or delayed menses. In 1902, a wishbone-shaped IUD was developed for contraception; it was implanted in the uterus. Some variations of this were supplied with instructions for self-insertion. Many complications resulted from their use, and they were quickly and unanimously condemned by the medical profession.

In the late 1920s, Dr. Ernest Gräfenberg developed a silver ring that was placed entirely within the uterus. In 1934, a ring with a center disc connected by three spokes was developed by Ota in Japan. The medical profession, aware of the problems of previous crude IUDs, did not accept the first generation IUDs of Gräfenberg and Dr. Ota. Gräfenberg subsequently abandoned his ideas, and the Ota Ring was banned by the Japanese government in 1936. Research in the late 1950s and early 1960s by physicians such as Margulies and Lippes finally encouraged reexamination of the theory of IUDs. Variations of the Gräfenberg Ring are still used today, and the Japanese lifted the ban on the Ota Ring in 1974. Today the IUD has an acknowledged place in the modern birth-control program.

How Does the IUD Work?

There is disagreement over exactly how the IUD prevents pregnancy. Some doctors maintain that it disrupts the dynamic muscular balance between the uterus, the cervix, and the fallopian tubes, interfering with the movement of the sperm up into the tubes and with the ovum's transport down toward the uterus. Fertilization would, thus, be prevented. Another theory maintains that the IUD causes cellular changes in the uterine lining, the endometrium. The development of the endometrium is disrupted, so even if the egg is fertilized, implantation is prevented.

Research has also shown high concentrations of *macrophages* in the uteri of women with IUDs. A macrophage is a normal cell which attacks invading cells, such as bacteria, swallowing and destroying them in a process called phagocytosis. What is most interesting is that macrophages do not normally exist in the uterus, and it is thought that they may destroy the fertilized egg in a process similar to phagocytosis.

Of course, uterine contractions increase with an IUD and this may prevent the normal implantation of a fertilized egg into the uterine wall. It has also recently been postulated that an IUD works simply by acting as a partition between the uterine walls. The highest contraceptive effect is obtained when the largest area of the uterine wall is covered. The more closely an IUD molds to the uterus, the more effective it is as a contraceptive.

Whatever the answer, an IUD does not work by causing early abortion or by creating a low-grade infection in the uterus. Both of these occur in a small percentage of women with IUDs, but they are not related to its contraceptive properties.

Types of IUDs

Intrauterine contraceptive devices are divided into two types: *inert* devices, usually most suitable for multiparous women (women who have given birth), and *bioactive* devices, which have a better acceptance rate in nulliparous women (women who have never given birth).

The inert devices depend largely on configuration and size for their contraceptive effectiveness. One of the most widely used devices of this type, the Lippes Loop, is a very effective contraceptive. The device is made of flexible plastic in a complex S-shape and measures little more than an inch across; it is available in several sizes to afford

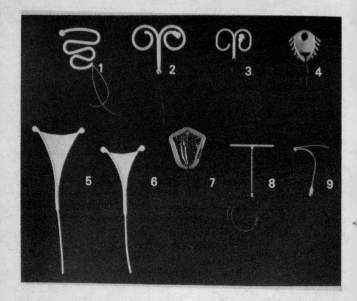

Fig. 9–8: Different types of IUDs. (1) Lippes Loop-D, the largest of the four sizes of this device; (2) Saf-T-Coil for a woman who has had children; (3) Saf-T-Coil for a woman who has never had a child; (4) Dalkon Shield, nulliparous size; the use of this IUD has been linked to septic spontaneous abortion; (5) Ypsilon, multiparous size; and (6) Ypsilon, nulliparous size, still under investigation; (7) Antigon-F, under investigation, chiefly effective in multiparous women; (8) Copper-T, still under investigation; (9) Cu-7, found to be very effective particularly in nulliparous women.

the best fit for the individual woman. The Lippes Loop has low expulsion and pregnancy rates combined with acceptable side effects. The Saf-T-Coil is constructed of plastic similar to the Lippes Loop, but is molded into a quite different shape. This device has a success rate similar to the Lippes Loop. The Antigon-F, a comparatively new inert device, is still being investigated in a limited number of institutions. Since it is a somewhat larger IUD and covers a greater area of the uterus, it appears to have a lower pregnancy rate than either the Lippes Loop or the Saf-T-Coil. These three devices are particularly well accepted as contraceptives by multiparous women.

There is one inert device which has, in initial testing, been shown effective and acceptable in both multiparous and nulliparous women; this is the Ypsilon. The Ypsilon, a Y-shaped IUD, has an inner core of stainless steel and is completely covered by silicone. The stainless-steel frame makes the device a bit rigid and more difficult to expel. In addition, the Ypsilon has a silicone web between the forks of the Y and, thus, covers a large area of the uterus. The Ypsilon has been tested for several years and has a good performance record, with a high acceptability rate and a low pregnancy rate, particularly in nulliparous women.

The bioactive IUDs are also acceptable by nulliparous women because they are usually smaller than the inert IUDs. Bioactive IUDs depend not so much on configuration for contraceptive effectiveness; instead, they act as delivery systems for certain material with contraceptive properties. The Copper-T and Copper-7 are small IUDs made of plastic with copper wire wound around the outside of their plastic stems. Copper has antifertility effects which are not completely understood, but which render these IUDs effective contraceptives. The devices are smaller than inert devices and therefore provide a better fit for the smaller uterus of the nulliparous woman. Of course, being small and flexible, they tend to be more easily expelled than some other IUDs. The copper is depleted from the device within two or three years after insertion, so the device must be replaced at least every three years.

A new bioactive IUD, Progestasert, contains progesterone, the hormone of pregnancy (see Chapter 5, The Reproductive Cycle). This IUD slowly releases the progesterone over a period of one year; thus, two methods of contraception are combined, the IUD and the minipill. The progesterone probably exerts its contraceptive effects by altering the cervical mucus, which interferes with the passage of sperm. It may also interfere with ovulation, but this has not been shown. Women who have the Progestasert have less cramping and bleeding during the menstrual period. This device has only recently been released, and, as yet, it does not appear to be appreciably more effective than copper-bearing devices. Since the progesterone is depleted one year after insertion, the device must be replaced yearly.

Who Can Have an IUD?

Most women can be fitted with and use an IUD. Multiparous women usually tolerate the IUD better than nulliparous women. After a woman has a child, an abortion, or a miscarriage, the cervix is slightly dilated, making it much easier to insert an IUD. Also, after childbirth, the uterus appears to be less irritated by the presence of an IUD, so multiparous women do not usually experience severe episodes of pain and bleeding with IUDs. Multiparous women can usually employ an IUD with good success and high acceptance rates.

Insertion into nulliparous women is more difficult because the cervical canal is narrower and the uterus is smaller. Postinsertion cramping and pain, are, therefore, more severe. Nulliparous women are more likely to have the device removed because of pain and cramping, and they have a higher rate of spontaneous expulsion than multiparous women. Many nulliparous women accept the IUD very well with a minimum amount of problems, but some are very sensitive and have persistent cramping and bleeding. Women with smaller uteri or women who have had a decrease in uterine size due to long-term use of oral contraceptives often have problems when fitted with a large IUD.

It is really impossible to predict how a woman will respond to the presence of an IUD before it is inserted. There are a few women with congenital uterine malformations who cannot use an IUD. If a woman is fitted with the proper size and type of IUD, as determined by her physician, and has a minimum number of side effects, she has found a very acceptable and convenient form of contraception. If, however, despite proper choice and fit of IUD, there is excessive pain and bleeding, the IUD should be removed and the woman must seek some other form of contraception.

Who Should Insert the IUD—Can the Doctor Make a Difference?

While there is a difference in the effectiveness and tolerability of various devices, a difference in performance can often be traced to the skill of the person inserting the device. To place the IUD properly, the doctor or technician must take into account the great differences in internal anatomy and position the device correctly for the location, size, and shape of a woman's uterus. Clinics or doctors with excellent follow-up programs for postinsertion examination and encouragement have much better success records, regardless of the device they are using. If you are considering an IUD, check into the technical skill, reputation, and rate of success for your clinic or physician. In this case, the doctor makes a big difference.

You Should Know How an IUD Is Inserted

The insertion of an IUD is a relatively quick procedure, but requires a skilled physician or paramedic. It usually entails a degree of discomfort. In general, it is wise to have an IUD inserted only by a competent physician familiar with IUDs.

An IUD can be inserted at any time during the cycle, but it is *best* done on the second to fourth day of menstrual flow. In this way, a woman can be certain the device is not interfering with an unsuspected pregnancy, since menstruation is the best evidence that a woman is not pregnant. Also, during the early part of the menstrual flow, the uterus is already contracting, and the cramps associated with the insertion of the device will be less severe. The IUD causes additional bleeding and spotting for several days following insertion, and this is less of a problem during menstruation. Most importantly, the cervical canal is slightly dilated during menstrual bleeding, so insertion is easier and less painful. The advantages of insertion of an IUD during the early part of the menstrual cycle are such that a woman should *only* have an IUD inserted during this period of the cycle, even if this entails an extra office visit.

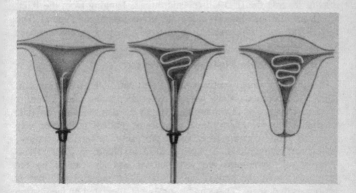

Fig. 9–9: The insertion of a Lippes Loop in three different phases. The loop unfolds inside the uterine cavity as it is inserted with the introducer. The cervix does not have to be dilated during the insertion. (Courtesy of Ortho Pharmaceutical Corporation, Raritan, New Jersey.)

Since insertion of an IUD is not without a degree of discomfort, it might be advisable for a woman to take a tranquilizer, such as Valium, and perhaps a painkiller, approximately an hour prior to the procedure. It is also advisable for a woman to take two aspirins. There is a theory that prostaglandin causes the cramps associated with IUD insertion; aspirin inhibits the synthesis of prostaglandin and, therefore, reduces the cramps. A woman's physician must be advised of the type, amount, and strength of any medication that is taken prior to the IUD insertion.

The insertion is preceded by a physical examination in which the physician determines the position, size, and shape of the uterus. It is important for a woman to get the IUD best suited to her body. Immediately prior to insertion, the IUD is threaded into a sterile, hollow instrument, an introducer. A vaginal speculum is used and the physician gently inserts the introducer through the cervical canal into the lowest part of the uterus. The physician may steady the uterus with a *tenaculum,* a special forceps, applied to the cervix. The application of the tenaculum may cause a minimum of pain, like a pinprick. The IUD is ejected from the introducer into the uterine cavity, where it regains its original shape. The introducer is withdrawn, leaving the IUD tail (plastic threads hanging from the IUD, which pass through the cervix into the upper part of the vagina). The threads are carefully trimmed so that only an inch or two remains visible.

The Immediate Postinsertion Period

A number of minor problems associated with IUDs occur immediately after insertion. Many women experience nausea and vomiting after insertion. For that reason, it might be advisable for an IUD candidate to avoid a heavy meal prior to the procedure. Women may also feel faint, become pale, sweat profusely, experience cramps, have heart palpitations, or have a drop in blood pressure. These "vaso-vagal" symptoms are well known and are caused by the manipulation of the cervix, but are transient and certainly not as serious as they seem. They can be somewhat alleviated by medication —tranquilizers, aspirin, and painkillers, as previously described. A woman should remain on the examining table for at least five minutes following insertion, and she should not get up until these symptoms have passed, even if she stays there an hour. Once a woman feels well enough to stand, she should sit in the doctor's office for a short time, or until she feels completely confident in venturing out into the street.

On the other hand, some women, particularly those who have had children, have no problems with the insertion and find the procedure as simple and benign as a routine pelvic examination.

A woman should not have any sexual intercourse for a few days after insertion. She should let the bleeding subside and allow the mucus of the uterus to form around the device, lowering the chances for infection. A woman should not use a tampon for several days following insertion, but should, rather, rely on a sanitary napkin. Foreign bodies should not be inserted into the vagina soon after the IUD.

During the first few months, a woman may experience some bleeding after intercourse. The penis may touch the uterus, causing contractions and bleeding from the irritated endometrium. In addition, the cycle might be shorter, so a woman might experience her menstrual period more often. Most low-grade infections that do occur can be treated quickly with antibiotics, and progesterone can be given to relieve cramping. A woman should, however, see a doctor about any severe cramping or pain.

The IUD should be checked by a physician after the first menstrual period following insertion, so that it can be ascertained that the device has not been displaced or expelled. The position of the IUD should be evaluated by a physician every six months.

The Pros and Cons of IUDs

The intrauterine device is probably the most effective form of contraception, after the oral contraceptive. The failure rate of the IUD ranges from 1.0 to 5 pregnancies per 100 woman-years of use and is dependent upon the type of device employed and the clinic or doctors who perform the actual insertion. IUDs provide extremely effective contraception without the introduction of drugs into the system (with the exception of the progesterone-bearing IUD). After the initial insertion and an occasional check that the IUD is still in place, a woman with an IUD is freed from continuous conscious concern over contraception; there is no need for daily medication or any type of device such as a diaphragm or a condom, and sexual intercourse can be completely spontaneous.

An IUD is usually an effective contraceptive from the moment of its insertion, but there is a marginal chance of pregnancy during the first month. It is usually advisable to use a spermicidal foam or a condom during the first month after insertion. If a woman is changing from an oral contraceptive to an IUD, it may be best for her to continue taking the birth-control pills for the first month after insertion. The pill prevents any accidental pregnancy and also helps reduce the amount of bleeding that normally accompanies the first month of IUD use. For some former users of oral contraceptives, this will not be possible. Since the birth-control pills have a tendency to diminish the size of the uterus, a woman's physician may suggest she stop taking oral contraceptives one or two months prior to insertion of an IUD to make the insertion somewhat easier.

The pregnancy rate with the IUD is higher in younger women, and declines with increasing age and decreasing fertility. In general, the greatest number of pregnancies occur during the first year after insertion. The pregnancy rate decreases with each succeeding year of use. The contraceptive effect is completely and immediately reversible simply by removing the IUD.

Can a Man Feel the Tail of the IUD?

Men occasionally say that they can feel the tail of an IUD during intercourse. This may be just the power of suggestion or, for the first time, they may notice they are touching the cervix. The cervical tails on the IUD can be cut shorter, and the doctor can check this to make certain the device has not actually slipped out of position. There is a greater chance that a man might feel the tail in the woman-dominant position, as the uterus does hang down slightly.

In general, however, a partner *cannot* feel the tail.

Bleeding and Pain

Many women with IUDs experience an increase in the amount and length of the menstrual flow for the first few periods after insertion. In some women, the menstrual cycle becomes temporarily shorter, so for a few months, a woman who has had a period every twenty-eight days may have her period every twenty-six days. Other IUD users experience bleeding and spotting between the menstrual periods soon after the insertion of the device. Since an increase in bleeding, both menstrual and intermenstrual, is not uncommon with an IUD, a woman must be aware of the possible development of a mild anemia. She might, therefore, find it advisable to take an iron supplement.

Increased uterine cramping at the time of the first few postinsertion menstrual periods is not uncommon. This cramping usually subsides as the uterus adjusts to the presence of the device. However, approximately one in ten women has the device removed within the first year of use because of side effects such as bleeding and pain.

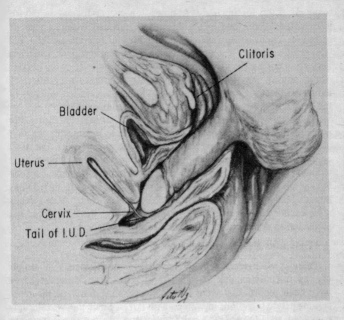

Fig. 9–10:   The relationship between the female and male genitalia during intercourse. An IUD is located inside the uterus. The tail of the IUD is located high in the vagina, behind the cervix, and should not be felt by the man during intercourse. The location of the clitoris is compared to the penis; friction between the clitoris and the penis does not occur in the male superior position.

Other effective forms of contraception are available and no woman should go to heroic extremes to retain an IUD if her body does not tolerate it. In fact, if an IUD is still causing trouble four to six weeks after insertion, you are either one of the ten percent who cannot use IUDs or you are using the wrong type for you. In such a case, demand the removal of the IUD.

Expulsion

The IUD is a foreign body within the uterus, and the increased cramping (increased uterine contractions) is an attempt by the uterus to get rid of this foreign body. At times, it is successful and the device is expelled. About one in ten devices is expelled within a year of insertion. There is no way to predict who will tolerate an IUD and who will expel one. If a woman has expelled her first IUD, there is a very good chance she will expel a second. The majority of expulsions occurs during the first months following insertion—the period of increased bleeding and cramping. The longer the device remains in the uterus, the less is the chance of spontaneous expulsion.

A woman with an IUD should be particularly observant during her menstrual period. She should return to her physician after the first postinsertion menstrual period to have the position of the IUD checked. During the first and all successive menstrual periods, a woman should check tampons or pads after removal to make sure the device has not been expelled with the menstrual flow. If an IUD has threads leading into the vagina, a woman should check these threads after each menstruation. If they cannot be felt, she should see her physician to determine if the device is still in place.

IUDs and Pelvic Infection

There is no evidence of an increase in the incidence of simple vaginal infections, such as monilia, in IUD users. However, there have been reports that there is an increased incidence of the more serious pelvic infections in women with IUDs. Since they are sterilely packaged and inserted, the pelvic infections do not come from the IUDs themselves. The infection usually comes from the vagina. It has been theorized that the presence of the IUD, and particularly the vaginal threads of the IUD, causes the cervical canal to remain slightly more dilated than it normally would. It is this minimal dilation of the cervix that permits passage of bacteria from the vagina, via the IUD threads and the cervical canal, into the uterus. The infection frequently spreads after menstruation. The occurrence of pelvic pain at this time should alert an IUD user to the possibility of pelvic infection.

The most common type of pelvic infection in IUD users remains localized in the uterus. This type of infection, called *endometritis*, results in discharge and severe pain which worsens during intercourse. Fortunately, this condition is usually successfully treated with antibiotics on an ambulatory basis. If it is left untreated, the infection can spread to the fallopian tubes, causing *salpingitis*. There appears to be an increasing number of infections in one fallopian tube, *single-sided salpingitis,* in women with IUDs.

If an IUD user feels a sharp pain on one side, she should immediately have this condition examined to determine if it is single-sided salpingitis, tubal pregnancy, or some other condition, such as appendicitis. If salpingitis is diagnosed, it can often be successfully treated with antibiotics without the removal of the IUD. However, if the physician determines that the response to antibiotics is not satisfactory, he must remove the IUD, which often speeds recovery. If the salpingitis is left untreated, tubal abscesses can develop, and can lead to sterility.

Salpingitis could also spread into the pelvic cavity and lead to pelvic inflammatory disease, PID (see Chapter 7, Venereal Disease). Mild PID can be treated on an outpatient basis with antibiotics. In severe cases, the patients must be hospitalized and treated with intravenous infusions of antibiotics, and the IUDs must be removed. The insertion of an IUD in a woman who has had a previous PID can cause a flare-up of symptoms if the previous infection is not completely under control. Women who have had PID can use an IUD, but their physicians must make certain that the previous infection has been totally eliminated. It is unfortunate, but almost all forms of PID, particularly gonorrhea, are more severe in women with IUDs. A woman with an IUD must be aware of her increased susceptibility and, thus, must be more vigilant concerning any signs of infection.

Perforation by the IUD

In rare instances, an IUD can pass through or perforate the wall of the uterus and travel into the abdomen. The reported incidence of uterine perforation varies from report to report and with the type of IUD used—from 0.5 in 1000 to as high as 5 in 1000 insertions. A major factor in the incidence of perforation appears to be the skill with which the IUD is inserted. Particular care must be taken with postabortion and postdelivery insertions of IUDs. Since the uterine wall is soft and thin, it is very easy for the device to be pushed through the wall at this time. An IUD with a less rounded edge tends to perforate the uterine wall spontaneously, perhaps as it is pushed out of the uterine cavity by contractions. Perforation by an IUD is not usually dangerous. The device is usually caught by the *omentum,* which encapsulates the device and prevents complication. However, if one of the copper-bearing devices perforates, there is a chance it will cause a dense adhesion in the peritoneal cavity; it should, then, be surgically removed. If there is suspicion that an IUD has perforated the uterus, its location should be determined by X-ray. An IUD which

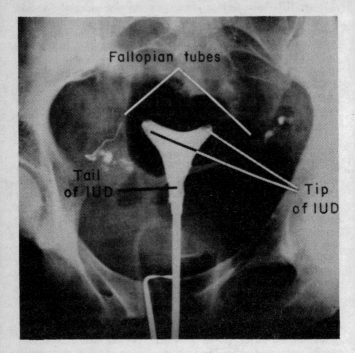

Fig. 9-11: This X-ray of the uterus and fallopian tubes (hysterosal-pingogram) illustrates how the Ypsilon conforms to the uterine cavity. The uterus and the fallopian tubes are completely normal. If a physician cannot see the tail of the IUD, he usually suggests an X-ray of the uterus to determine if the IUD is still in place.

has perforated can usually be removed with the aid of a laparoscope (see Laparoscopy, in Chapter 10).

Pregnancy and the IUD

If an IUD user becomes pregnant, she has a relatively higher chance for an ectopic (tubal) pregnancy than a woman who becomes pregnant without an IUD. There are two possible explanations for this. In general, the incidence of tubal pregnancy ranges from 1 in 120 to 1 in 200 pregnancies. The presence of an IUD usually prevents implantation of the fertilized egg in the uterus, but may have no effect on implantation in the fallopian tube. Therefore, while preventing most uterine pregnancies, the IUD is not able to prevent extrauterine pregnancy. Secondly, since an IUD renders the wearer more susceptible to tubal infection, the normal passage of the egg down the fallopian tube can be impeded by tubal inflammation. An ectopic pregnancy can result. An IUD user should be aware of these possibilities and alert to any delayed period, particularly when accompanied by one-sided pain. She should seek immediate attention with the onset of any such symptoms.

If uterine pregnancy occurs in a woman using an IUD, there is about a 50 percent chance that she can carry the infant to term and deliver without any ill effects either to herself or the infant. Approximately half of all IUD wearers spontaneously abort uterine pregnancies.

There have been a number of cases of septic abortion among IUD users, some associated with *septicemia* (severe infection in the blood), septic shock, and even death. Septic abortion has been particularly related to the Dalkon Shield, perhaps due to its particular configuration and its braided vaginal strings, which may render it a more efficient vehicle for the transmission of infection. There have been reports of severe infection and even death due to septic abortion with other IUDs, but to a lesser degree. It is estimated that 15 in 1000 pregnancies occurring with the IUD result in death from septic abortion.

It is strongly suggested that an IUD be removed as early as possible in any woman who becomes pregnant with the IUD. The fertilized egg in an IUD pregnancy usually implants higher up in the uterus than the IUD. Because of this, an IUD can usually be removed easily without disturbing the developing pregnancy. This is particularly true if the vaginal strings are visible. If the strings are not visible, the IUD may have to be removed under general anesthesia and, perhaps, in combination with termination of pregnancy.

Cancer and the IUD

There has been some concern that because the IUD is a foreign body within the uterus it might act as a constant irritant to this organ and increase the user's chances of developing cancer. However, there is no difference in the incidence of cervical cancer among women with IUDs, women on oral contraceptives, and women who use no form of birth control. Women who regularly use a diaphragm have a somewhat lower incidence of cervical cancer. Recent studies have shown the development of abnormal Pap smears in some women who are long-term IUD users. In such cases, the Pap smears should be repeated, and if the results have not spontaneously reverted to normal, the IUD should be removed.

Removal of the IUD

The removal of an IUD is much easier than its insertion, particularly if the string is visible and the IUD is not imbedded in the uterine wall. The Dalkon Shield appears to have a propensity for imbedding and, on occasion, has to be removed under general anesthesia. The majority of other IUDs have a smooth surface and are easy to remove. The removal is usually associated with cramping, which subsides within a few minutes after the procedure. It is probably better for the device to be removed during the menstrual period. If the threads are not visible, removal is somewhat more difficult and is accomplished with a long, narrow metal device, similar to a uterine sound, with a smooth hook at the end.

Summary

An intrauterine contraceptive device is recommended for women who do not want to take oral contraceptives but wish to have a contraceptive technique more effective than barrier methods such as the diaphragm and the condom. The IUD offers the added advantage of contraception without the need of conscious control. Not every woman can tolerate the presence of the IUD in the uterus, and there is no way to predict who can tolerate an IUD and who cannot. IUDs are generally a more successful form of contraception for multiparous women (women who have already given birth). These women seem to have fewer problems with irritation and contractions of the uterus and are less likely to expel an IUD. If a nulliparous woman (one who has not given birth) is fitted correctly with the appropriate IUD and does not expel the device, this can offer an excellent method of contraception. As a general rule, IUD users are somewhat older than users of oral contraceptives. An IUD is not recommended as the contraceptive of choice for a young woman, who has not borne children and has multiple sex partners. This woman is a prime candidate for pelvic infection with resultant infertility problems in later life.

If you decide to use an intrauterine device, be sure to ask your physician what type of device is to be used. Once your device is inserted, *remember its name*. If it has to be changed periodically, as with the copper and progesterone-bearing devices, if any type of complication should occur, or if you simply wish to have it removed, it is imperative that you know what device you are using.

ORAL CONTRACEPTION

The development of the oral contraceptive is one of the most far-reaching and socially influential discoveries of modern science. Birth-control pills are the most widely prescribed drugs, currently used by more than fifty million women throughout the world. Their popularity is evidence of their general acceptance and enormous social impact.

It is easy to see why oral contraceptives are so popular. Short of sterilization, they are the most effective way to prevent unwanted pregnancy; they are nearly 100 percent effective. In fact, far more pregnancies result from forgetting to take the pill than from an actual drug failure. Although there are still many unanswered questions, oral contraceptives appear relatively safe. The contraceptive effects of the pill are usually reversible, making it useful for family planning. Women do not have to rely on either the promises of their partners or tedious preparations. Although some have called the pill an insult to the physiology of a woman's body and have proved its serious, and sometimes fatal, consequences, the benefits of this form of contraception still seem to outweigh its admitted dangers.

History of Oral Contraceptives

The search for an effective oral contraceptive is centuries old. Hundreds of years ago, women took arsenic and strychnine to prevent pregnancy. More women probably died from ingesting these poisons than would have died from the resulting pregnancies.

The discovery of the modern oral contraceptives is based on a simple but obvious fact of nature: Once a woman is pregnant, she will not become pregnant again during this pregnancy. Hormones produced in the ovaries are responsible for the development of a woman's secondary sexual characteristics. The possible role of these hormones in the maintenance or the prevention of pregnancy was clarified in the 1900s. It was then observed by a German scientist that if the corpus luteum, which secretes progesterone, was removed from the ovary following ovulation, implantation of a fertilized egg would not occur. On the other hand, if the corpus luteum was left intact, the egg would implant, but the development and release of other eggs from the ovary was prevented.

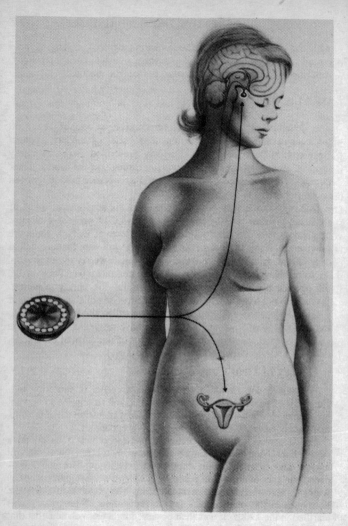

Fig. 9-12: Birth-control pills affect both the brain hormones and the uterus. The hormones in the birth-control pills suppress the body's hormones and, thus, control the menstrual cycle and prevent ovulation. (Courtesy of Ortho Pharmaceutical Corporation, Raritan, New Jersey.)

American investigators in the late 1920s identified progesterone as the active ingredient in the corpus luteum that maintained the pregnancy of a released and fertilized egg. In 1929, the hormone estrogen was isolated from the Graafian follicle of the rat ovary. Initially, progesterone was obtained in limited amounts only from animal sources and then purified. This made it a relatively expensive substance which was active only in an injectable form. The discovery, in 1944, that progesterone could be synthesized from plant steroids found in the root of the wild Mexican yam made an orally active and relatively inexpensive synthetic progesterone available.

Once these hormones were available, their effects on menstrual disorders and the inhibition of ovulation were investigated. In 1953, Dr. Pincus reported that ovulation could be inhibited in animals with a synthetic progestin. These results were confirmed in a group of volunteer women in the Boston area by Dr. Rock. In 1956, the famous Puerto Rican studies were undertaken with Enovid, an oral contraceptive containing both estrogen and progesterone. Their effectiveness as contraceptives·was proven and the first birth-control pill, Enovid-10, was released in the United States four years later.

How Does the Pill Work?

Most simply, oral contraceptives produce a state of pseudo-pregnancy, which prevents the development and release of an ovum. This state of pseudopregnancy is produced by interference with the delicate balance of hormones produced in the brain and in the ovary during the normal menstrual cycle (see Chapter 5, The Reproductive Cycle).

Ingestion of the *combined oral contraceptives,* those containing both estrogen and progesterone, produces a constant level of estrogen and progesterone in the blood, which, in turn, replaces the normal hormonal variation during the menstrual cycle. The combined oral contraceptives exert their contraceptive influence at two different points, making them particularly effective. Primarily, the steady level of estrogen inhibits the release of FSH (follicle stimulating hormone) from the pituitary. FSH stimulates the maturation of eggs in the ovary; by inhibiting FSH, the estrogen inhibits ovulation. The progesterone in the combined pill produces changes in the cervical mucus, which prevent the passage of sperm into the uterus. The progesterone makes the mucus thick and acts almost as a natural diaphragm.

The steady level of estrogen-progesterone produced by the combined birth-control pill causes a change in the lining of the uterus. The endometrium does not build up under the steady level of hormones from the pill, as it does during the normal menstrual cycle. The bleeding experienced by a woman on oral contraceptives is a withdrawal bleeding, resulting from the drop in the estrogen-progesterone blood level when the pills are not taken for seven of the twenty-eight days. It is not a true menstruation, and this withdrawal bleeding is usually less than that experienced with normal, or true, menstruation.

The sequential oral contraceptives reflect an attempt to produce an effective contraceptive that more closely mimics the flow of hormones during the normal menstrual cycle. Estrogen alone is taken for fourteen days; this prevents ovulation. Progesterone is then taken with the estrogen for seven days to cause a buildup in the endometrium similar to the buildup following ovulation. No pills are taken for the next seven days, during which menstruation occurs.

The sequentials, which are no longer available in the United States, were particularly attractive to women with low tolerance for progesterone, but they were less effective than the combined pills, because the secondary contraceptive effect of progesterone on the cervical mucus was absent for the first two weeks of the cycle. Also, if a single pill of the sequential series was forgotten or missed, ovulation could occur.

The minipill contains no estrogen, only progesterone. It exerts contraceptive effectiveness primarily by causing the cervical mucus to thicken and act as a natural diaphragm or barrier to the passage of sperm. The progesterone also interferes with the normal buildup of the uterine lining; thus, if fertilization does take place, the endometrium will not be receptive to implantation. It is believed that the minipill does not interfere with ovulation. For that reason, the pregnancy rate with this oral contraceptive is higher than with the other birth-control pills.

Types of Oral Contraceptives

The first oral contraceptives released in the United States in 1960 contained ten to twenty times more progestin and two to three times more estrogen than needed. The reported severe side effects related to the oral contraceptives were, in most cases, related to the high-dose contraceptive initially released. As the estrogen level in birth-control pills was lowered, there was a decrease in occurrence of severe side effects. A woman should know which birth-control pill she is taking

Name	Year Released	Estrogen	(in micrograms)	Progestin	(in milligrams)
Enovid-E	1964	Mestranol	100 mcg	Norethynodrel	2.5 mg
Ortho-Novum-2	1963	Mestranol	100 mcg	Norethindrone	2.0 mg
Norinyl	1964	Mestranol	100 mcg	Norethindrone	2.0 mg
Ovulen	1966	Mestranol	100 mcg	Ethynodiol diacetate	1.0 mg
Ortho-Novum 1 + 80	1968	Mestranol	80 mcg	Norethindrone	1.0 mg
Norinyl 1 + 80	1968	Mestranol	80 mcg	Norethindrone	1.0 mg
Enovid-5	1962	Mestranol	75 mcg	Norethynodrel	5.0 mg
Ortho-Novum-10	1963	Mestranol	60 mcg	Norethindrone	10.0 mg
Norlestrin-2.5	1964	Ethinyl estradiol	50 mcg	Norethindrone acetate	1.0 mg
Demulen	1970	Ethinyl estradiol	50 mcg	Ethynodiol diacetate	1.0 mg
Norlestrin 1 + 50	1967	Ethinyl estradiol	50 mcg	Norethindrone acetate	1.0 mg
Zorane 1 + 50	1974	Ethinyl estradiol	50 mcg	Norethindrone acetate	1.0 mg
Ortho-Novum 1 + 50	1967	Mestranol	50 mcg	Norethindrone	1.0 mg
Ortho-Novum 1 + 35	1979	Mestranol	35 mcg	Norethindrone	1.0 mg
Norinyl 1 + 50	1967	Mestranol	50 mcg	Norethindrone	1.0 mg
Norinyl 1 + 35	1980	Mestranol	35 mcg	Norethindrone	1.0 mg
Ovral	1968	Ethinyl estradiol	50 mcg	Norgestrel	0.5 mg
Ovcon-50	1976	Ethinyl estradiol	50 mcg	Norethindrone	1.0 mg
Brevicon	1975	Ethinyl estradiol	35 mcg	Norethindrone	0.5 mg
Modicon	1975	Ethinyl estradiol	35 mcg	Norethindrone	0.5 mg
Ovcon-35	1976	Ethinyl estradiol	35 mcg	Norethindrone	0.4 mg
Loestrin 1.5 + 30	1973	Ethinyl estradiol	30 mcg	Norethindrone acetate	1.5 mg
Zorane 1.5 + 30	1974	Ethinyl estradiol	30 mcg	Norethindrone acetate	1.5 mg
Lo-ovral	1975	Ethinyl estradiol	30 mcg	Norgestrel	0.3 mg
Loestrin 1 + 20	1973.	Ethinyl estradiol	20 mcg	Norethindrone acetate	1.0 mg
Zorane 1 + 20	1974	Ethinyl estradiol	20 mcg	Norethindrone acetate	1.0 mg

and how much estrogen is in that pill. If her oral contraceptive contains more than 50 micrograms of estrogen, she should request a lower dose from her physician. If a woman is new to the pill, she should start on a low-estrogen dose; if side effects occur, the estrogen can then be altered accordingly. A list of the presently available combined oral contraceptives follows.

Oral contraceptives contain one of two types of estrogen, either *ethinyl estradiol* or *mestranol*. Ethinyl estradiol is slightly more potent than mestranol.

There are basically five different types of progestin currently used in the combination oral contraceptives: *norethynodrel, norethindrone, norethindrone acetate, ethynodiol diacetate*, and *norgestrel*. These synthetic progestins, with the exception of norgestrel, have some estrogenic effect. On a weight-for-weight basis, norgestrel is the most potent progestational agent, and, in addition, it has the highest androgenic activity of all the progestins.

It is both the amount of estrogen and the characteristics of the progestin in the oral contraceptive that contribute to the effects of the pill on a woman's system. If the oral contraceptive produces nausea, breast soreness, and water retention—the estrogen-related symptoms —a pill with lower estrogen should be taken. On the other hand, if side effects such as amenorrhea or acne occur, it is advisable to change to a pill with higher estrogen or a progestin with less androgenic activity. The option in relation to what type of oral contraceptive to use when side effects occur will be discussed more fully under the individual side effects.

These sequential birth-control pills were taken by approximately one million women in the United States in 1976:

Name	Year Released	Estrogen	(in micrograms)	Progestin	(in milligrams)
Oracon	1965	Ethinyl estradiol	100 mcg	Dimethisterone	25 mg
Ortho-Novum SQ	1966	Mestranol	80 mcg	Norethindrone	2 mg
Norquen	1967	Mestranol	80 mcg	Norethindrone	2 mg

These pills all contain more than the recommended 50 micrograms of estrogen and have a failure rate of 2 pregnancies per 100 woman-years of use. For years, many physicians have not recommended sequentials and, because of their high levels of estrogen and high failure rates, they have been banned from some European countries. Recently, there was evidence of a link between uterine cancer and the sequential oral contraceptives. The FDA subsequently recommended that drug companies withdraw these pills from the market. Any woman still taking sequentials should consult her physician and change to a combined contraceptive.

The *minipills* contain no estrogen and have a high rate of irregular bleeding. The three minipills presently marketed are:

Name	Year Released	Progestin	(in milligrams)
Micronor	1973	Norethindrone	0.35 mg
Nor-Q.D.	1973	Norethindrone	0.35 mg
Ovrette	1973	Norgestrel	0.075 mg

The failure rate on the minipill is higher than with the combined pills, ranging from 1.1 to 3.7 pregnancies per 100 woman-years of use. Women who cannot tolerate estrogen should be the only users of the minipill. It should not be taken by women who experience irregular menses.

Who Can Take the Pill?

The majority of women can take oral contraceptives. Women who use oral contraceptives must be sufficiently motivated to take the pill day after day and must be free of certain health problems. Oral contraceptives are particularly attractive to women who strongly wish to avoid pregnancy and would be adverse to abortion in the case of contraceptive failure. They are an excellent form of contraception for women who have active sex lives, as well as for women who suffer from dysmenorrhea or premenstrual tension.

If a woman wishes to use birth-control pills, she must first undergo an interview and an examination, either by her physician or in a family-planning clinic. The purpose of the interview is to reveal past medical and family history of any condition that might be a contraindication for the use of oral contraceptives. If there are contraindications, the physician should suggest another, more appropriate, method of contraception. However, if the medical history is benign, the physician performs a complete physical examination, including blood pressure, to rule out hypertension, a pelvic examination to exclude uterine abnormalities such as fibroid tumors, and a breast exam to determine any form of breast tumors. All are contraindications to the pill. A urine specimen should be obtained for analysis of sugar and protein levels to rule out diabetes or any kidney condition.

If a woman is placed on birth-control pills, she should see her physician at least twice a year. At this biannual visit, blood pressure should be checked, breasts examined, and urine analysis performed. A Pap smear should be taken once a year.

Absolute Contraindications to the Pill

Women who have any of the following conditions *must not* take oral contraceptives:

Thrombophlebitis. The formation of a blood clot within a vein, which then breaks loose and travels to another part of the body (such as the lung or the brain), with the potential of causing extreme damage and even death.

Cerebral Vascular Disease or Accident. A history of stroke, aneurysm, or any other form of intracranial bleeding.

Cardiovascular Disease. Abnormalities in the vascular system, such as a history of *myocardial infarction* (heart attack) or congenital heart abnormalities.

Markedly Impaired Liver Function. Liver damage subsequent to conditions such as severe hepatitis or cirrhosis.

Malignancy of the Reproductive System. Suspected or treated cancer of the breast or uterus.

Pregnancy. The hormones in the oral contraceptives can cause congenital malformation in the fetus.

Other Conditions that Usually Prohibit the Pill

Women who have the following conditions *should not* take oral contraceptives:

Hypertension. Women with severe high blood pressure who are on antihypertensives should not take oral contraceptives. Women with mild hypertension can take the pill, but they should be placed on a low-estrogen pill. These women must be carefully monitored and should be seen every three months for blood-pressure checks.

Diabetes. Oral contraceptives can interfere with carbohydrate metabolism. Therefore, women with diabetes who require daily insulin administration should not use oral contraceptives. Pre-diabetic women and women in whom the diabetes can be controlled by diet alone can take birth-control pills. These women should be placed on a low-dose estrogen pill and must be closely followed by their physicians with annual or semiannual glucose-tolerance tests.

Fibroid Tumors. The growth of fibroid tumors can be stimulated by estrogen. If a woman with fibroids insists on oral contraceptives, she should be placed on the lowest-dose estrogen or on the minipill.

Conditions that Limit the Pill

Oral contraceptives are potent drugs which cause profound effects throughout the body. When deciding on the value of birth-control pills, a woman must weigh the advantages against the problems in order to make an intelligent and informed decision. There are a number of conditions that appear to be affected by oral contraceptives, and women with these conditions must be aware of the possible adverse effects of the pill. These conditions are epilepsy, migraine headaches, and significant psychological disorders, such as severe depression. Women with these conditions should be on a low-estrogen dose and should be aware that if the condition becomes worse, oral contraceptives should be terminated. Women suffering from severe asthma should probably not take oral contraceptives, since any water retention may adversely affect the lungs. Women who are over thirty-five and heavy smokers should use an alternative form of contraception, because of a significant increase in cardiovascular problems. Women with varicose veins can take oral contraceptives, but they should be particularly alert to any occurrence of leg pain indicative of blood-clotting disorders. Women who have sickle cell anemia or who are breast-feeding should also refrain from the pill. Sickle cell trait is not, however, a contraindication.

Age and Oral Contraceptives

The years between about sixteen and thirty-five are the most fertile time of a woman's life. During these years, the birth-control pill is a most attractive form of contraception because of its great effectiveness. Because women who have not had children usually have a harder time adjusting to an IUD, oral contraceptives are particularly acceptable to younger women. Women who have a number of sexual partners usually would rather depend on the great protection afforded by birth-control pills rather than worry about less effective techniques such as barrier methods. Finally, women at this age have, as a group, a lower incidence of those medical problems which contraindicate the use of oral contraceptives.

Women under eighteen who are sexually active can take birth-control pills, since the risk of the pills is probably less than the risk of an abortion. As with older women, a teenager experiencing only intermittent sex, perhaps once every few months, might be better off with some other contraceptive technique. If a teenager is having very irregular periods, early use of oral contraceptives is not strongly recommended.

There has been some concern that early use of oral contraceptives stunts growth, but this is *not* true. Estrogen must be given in *very* high doses—amounts that far exceed the amount in birth-control pills—for a long period of time immediately following puberty to have even a 50 percent chance of limiting growth. A teenager who assumes the adult responsibility of sexual intercourse must also realize her responsibility to protect herself from unwanted pregnancy. Oral contraceptives should be available to her.

After the age of forty, the risks involved with oral contraceptives, particularly the risks of myocardial infarction (heart attack), must be carefully weighed against the risk of pregnancy and the acceptability of other forms of contraception. For women over forty, the excess risk of developing a fatal heart attack is 27.6 per 100,000 women on the pill. However, the risk of death is 124.1 fatalities per 100,000 pregnancies in women between 40 and 44. Pregnancy is still more of a risk than the pill, but since fertility is lower in this age group, other contraceptive techniques should be closely examined. If a woman over forty elects to use oral contraceptives, she should take a pill containing less than 50 micrograms of estrogen and must be carefully followed by her physician.

Smoking and the Pill

Heavy smoking, increasing age, and the pill do not make a healthy combination. Smoking increases a woman's chances of developing cardiovascular problems as she gets older, and these chances are again increased if the woman takes oral contraceptives. Smoking fifteen or more cigarettes per day will result in increased risk; age becomes a significant risk factor after thirty-five, if a woman smokes. A woman of thirty-five must make the choice to either smoke heavily or use oral contraceptives and realize that if she does both, she is placing herself at high risk.

How to Take the Pill

Once a woman and her physician determine she is a candidate for oral contraception, she can take the pills on the following schedule:

Combined Oral Contraceptives. A woman counts the very first sign of menstrual bleeding as day 1 of her cycle. On day 5, she starts taking the combined estrogen-progesterone pills for twenty-one days. If she has a twenty-eight-day pill packet, she takes a placebo for seven days. After these seven placebo or pill-less days, no matter when withdrawal bleeding has initiated, she will restart her pills. In other words, if a woman starts taking the combined birth-control pills on a Sunday, she takes her last effective pill twenty-one days later on a Saturday. She then takes either a placebo for seven days or no pill for seven days. She starts her new packet of pills on Sunday again. From that day forward, she always starts a new packet every twenty-eight days on Sunday. The pill packets are usually designed so the pills are matched with the days of the week. In this way, it is easy to determine if a pill has been taken or forgotten.

Sequentials. The instructions for the proper administration of the sequential oral contraceptives are omitted, since these drugs have been removed from the market.

Minipills. As with the combined birth-control pills, a woman originally starts the minipill on day 5 of her cycle. However, the minipills are taken constantly, day after day, with no interruption in the medication.

Most women on oral contraceptives try to incorporate taking the pill into their daily schedule to minimize the chance of missing a pill and in any way diminishing protection. An attempt should be made to take the pill at the same time every day to keep a steady level of drug in the body. A number of women find that the side effects are fewer if the pills are taken after the evening meal or right before bedtime. A woman should have an extra packet of oral contraceptives at her place of work or in the purse she uses every day just in case she forgets to take the pill at home.

What If a Pill Is Forgotten?

If a pill is forgotten, a woman should take that pill as soon as she remembers it and the next pill at its regular time, even if it means taking two pills during the same twenty-four-hour period. If a woman forgets to take the oral contraceptives two days in a row, she should take two pills as soon as she remembers and two pills the following day. She should also employ some additional form of contraception, such as a spermicidal foam or condom, for the remaining part of the cycle. If the pills are forgotten for three or more days, no further pills should be taken from that packet. In that case, a woman should stay off the pills for seven days and then start a new packet. During this time, and for the next cycle on the pills, there is a chance that ovulation will occur, and additional contraception must be employed. A second school of thought lets a woman who has missed three consecutive pills continue taking the pill by starting the new packet of pills immediately. This may, however, cause some irregular bleeding.

If a woman forgets two or more pills during a cycle and her period is delayed, she should have a pregnancy test prior to initiating a new pill packet. If any *minipills* are forgotten, a woman must immediately double up on the pill. Since there is a high failure rate with the minipill, an additional form of contraception should be used for three to four weeks even if a single pill is missed.

How Long Can a Woman Stay on the Pill?

A woman can use oral contraceptives for as long as she wishes. There are at the present time no contraindications for taking the pill for ten or even twenty years. A woman must see her physician at least annually, and biannually after age thirty-five, when she is on birth-control pills. However, the prolonged administration of pills is directly dependent on the absence of any adverse reaction or the occurrence of any of the conditions previously described as absolute contraindications to the pill.

In the past, it was routine for a woman to stop the pills every two or three years to let the body "recycle." A woman stopped taking the pills until she experienced three menstrual cycles and then would start them again, leaving herself unprotected for a period of up to six months. It was theorized that such a routine recycling acted as a check of the normal interaction of the pituitary and the ovary. This theory is given little credence today. A woman need *not* stop the pills to recycle.

Vitamins, Iron, and the Pill

There is an increased need for vitamins B_1, B_6, B_{11}, B_{12}, and vitamin C when oral contraceptives are used. Of these vitamins, the need for vitamin B_6 seems to be the greatest. The birth-control pill creates a pseudopregnancy; it is, therefore, easy to understand why a woman needs extra vitamin intake. The requirement for iron might, however, be slightly reduced; women on oral contraceptives tend to bleed less, and thus lose less iron. There is also an increase in iron absorption when a woman is taking the pill. It is suggested that women take at least one multiple vitamin daily, preferably a vitamin with a high concentration of vitamin B_6. Several such pills are now available (for example, the Feminins tablets). Instead of a multiple vitamin, an extra vitamin-B complex, possibly in combination with vitamin C, can be taken, especially for women who feel tired and run down. The extra intake of vitamin B_6 might also help prevent acne and depression.

The Pros and Cons of Oral Contraceptives

The combined oral contraceptives are usually effective in the prevention of pregnancy from the taking of the first pill. During the first month, there is a minimal chance of escape ovulation, and some backup form of contraception such as a condom or spermicide should be used. The failure rate of the combined birth-control pills is estimated at 0.1 pregnancy per 100 woman-years of use if the oral contraceptives are taken according to schedule. However, since human error cannot be eliminated and pills can be forgotten, the actual failure rate is from 2 to 5 pregnancies per 100 woman-years. Any woman who consistently has difficulty remembering to take her birth-control pills on schedule should examine her attitude toward the pills and contraception in general.

Freedom from the fear of pregnancy is the greatest benefit of the oral contraceptives to many women. Sexual intercourse may be enjoyed spontaneously, without the need for concern or for any preparation. Still, oral contraceptives have advantages other than effective birth control. Combination pills help regulate a woman's menstrual period, ease painful menstruation (dysmenorrhea), and decrease excessive bleeding from 50 to 75 percent. They prevent the cyclic buildup of hormonal peaks, which reduces the amount of uterine lining and subsequent menstrual flow. This helps women with anemia. The pill is valuable for women who tend to develop ovarian cysts, because it prevents formation of the Graafian follicle where the cysts can develop.

In addition, the Walnut Creek contraceptive-drug study, a ten-year investigation by Dr. Howard Ory, of the Center for Disease Control in Atlanta, on the effects of oral contraceptives in more than 16,600 women, has helped put the risks and advantages of the pill in proper perspective. The results of this study have shed a more optimistic light on oral contraceptives. The risk for the development of breast cancer was not increased by the pill and the risk of benign breast disease was significantly reduced. Pill users experienced less iron deficiency, anemia, and rheumatoid arthritis. The use of oral contraceptives did not increase the chances of developing either endometrial or ovarian cancer and may have actually had some protective effect against these serious disorders. Finally, the incidence of pelvic inflammatory disease (PID) among pill users was found to be half that of women who used other forms of contraceptives.

The pill is *not* intended to provide protection from venereal diseases. New regulations by the FDA require this warning information to be on all prescriptions for the pill in the United States. Additional information about possible side effects is also required.

The sequential birth-control pills have a theoretical failure rate of 1 to 2 pregnancies per 100 woman-years of use, even when taken faithfully. The minipill has a theoretical failure rate of 1 to 4 pregnancies per 100 woman-years when taken every day. The chances of escape ovulation are high if even a single minipill is forgotten. The majority of women who become pregnant on the minipill do so during the first six months. Some secondary form of contraception should be employed during this period to provide additional protection.

There are about twenty-five to thirty different brands of oral contraceptives currently available. The pill, especially the new low-estrogen type, is perhaps most popular in northern Europe. In the Netherlands, for example, nearly 35 percent of women use the pill in their birth-control programs. In the United States and Great Britain, the pill is taken by about 20 percent of women. The use of combination pills has been growing steadily, while, fortunately, the less effective and more dangerous sequentials have been removed from the market.

Side Effects of Oral Contraceptives

The rise and fall of estrogen and progesterone experienced with a normal menstrual cycle are replaced by steady levels of these hormones furnished by the combined birth-control pills. These artificial (pill-produced) steady levels of estrogen and progesterone give the pill its contraceptive effectiveness, but they are also responsible for its side effects. The side effects can be attributed to estrogen excess, progesterone excess, and, conversely, estrogen deficiency and progesterone deficiency. Some of the synthetic progestins have a degree of androgenic activity and can also be a source of pill-related side effects.

Minor "Estrogen Excess" Side Effects

Probably the most common side effects related to estrogen excess are nausea and vomiting, which usually occur only at first and subside after a while. Some women find these gastrointestinal side effects are minimized by taking the pill either following the evening meal or at bedtime. Dizziness is reported by about 2 of every 100 women. Headaches can occur at the beginning of the cycle, but if they persist from cycle to cycle, an alternate form of contraception should be found. Water retention is reflected in a number of possible symptoms —edema of the legs accompanied by leg cramps or cyclic breast enlargement and difficulty with the fit of contact lenses, caused by water retention swelling the entire eye. Water retention is usually mild and can be controlled by carefully watching salt intake and drinking adequate amounts of water to dilute sodium in the system. If the symptoms of water retention are more severe, diuretics might be taken for the last few days of the cycle prior to withdrawal bleeding.

An increase in breast size due to an increase in "female fat" deposition is also caused by estrogen excess. This condition is often considered a side benefit. *Leukorrhea*, a clear, nonodorous vaginal secretion, can also be an estrogen-related side effect, and while it may be a minor annoyance, it presents no medical problem.

One of the rare side effects related to estrogen excess is the appearance of freckles on the brow, across the bridge of the nose, and under the eyes; this is *chloasma*, the so-called mask of pregnancy. Chloasma most often appears after exposure to strong sunlight. Chloasma, while completely benign, is understandably disturbing from a cosmetic viewpoint. It usually is an indication that the birth-control pills should be replaced by some other form of contraception.

If any of the estrogen-excess side effects become difficult to tolerate, a woman should change to a pill with lower estrogen content or consider the minipill, which is estrogen-free.

Minor "Progesterone Excess" Side Effects

One of the most commonly reported side effects, occurring in almost 13 percent of oral contraceptive users, is depression. This change in mood is attributed to "progesterone excess." Levels of some vitamins are lowered by the use of oral contraceptives, and a dietary supplement containing vitamin B_6 may alleviate any pill-related depression. Progesterone excess sometimes causes an increased appetite, which can result in weight gain. Fatigue and tiredness can be the result of progesterone excess and can be partly eliminated by supplementary vitamins, particularly B_6. Progesterone excess, particularly in combination with estrogen deficiency, can alter the vaginal milieu and cause *monilia vaginitis*. If this condition persists even after local administration of antiyeast medication, a change to birth-control pills with lower progesterone or higher estrogen might be necessary.

A few women complain of decreased libido. If this occurs, change to another pill, perhaps one with a different type of progesterone, like norgestrel, which has a more androgenic or male-hormone effect. If this does not increase the libido, change to a pill with a higher estrogen content.

Oiliness of the skin or acne are usually caused by pills having a progesterone with stronger androgenic effects, particularly in combination with low estrogen (Lo-ovral, for one). These problems can usually be alleviated simply by changing to another brand with a less androgenic progesterone and a higher estrogen content.

Progesterone excess in combination with estrogen deficiency can cause irregular or no uterine bleeding. This is more common in women with a history of irregular bleeding, and occurs when the lining of the uterus does not build up sufficiently to be sloughed off during the seven days the pills are not taken. Pill-induced amenorrhea is not a serious condition per se, as it only indicates that the uterine lining is at rest. This can be beneficial, particularly for women who suffer from severe menstrual cramps. If a woman is concerned about absent or irregular bleeding, she should change to a pill with a higher estrogen content or a different progesterone. If amenorrhea occurs after the first pill cycle, particularly with the minipill, a woman should have a pregnancy test performed. Amenorrhea after three months on the pills, especially if no pills have been forgotten, is very seldom a sign of pregnancy. Regular menstrual bleeding usually starts again spontaneously once the pills have been discontinued. If the amenorrhea persists, the physician administers either a progesterone or an estrogen to trigger the cyclic hormone changes.

Minor Side Effects Related to Estrogen Deficiency

Side effects related to estrogen deficiency are most commonly found among users of the minipill. Estrogen deficiency can result in inadequate endometrial buildup. Spotting and breakthrough bleeding are common phenomena. Because of this, the minipill cannot be recommended to women who have histories of irregular bleeding.

Other symptoms of estrogen deficiency are fatigue, loss of libido, and acne. If any of these symptoms occurs, a woman should increase intake of vitamins, particularly B_6. If this does not help, she should change to a pill with more estrogen.

Minor Side Effects Related to Progestin Deficiency

If the level of progesterone provided by the pill is insufficient, the development of the endometrium can be overstimulated, which can result in profuse bleeding that is often irregular in character and not cyclic. These symptoms are best treated by changing to another brand of pill which contains more progesterone in relationship to the estrogen.

Breakthrough Bleeding

Breakthrough bleeding is the term used to describe the occurrence of either vaginal bleeding or spotting at any time during the oral contraceptive cycle, other than the time of withdrawal or cyclic bleeding. This condition is a minor, but frequent, side effect of oral contraceptives. It is usually encountered during the first three cycles and may be caused by both estrogen and progesterone deficiency. A woman need not be concerned about *mild* vaginal spotting for the first few cycles, but if this persists after three cycles, she should inform her physician.

If a woman experiences true breakthrough bleeding, she should take two pills a day either until the bleeding stops or, preferably, until the end of the cycle. If bleeding persists at two pills per day, a third pill may be taken without worry. If breakthrough spotting or bleeding persists for more than three cycles, a pill with higher estrogen and progesterone should be considered.

Serious Side Effects Related to Oral Contraceptives

The serious side effects related to oral contraceptives are those that so profoundly disturb the normal functioning of a woman's body that they can lead to permanent damage or even death.

Thromboembolic Disorders. Thromboembolic disorders are the result of the abnormal formation of a blood clot within either a superficial (near the skin surface) or a deep vein. The increased incidence of thromboembolic disorders among women using contraceptives has received widespread publicity. Oral contraceptives increase the chances of developing some type of thromboembolic disorder by five to ten times. However, these statistics must be taken in perspective. Normally, each year 200 of 100,000 women of childbearing age develop *superficial thrombosis* (phlebitis) in the leg; among women taking oral contraceptives this number is increased to 300. The risk of *deep-vein thrombosis,* which is much more serious and potentially life threatening, is increased from 20 to 110 per 100,000 women per year. The risk of *thrombotic strokes (cerebral thrombosis)* is increased from 10 to 40 per 100,000 women per year. The presence of a number of pre-existent health problems such as hypertension, vascular problems, diabetes, and obesity appears to predispose women taking oral contraceptives to the development of clotting disorders. Smoking is a particularly potent factor in predisposing pill users to cerebral thrombosis. The clotting abnormalities appear to be related to the estrogen component, because the incidence of deep-vein thrombosis is reduced by 25 percent when estrogen is reduced to 50 micrograms. Thus, again and again the indications for low estrogen—below 50 micrograms—content in birth-control pills become stronger. Women are also advised to increase their fluid intake to help keep a good fluid balance. The effects on blood clotting exist only while the pills are being taken. Once a woman stops taking the oral contraceptives, the hormones rapidly metabolize and the increased risk disappears. Women scheduled for surgery should not take the pills for at least ten to fourteen days prior to the operative procedure. This reduces the chance of abnormal postoperative blood clotting.

The symptoms of early superficial phlebitis are tender and swollen leg veins. For deep thrombophlebitis, there is usually pain deep in the back of the legs. As the condition becomes more advanced, the leg swells.

The symptoms of cerebral thrombophlebitis are severe one-sided headaches and disturbance of vision. If any of these symptoms occurs, a woman should immediately stop taking the pill and contact her physician. Superficial phlebitis can usually be treated by local heat applications and aspirin. Deep-vein phlebitis and cerebral phlebitis require hospitalization and closely supervised anticoagulation treatment.

Heart Attack. The use of oral contraceptives increases a woman's chances for heart attack (myocardial infarction), particularly as her age increases, and even more so if she smokes. The incidence of fatal heart attack among nonusers between thirty and thirty-nine years old is less than 2 per 100,000 per year. This increases among users to 5.4 per 100,000 per year. Between ages forty to forty-four, risk of fatal heart attack among nonusers is approximately 3 per 100,000 per year and among users the risk is 20 per 100,000 per year. Although the risk of heart attack increases as age increases, particularly above forty, it must be remembered that these are the women who would be most at risk from the strain of pregnancy and/or delivery. The risk of the pill must be weighed against these risks. Still, if a woman over forty wishes to take the pill, she should take a very-low-estrogen pill.

Hypertension.   Mild elevations in both *systolic* and *diastolic* blood pressure are seen in women who have taken the birth-control pills over a period of years. In general, these elevations are quite small and do not elevate the blood pressure beyond normal levels. However, in 5 percent of women who take the pill for five years, the development of hypertension with blood pressure reading beyond 140/90 has been observed. Unfortunately, there is no way to predict in advance who will develop hypertension and who will not. In some women, the development of hypertension has been linked to some underlying medical problem, such as chronic kidney disease or the absence of a kidney, which would normally predispose a patient to hypertension.

The hypertensive effects in women who do not have any underlying disease processes are reversible, and blood pressure usually returns to normal once the pills are discontinued. It is essential to have blood pressure checked every six months, since hypertension is asymptomatic in its early stages. If a woman's physician fails to check her blood pressure, she should firmly request that readings be taken and perhaps consider another doctor. Women on oral contraceptives should limit their intake of salt, and, if they notice water retention, diuretics might be taken; these two measures can have antihypertensive effects.

If hypertension, or high blood pressure, occurs while a woman is on the pill, she should immediately stop taking oral contraceptives. Blood pressure should return to normal within a few months. It is interesting to note that women who develop high blood pressure on the pill have an increased risk of toxemia in pregnancy. If you become hypertensive on oral contraceptives, you should mention this fact to your obstetrician when you become pregnant.

Gallbladder Diseases.   Gallstones occur about twice as frequently among users of birth-control pills. The hormones may cause the formation of gallstones by decreasing the amount of bile and increasing the cholesterol concentration in the bile. There also appears to be an increased incidence of *cholecystitis* (gallbladder infection) among pill users. Although these conditions may require surgery, they are rarely fatal.

Liver Tumors. Adenomas of the liver (liver tumors) are extremely rare. Forty-two cases have been reported in the last six years, and a statistical correlation between this condition and oral contraceptives has been established. There has been a further correlation between the types of estrogen used—a greater number of tumors occurred in women taking *mestranol* as opposed to *ethinyl estradiol*. Although the majority of these tumors have been benign, death from intra-abdominal bleeding has been reported. The tumors are diagnosed by the discovery of abdominal masses. Women with such masses should see their physicians.

Pregnancy and the Pill

There is mounting evidence that if either progestins alone, such as in the minipill, or progestin-estrogen combinations, such as in the combined birth-control pills, are taken during the early part of pregnancy, congenital malformations may occur in the developing fetus. If a woman becomes pregnant while taking oral contraceptives, she should stop taking the pills the moment pregnancy is *confirmed*. There is no way to determine prior to birth whether the fetus has been severely affected by the pill, so early termination of pregnancy may be considered. The effects of the pill on the developing fetus can last even when conception has occurred after the pill has been stopped. There was an increased incidence of severe malformations among the spontaneously aborted fetuses of women who became pregnant soon after they had stopped taking high doses of oral contraceptives (estrogen above 50 mcg.). Although there is no such evidence indicting the low-dose oral contraceptives, a woman who wishes to conceive should stop taking the pills for at least three months prior to conception. This gives the body a chance to resume normal cyclic menstruation. Another form of contraception should be used in the interval.

Cancer and the Pill

There is no evidence that a woman who takes oral contraceptives increases her chances of developing breast cancer. In fact, the incidence of benign breast diseases, such as fibrocystic disease and chronic cystic mastitis, is less among pill users. Since the pill helps protect a woman against these benign breast diseases which are thought to predispose a woman to the development of breast cancer, it might protect her against breast cancer, although this has not been proven.

There is, similarly, no evidence that a woman who takes oral contraceptives increases her chances of developing cervical cancer. However, the portrait of the woman who runs the highest risk of cervical cancer (a woman who is sexually active at a young age, has a number of sexual partners, and has a child early in life) is probably the very woman who will opt for contraception via birth-control pills. One study showed that women who used the diaphragm rather than the pill for contraception had a lower incidence of cervical cancer, but this was attributed to the protective properties of the diaphragm rather than the direct effect of the pill.

There is some preliminary evidence that oral contraceptives increase the risk of developing endometrial cancer. In the spring of 1976, twenty-one cases of endometrial cancer were reported in women under the age of forty who used oral contraceptives. Thirteen of these women used the sequential birth-control pills, which have since been withdrawn from the market. Although the incidence of cancer is very low, women who experience irregular bleeding that is neither controlled by increasing the dosage of the pill nor subsides after the first three cycles should have an endometrial biopsy.

Summary

There is no perfect form of contraception. It seems that as the effectiveness of the contraceptive increases, the risk inherent in its use also increases. However, the benefit-risk ratio is very favorable for oral contraceptives. Besides their extreme effectiveness, oral contraceptives relieve severe dysmenorrhea, decrease the amount of blood lost during menstruation by 50 percent, and alleviate premenstrual tension. Women with chronic cystic mastitis and fibrocystic breast disease receive some symptomatic relief from taking oral contraceptives. Oral contraceptives produce a decreased incidence in ovarian cysts, duodenal ulcers, sebaceous cysts, and acne. There is even a 25 percent decrease in ear wax production!

There are risks involved in oral contraceptives, but they are not as great as the risks involved in pregnancy. Women should be aware that the pill can have serious side effects. The risk involved in oral contraception is magnified for women who smoke. They should protect themselves by notifying physicians of the appearance of any symptoms. It has been said there are no safe drugs, only safe physicians. This could be changed to: There are no safe pills, only informed women.

The pill has changed the life-style of almost an entire generation of women. It has given them a new freedom of expression in their sexual, academic, and financial lives. Perhaps most importantly, it has given them the expectation that a reliable method of birth control is their right. The pill may not be the ultimate method of contraception, but if that ultimate method is ever discovered, it will be based on the expectations raised by the pill.

THE "MORNING-AFTER" PILL

The so-called morning-after pill should not be considered a routine method of contraception but used only as an emergency measure. It is used in extreme cases such as rape and contraceptive failure. The theory behind the morning-after pill is that extremely high doses of estrogen over a period of days prevent implantation of a fertilized egg. The administration of this hormone must be started within seventy-two hours of unprotected intercourse. The dose schedule is 25 milligrams of diethylstilbestrol twice a day for five days, or 5 milligrams of ethinyl estradiol (administered in ten tablets of 0.5 mg.) for five days. Some physicians administer a type of estrogen at a dose of 1.25 milligrams three times a day for five days. These very high amounts of estrogen often produce severe side effects: constant nausea, vomiting, and water retention. If the morning-after pills fail to interrupt the pregnancy, abortion is usually indicated. The high dose of estrogen has been found to cause abnormalities in the fetus and diethylstilbestrol has been found to cause vaginal cancer in the daughters and genital abnormalities in the sons of treated women.

It must be emphasized that the morning-after pill should only be used for emergency situations and not as a routine contraception. The effects of its long-term and continued usage have not been estimated. Recent studies indicate that an IUD inserted immediately after intercourse has been effective morning-after treatment for unprotected intercourse and may be considered an alternative to the morning-after pill.

PROGESTERONE INJECTIONS FOR CONTRACEPTION

An injectable progesterone contraceptive, Depo-Provera, is being used by nearly a million women around the world. It works by inhibiting ovulation, making the cervical mucus impenetrable to the sperm and the lining of the uterus unreceptive to a fertilized egg. It has an apparent effectiveness rate of about 99 percent.

The administration of Depo-Provera consists of a simple shot of 150 milligrams of injectable progesterone once every three months. Though the contraceptive works well, there are several side effects, including irregular bleeding, amenorrhea, and weight gain. The irregular bleeding usually straightens itself out after a few months. If there is no change in the amenorrhea, the injections may have to be discontinued. The average time for conception after discontinuing Depo-Provera has been about a year, although menstruation begins in about three months. Animal studies in the United States showed Depo-Provera may lead to breast cancer in beagle dogs. As beagles do not metabolize hormones in the same manner as humans, the studies do not necessarily prove that there would be similar side effects in women. Depo-Provera might soon be released by the Food and Drug Administration for contraceptive use in the United States.

BREAST-FEEDING AS A FORM OF CONTRACEPTION

If a woman fully breast-feeds her newborn child, she is usually protected from pregnancy for two to four months after delivery. However, as soon as she shows any sign of menstruation, even minimal vaginal spotting, or starts giving her child a supplementary bottle, she must seek some other form of contraception. Oral contraceptives are contraindicated in a breast-feeding woman because the synthetic hormones could be passed to the infant via the milk. An IUD, a diaphragm, or contraceptive jellies are all acceptable alternatives.

DOUCHING FOR CONTRACEPTION

Many people still believe that a quick douche after intercourse prevents pregnancy. In fact, sperm swim so fast, they can reach the uterus and the fallopian tubes within three to five minutes after coitus, or often before you get to the bathroom. Douching, therefore, has absolutely no effect as a contraceptive. Too frequent douching may wash away the normal defensive bacteria of the vagina. It may even push the sperm into the uterus. Postcoital douching may be of some undetermined benefit in reducing the chance of contracting venereal disease, but it has no value as a contraceptive.

One of the prevailing myths among teenagers in the United States is that Coca-Cola is a particularly effective douche. Girls who do not get pregnant after a Coke douche are simply lucky; the Coke is about as effective taken vaginally as it would be taken orally.

THE FUTURE OF CONTRACEPTION

There is a continuing search for safe, effective, and reversible forms of contraception. The major thrust of this research has been aimed at women. There has been research focused on the inhibition of sperm production in the male, but it seems easier to interrupt the mechanism involved in the production of a single egg a month, compared to blocking the millions of sperm which are produced in a man every day.

Silastic Implants

There has been research in a number of foreign countries into the contraceptive effectiveness of progesterone released slowly from a silastic device implanted under the skin of the arm. These silastic devices are "injected" under the skin with special instruments and usually have to be replaced every year, although some devices release progesterone for a period of three years. The major side effect is extremely irregular bleeding. There have been reports of break-through bleeding, weight gain, and, on occasion, irritation from the site of the injected silastic capsule.

Vaginal Rings

Doughnut-shaped vaginal rings that slowly release progesterone have been developed. These steroid-releasing devices are placed in the vagina for three weeks, then removed for one week to allow cyclic bleeding. They are then replaced. It is believed that these devices act like the minipill in that they do not inhibit ovulation but prevent fertilization and implantation. Devices are also being tested that are left in the vagina for more than three weeks.

The advantage of such a device over the pill is that it requires insertion only once every month, eliminating the need for daily medication. The major disadvantage is that it is a foreign body within the vagina and might predispose the user to vaginal infections.

Once-a-Month Suppositories

A woman with an active and unprotected sex life would, on the average, become pregnant every three to four months. Even without contraception, a woman would not get pregnant every cycle. Women who try to become pregnant find that it is almost impossible to pick the exact month in which they will conceive. A delayed menses is often one of the first signs of pregnancy. Vaginal suppositories comprised of *prostaglandin analogs* are being studied for the induction of uterine contractions and menses in the nonpregnant woman, and contractions causing a very early abortion in the pregnant patient. More than one hundred women with confirmed pregnancies of under seven weeks have received these prostaglandin suppositories and successfully aborted in Sweden.

In this country, similar research is being performed with two prostaglandin vaginal suppositories, inserted in the doctor's office as an out-patient procedure. It is hoped that these new therapies will permit the induction of menses and very early abortion in a manner almost identical to spontaneous abortion, thus minimizing the need for *mechanical* interruption of pregnancy.

New Oral Contraceptives

Recent drug research has yielded a promising new agent, *danazol* (Danocrine). By inhibiting the release of LH and FSH from the pituitary gland, danazol suppresses stimulation of ovulation. Danazol has been effective in the treatment of endocrine disorders, as well as pelvic endometriosis and chronic cystic breast disease. Since it has a further advantage of containing no estrogen, work is being done to determine its use as a birth-control pill. Additional research is needed before any affirmative statement can be made about danazol as an oral contraceptive.

The contraceptive effectiveness of an *antiprogesterone drug* is being investigated. The progesterone produced after ovulation is necessary for the maintenance of pregnancy once an egg is fertilized. Any drug that inhibited progesterone production would also prevent pregnancy. This antiprogesterone would not have to be taken throughout the cycle, only during the immediate postovulation days. Such an antiprogesterone has been developed and has been tested in 160 women in Haiti, but the pregnancy rate on it is still too high. The concept, however, is valid, and more work is being done.

Vaccination for Contraception

Vaccines have been used to protect the body against a variety of diseases from measles to polio. Perhaps a vaccine could be developed that would interfere with normal conception. When a person is vaccinated against any disease, a small amount of material resembling the disease is injected into the body—briefly, the person is given a very, very mild case of the disease. The body's natural defenses rally to destroy the injected material by producing antibodies. These antibodies then continue to circulate in the blood, giving prolonged protection against future invasion by a similar germ. In some diseases the protection is lifelong. With other diseases, the antibodies need renewing and booster shots are needed at periodic intervals.

For years, it has been hoped that the ability of the body to produce antibodies against foreign substances could be used for contraceptive purposes. It is well known that prostitutes are usually extremely infertile. They produce antibodies against sperm, and it is believed that their overexposure to sperm is the basis for this condition. A woman's production of antibodies to her partner's sperm is one of the causes of infertility. Attempts have been made to isolate and synthesize these sperm antibodies, but there has been little success in this area.

Another approach in the search for a contraceptive vaccine is far more subtle and involves stimulating the body to produce antibodies against *hormones* involved in conception. In other words, the body is asked to raise antibodies against a natural substance rather than against a foreign invader. Vaccinations against the gonadotrophins LH and FSH have been studied in both female and male animals. In female animals, antibody inactivation of LH and FSH prevented ovulation and also severely affected the menstrual cycle, while decreasing the production of female hormones. In male animals, antibodies raised against LH caused testicular atrophy, and a severe drop in testosterone caused a decreased libido. This change was so exaggerated that these male animals were rejected by the other inhabitants of the animal colony.

It was concluded that disruption of the normal process of reproduction by antifertility vaccines is more feasible in women, since women can be immunized to placental hormones or proteins. Thus pregnancy might be prevented without interfering with the normal female hormones, ovulation, or menstruation. In men, there are few substances that can be inhibited with antibodies without disturbing vital hormone production as well as other organs.

Complex proteins which appear to play a necessary role in the maintenance of pregnancy have been isolated from the placenta. Antibodies have been produced against these proteins in rabbits and sheep. These antibodies have produced abortion in pregnant monkeys.

There is a very particular type of HCG (human chorionic gonadotrophin), called *beta-subunit HCG*. This is only found during pregnancy, and the maintenance of pregnancy might be prevented by a vaccine against beta-subunit HCG. Antibodies that destroy the biologic activity of beta-subunit HCG have been raised in laboratory animals and, when injected into other animals, these antibodies have caused interruption of a pregnancy by preventing, if conception occurred, the formation of the placenta. Researchers in India and Sweden have vaccinated women volunteers with the beta-subunit HCG antibodies. This single vaccination appears to have prevented the maintenance of pregnancy. The vaccine seems to be without other significant side effects, but the women seem to be irreversibly immune and unable to conceive for the rest of their lives.

There are enzymes normally present on the surface of the sperm. One of these enzymes, *lactic dehydrogenase* (LDH-X), has been isolated from the surface of mouse sperm and found to cause a cross-reaction with the similar enzyme in several species, including humans. Female mice and rabbits who were injected with the purified lactic dehydrogenase developed antibodies against this sperm enzyme, with a consequent reduction in fertility of up to 80 percent, *and the effects were reversible*. Studies of this type of active immunization are being carried out in monkeys, but the antifertility effects of the injected enzyme must be improved. The mouse lactic dehydrogenase was also injected into male rabbits, and fertility was decreased in direct relation to the amount of antibody in the blood, without any effects on libido. Again, the antifertility effect of the vaccination was reversible. A number of other sperm enzymes are also being investigated for their antifertility effects.

The Male Pill

Contraceptive research has not been limited to methods of female fertility control; there have been a number of studies into the efficacy of agents which will inhibit sperm production in the male or render the sperm incapable of fertilizing the ovum. High doses of female hormones such as estrogen may decrease sperm production, but would have a number of side effects such as decrease in libido and the development of female secondary sex characteristics. Administration of high doses of estrogen is a primary step in a male-to-female transsexual operation.

The antifertility effect of a new drug, danazol, on men has shown some promise. This potent drug, which inhibits the gonadotrophins (LH, FSH), has recently been released by the Food and Drug Administration under the name of Danocrine for the treatment of pelvic endometriosis. Danazol is also being tested in women as an oral contraceptive. When danazol alone was given to a group of male volunteers, the reduction in sperm count was not consistent and the men complained of decreased libido. In later trials, 600-milligram doses of danazol daily were given in association with a monthly intramuscular injection of testosterone. This combined therapy resulted in a striking drop in sperm count—to infertile levels—within four to eight weeks. More than fifty men have been treated with danazol and testosterone with no apparent side effects and no decrease in libido or sexual potency. The antifertility effects of this combined treatment are reversible, and sperm count returns to fertile levels eight to ten weeks after discontinuation of the danazol. Widespread and long-term studies are needed to determine the full antifertility effects of danazol in the male.

Even if a male pill is developed, there is some doubt that women would actually trust the man to take it. A male pill would be acceptable in an established relationship where both partners assume responsibility for contraception, but there may be little acceptance among people practicing casual sex.

The Chinese claim to have developed an effective male oral contraceptive—*gossypol*. A derivative of the cotton plant, gossypol is said to interfere with sperm maturation. This agent has been given to tens of thousands of men in China with anticontraceptive effectiveness approaching 100 percent. These results are being carefully scrutinized in this country in an effort to establish the drug's effectiveness and also to determine its side effects, which may prove to be serious.

Heat as a Male Contraceptive

One approach to birth control has been to increase the temperature of the testes. In both humans and animals, sperm must be stored at a temperature a few degrees lower than body temperature to maintain their fertility. This is why the testicles are outside the body, with their own specialized circulatory system. The effect of heat on the inhibition of sperm is consistent throughout the animal kingdom; no animal has hair or fur on the testicles. If the temperature of the testicles is raised a few degrees, the fertility of the sperm drops. The contraceptive effects of hot baths have been tested by the Japanese. Other researchers have developed a "testicle warmer" to be worn constantly. Although these somewhat bizarre methods appear effective, they have very little general appeal.

WHICH CONTRACEPTIVE METHOD IS BEST FOR ME?

It has been demonstrated that there is a safe method of contraception for every woman, although the same method cannot be used by every woman throughout her fertile age. If a teenager decides she is ready for sex, she should also be ready to assume the responsibility of obtaining contraception; a doctor or family-planning clinic can help her choose the method best suited to her needs. Recent studies conducted in Great Britain and the United States have shown that birth-control pills containing less than fifty micrograms of estrogen when used by healthy, informed women are relatively risk free. No late ill effect of these low estrogen birth-control pills has been found, and it is believed that this type of oral contraceptive is particularly suited to young women who have not borne children and in whom pregnancy would be a catastrophe. Young women are much more fertile and they need an extremely effective method of contraception. An intrauterine device might be more appropriate for a woman who has already borne a child and wishes to conceive again at planned intervals. It would be less advisable for a woman who is prone to pelvic infections or who is sexually active with several partners. However, the pill can still safely be used by motivated women after their teens. There has been a reported higher incidence of cardio-vascular side effects among pill users who smoke. The difference between smokers and nonsmokers, though, is not significant until the age of 35. Women who don't smoke could continue taking the pill until age 40, but should then use another method. The barrier methods —diaphragm, cervical cup, foam, creams or jellies—are all effective for women at any age; however, the effectiveness greatly depends on a woman's motivation to use them and on her understanding of her own body. Finally, the condom, easily available over the counter, should always be kept in mind as an effective alternative that provides an added bonus of prophylaxis against VD.

chapter 10

VOLUNTARY STERILIZATION

In the wake of society's ongoing concern over birth control, an age-old procedure, improved by modern techniques, still provides a great number of women and men with a safe and reliable method of contraception. That procedure is sterilization, a viable and voluntary alternative to other contraceptive methods.

Voluntary sterilization has been the victim of some very unfair attacks and myths. Many people associate it with castration and/or any one of a number of cruel punishments. Still others think it desexes a person.

In fact, voluntary sterilization is one of the greatest aids to the world community. It helps rich countries and Third World nations alike. It's no wonder that it has become the world's leading method of final and definitive contraception.

The United States arrived late at full acceptance of voluntary sterilization. Just ten years ago, only a few hospitals in the country allowed women to undergo the procedure voluntarily. Even then, women had to have four or five children and submit to a hospital committee before gaining approval for the operation. This was the subject of many lawsuits in the late 1960s.

When New York State passed its Abortion Law in 1970, it was a major breakthrough for the advocates of voluntary sterilization. That law, supported by recent Supreme Court rulings, effectively gave women control over their own bodies. No longer could doctors or society dictate to women or rule their bodies. For the first time in history, a woman could choose what to do with her body—to have a child or not. Of course, this ethical and legal concept naturally extended to the area of sterilization.

Today, people all around the nation and world can volunteer for sterilization. Some hospitals still require a woman to have her husband's consent, which seems unjust, because, after all, a man doesn't need his wife's consent to have a vasectomy.

Fig. 10–1: The female and male sterilization symbols. The female is to the left and the male to the right. These are the classic sexual symbols, with a portion removed from the circle. Some men who have undergone vasectomy wear pins bearing the male sterilization symbol; these are called vasectomy pins.

PROS & CONS OF STERILIZATION

Voluntary sterilization protects not only against unwanted pregnancies, but against "accidents" as well. Accidents happen to everyone. A woman can forget to take her pill. A diaphragm can be inserted improperly. An IUD can lose its chemical effectiveness. A man can have a condom slide off at just the wrong moment. These are not uncommon events; they are altogether human. While these contraceptive methods are relatively effective, it is interesting to note that the failure for each is composed largely of such accidents. These are prevented by sterilization.

The virtual certainty of pregnancy prevention brings many side benefits. It relieves the anxiety of unwanted pregnancy, while allowing a couple their choice of family size. It allows the retarded to marry and lead normal lives. It prevents the transmission of hereditary abnormalities. It also relieves the family and society of a financial burden.

In general, the systemic effects of sterilization should be minimal, and it should not interfere with sexual pleasure. In fact, many people find sex more pleasurable when the anxieties surrounding unwanted conception are relieved.

Problems with Sterilization

Sterilization is not completely without side effects. As voluntary sterilization has become the most popular form of contraception in the United States, new and previously unrecognized problems with female sterilization have emerged. Tubal sterilization in a woman involves destruction of part of the fallopian tube. If this destruction is too extensive, interference with ovarian blood flow may occur and systemic effects can follow. A woman might experience certain menopausal symptoms such as "hot flashes." A change in the pattern and amount of menstrual bleeding may occur, and there is some indication of increased susceptibility to the development of ovarian cysts. Adhesion formation is also possible. These adhesions can cause pain, and in rare cases, necessitate a hysterectomy.

Problems with male sterilization have also been more fully recognized and will be discussed later in this chapter in the section on male sterilization techniques.

FEMALE STERILIZATION

Sterilization for a woman is called *tubal ligation*. It is a procedure in which the continuity of the fallopian tubes is interrupted. There are many new and emerging techniques, but this surgery is basically separated into two categories: (1) sterilization through the abdomen; and (2) sterilization through the vagina. In both, the tubes are either cut, tied, or clamped so that the egg will not meet a sperm and pass into the uterus. There is, of course, no pregnancy if the egg does not meet the sperm.

Postpartum Sterilization (Sterilization after Childbirth)

An ideal time to perform female sterilization is immediately after childbirth, usually within one or two days. At that time, the uterus is enlarged, making it much easier to find the fallopian tubes. The woman is usually placed under a general or spinal anesthetic. An incision approximately one and a half inches long is made immediately underneath or inside the navel. One finger can usually sweep over the fundus (top) of the uterus and reach the fallopian tubes, or the surgeon can use a small instrument to pick up the tubes. With the tubes in direct vision, the sterilization can be performed very easily.

By having the so-called *postpartum* tubal sterilization done, a woman does not need a second hospitalization; she can recuperate

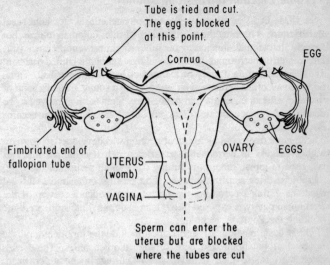

Tube is tied and cut.
The egg is blocked
at this point.

Cornua

EGG

Fimbriated end of
fallopian tube

OVARY   EGGS

UTERUS
(womb)

VAGINA

Sperm can enter the
uterus but are blocked
where the tubes are cut

Fig. 10-2: Locations in which tubal ligations have been performed. Ovulation can occur, but the egg is blocked where the tube has been tied and cut. The egg, therefore, dies and is reabsorbed in the tube. The sperm can freely swim into the uterus, but cannot reach the egg, since the sperm are blocked where the tube has been tied and cut.

The fimbriated ends of the fallopian tubes are also shown. A *fimbriaectomy* is a form of sterilization in which the fimbriated ends on both sides are removed. A *cornual resection* of the tubes is a complete removal of the fallopian tubes from the cornua area of the uterus (indicated by arrow).

from the delivery and the surgery at the same time. She also does not have to worry about leaving the child alone if she should be readmitted for a tubal ligation.

The abdominal approach is also applied when sterilization is performed at the time of Caesarean birth. As that area is open during the bearing, it is a good time to perform tubal ligation.

It should be kept in mind that a woman *must be certain* this will be her last childbirth before undergoing sterilization. A woman carrying an unwanted pregnancy should not hastily choose to have her tubes ligated.

Tubal Ligation during Laparotomy

In 1834, Dr. Von Blundell, the first physician to write about tubal sterilization, suggested total resection of the fallopian tubes, but thought that simple division of the tubes might prevent pregnancy. A Dr. Lundgren performed the first tubal ligation in the United States in 1881. Since then, a variety of techniques has been described. Tubal ligation was often performed by just placing a suture around a loop of the tube without cutting a part of the tube. This method proved to be unsuccessful, since the tie often slipped off and the woman became fertile again.

The Pomeroy technique of tubal ligation was developed to ensure a higher success in permanent sterilization. This technique involves tying the fallopian tube, plus cutting out a small section of the tube, thereby ensuring sterilization even if the tie slips off. Almost all tubal ligations during laparotomy (an operation in which a section of the abdominal cavity is exposed through an abdominal incision) are done utilizing the Pomeroy technique.

Other basic methods of sterilization include the fimbriectomy, the removal of the fimbriated ends of the fallopian tubes. These ends catch the egg, so their removal allows the egg to go unfertilized. Fimbriectomy is performed through an abdominal incision.

Also performed abdominally is a cornual resection of the uterus. The entire cornual area (the upper corners of the uterus) is excised. This, however, is an extensive and rather unnecessary operation. The Pomeroy technique seems to be the most efficient operation, with an almost 100 percent success rate. Tubal sterilization by exploratory laparotomy is performed in vast numbers, but its popularity has decreased in the past few years because it requires a postoperative hospitalization of five to seven days.

Voluntary Sterilization by Minilaparotomy

A mini-lap is an operation through a very small incision. This technique is less complicated and faster than a regular laparotomy (abdominal operation). It is done under general, spinal, or local anesthesia. The operation takes twenty to thirty minutes and is, basically, a simplification of a laparotomy. This procedure is often done for postpartum sterilization. The mini-lap is done the world over and is, in several countries, the preferred mode of sterilization. More importantly, it can be performed on an outpatient basis—if the patient tolerates the procedure, she can go home the same day. In the United

States, a woman usually stays in the hospital for a few days, but in other countries, it is a same-day procedure.

Very similar to the laparotomy, an incision only one-third the size of a normal laparotomy incision is made just above the pubic hairline. The one-inch incision allows the doctor to insert small instruments and bring the tubes into direct vision. He can then tie the tube and excise a small segment in a modification of the Pomeroy technique. The tubal ligation can also be done by placing a special clip on the tube. This method is relatively new but makes reversibility more possible.

The complication rate with this technique seems extremely low, although if a woman is very obese, the procedure becomes more difficult. For example, in 2,800 procedures performed recently by 112 surgeons at fifty different hospitals in Thailand, complications ranged from only 0.4 to one percent.

Sterilization Via the Band-Aid Procedure (Laparoscopy)

Laparoscopy is presently the preferred technique in this country. The *laparoscope* is a periscope-type instrument that is inserted through an incision in the navel. It makes readily visible all parts of the abdomen—most importantly, the uterus, the ovaries, and the tubes. This slender, tubular instrument has many advantages. Primarily, it has a fiber optic light source which allows the physician to visualize the internal organs. Fiberoptics (a cold, nonburning source of light) have improved almost all *endoscopic*, or internal, instruments. Infections can be spotted through the laparoscope, tube endings can be checked for infertility problems, and fibroid tumors can be detected on the uterus.

For a sterilization using the laparoscope, a woman is placed under a local or general anesthetic. She is then placed in the Trendelenburg position (a tilted position in which the head is lowered and the legs are elevated). A small incision is made in the navel. In order to get a better visual field and push the bowels toward the diaphragm during the operation, carbon dioxide (CO_2) is first injected into the abdominal cavity. The laparoscope is then inserted and the light source attached. The physician first closely observes the bowels, and maybe the appendix. His attention is then focused on the uterus, the tubes, and the ovaries.

The sterilization can be performed through the laparoscope itself by insertion of an abdominal forceps through the instrument. More often a second incision is made near the pubic hairline and the abdominal

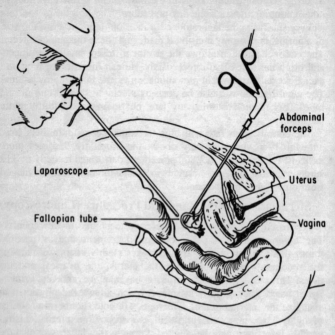

Fig. 10–3: A tubal ligation performed through a laparoscopy (the Band-Aid operation). If a tubal sterilization is performed, abdominal forceps can be inserted through a small hole in the lower abdomen (as shown in figure). The forceps can also be inserted through the laparoscope.

forceps is inserted through that incision. From here, a variety of techniques can be effected; the most common is tubal cauterization. During this procedure, the fallopian tubes are picked up by the abdominal forceps and are then cauterized (burned), and a piece of the tube is removed. This is quite effective, but if cauterization of the tube is excessive, the result can be interference with ovarian blood flow; there is also a possibility of burning the bowels. It should, therefore, only be done by physicians who are familiar with the procedure.

Recently there has been some experimentation with clips and rings.

A device called the *tantalum wick hemoclip* can be inserted through the laparoscope and attached to the tubes. The portion of the tube between the clips is then removed.

Also, the *silicone ring* (fallopian ring) is experiencing recent success. The "ring" is squeezed down on the tubes during laparoscopy, cutting off canalization of the tubes. An advantage to this technique is that reversibility is more feasible, since only a small portion of the tubes has been damaged.

After the actual sterilization, the physician checks through the laparoscope to see that no bleeding has occurred. The instrument is then pulled out, the CO_2 is expelled, and one or two sutures are placed underneath the skin. A small Band-Aid is placed over the incision. It takes only about thirty to fifty minutes, and the patient who has been under a local anesthesia can go home the same day; the patient who has general anesthesia can usually be discharged the following day.

There are contraindications to laparoscopic sterilization. Prime considerations are previous appendectomy or other previous abdominal surgery causing adhesions. Cardiac disease might make the operation dangerous, since the abdomen is distended with the CO_2, causing pressure on the lungs. Obesity is another factor. In the case of an overweight woman, it is almost impossible to insert the laparoscope correctly. One final caution: Make certain the physician is trained and experienced in laparoscopy. The laparoscope is a delicate instrument, and one with which not all doctors are familiar. A physician can easily perforate the bowels and burn organs if he is not expert. If a large portion of the tubes are damaged by coagulation, there could be a decreased blood supply to the ovaries resulting in abdominal pain and future irregular bleeding.

Culdoscopic Tubal Sterilization

Another means of female sterilization is via a *colpotomy,* an operation in which the abdominal cavity is entered through a small incision in the vagina. The *culdoscope* is a periscope which is inserted through the vaginal wall rather than the abdomen (see Fig. 16–7). The woman is placed in the knee-chest position, which is a position in which she sits on her knees, hands forward, resting her chest on a table (see Fig. 16–6). The operation is always performed using only local anesthesia. A speculum is inserted into the vagina and pulled backward to increase the physician's ability to see the area. The cervix is then held with a tenaculum (special forceps) and a small incision is made behind the cervix, through which the culdoscope is inserted. A fiberoptic light source attached to the culdoscope enables the physician to see the pelvic organs. After visualization, the tubes are picked up through the culdoscope by a small instrument. The fallopian tubes are ligated, most likely with the use of a special hemoclip, which is squeezed around the tubes. A portion is then excised between two clips.

The infection rate has been high after this type of operation. Yet if a doctor is familiar with colposcopy this poses no real problem. Actually, this operation has no really deterrent factors, as there is no need for gas insufflation in the abdominal cavity. In skilled hands, this is a twenty-minute operation and a good method. The woman can be discharged the same day. The operation is, however, associated with considerable discomfort because of the position in which the woman must be and because only local anesthesia is used. In this country, culdoscopy is used only in rare cases for sterilization.

Hysteroscopic Sterilization

The final internal instrument to be discussed is the *hysteroscope*. The hysteroscope is another periscopic-type tool passed through the vagina and the cervix on its way to visualizing the uterine cavity. It has been considered valuable for inspecting and diagnosing cancer of the uterus.

The major difficulty with the hysteroscope is that the uterine cavity has to be distended to get a clear view. Different types of hysteroscopes have been developed. The first type had a balloon on the tip, which was blown up inside the uterus to expand the cavity. The more recent ones use Dextran (a highly viscous solution) or CO_2 to distend the uterine cavity to give a better view. When the cavity is distended, it can be carefully inspected through hysteroscope and the opening of the tubes can be seen. A fine operative instrument can then be placed through the hysteroscope. Biopsies from the uterus can be obtained and various types of tubal sterilizations can be performed.

Recently, means of closing the fallopian tubes through the hysteroscope have been investigated. As yet there is no definitive technique, but cauterization of the cornual area of the fallopian tubes is being attempted, as is the placement of various types of plugs into the tubes to prevent sperm migration.

A method is being examined in which a solution is injected directly into the tubes through the hysteroscope. Research is being done on just this kind of solution, which would block off the tubes permanently, or at least for a long period of time. If hysteroscopic

Hysteroscopy

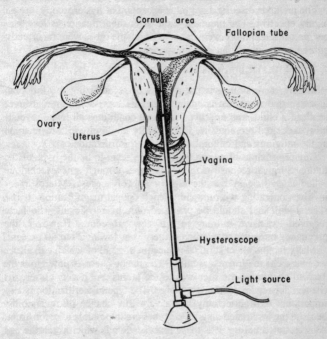

Fig. 10-4: Hysteroscopy is a procedure in which a hysteroscope (a periscope-type instrument) is inserted into the uterine cavity to enable the physician to look into the uterus. The hysteroscope is inserted through the vagina and the cervix into the uterus without any need for an abdominal incision.

sterilization one day becomes readily available and the technique is improved, this would be a highly recommended method, since the sterilization could be done on an outpatient basis and would result in only minimal pain and discomfort.

A few researchers are exploring the possibility of inserting "plugs" into the fallopian tubes via the hysteroscope. These plugs would block the tubes while they were there, but could be removed if pregnancy was desired. A new form of *reversible* sterilization will be born if this technique proves safe and feasible. It is now still in a developmental stage.

The methods discussed, with the exception of hysteroscopy, are all highly effective. The pregnancy rate after tubal ligation is less than one percent, and those were cases in which the tubes were incorrectly burned or the physician was inexperienced.

Are Tubal Ligations Reversible?

Simply, reversibility is the process of recanalizing the fallopian tubes so that a woman is again fertile. Factors such as remarriage, death of a child, and improved financial conditions all make reversibility a desired prerequisite. Reversibility might also eliminate some of the religious and cultural objections to sterilization.

Devices such as clips and silastic rings seem to be the hope of the future. Surgical reconstruction of the tubes through a new technique called *microsurgery* has the highest rate of success. Microsurgery involves operating with the aid of high optical magnification. It is a special skill and should be practiced *only* by physicians who have received extensive training in this new procedure. However, the pregnancy rate even after microsurgery is as low as 20 to 40 percent.

Many factors affect surgical reconstruction, all of which can alter a woman's chance for reversibility. The major factor is how close the excised portion of the tube was to the uterus. As it gets closer, the chances for reconstruction get higher. The type of sterilization is also important. A fimbriectomy has a very low chance of reversibility because the fimbriated ends of the tubes are impossible to reconstruct. As was stated before, it is these fimbriated ends which catch the egg and determine fertility.

If a woman decides to attempt reversibility, she should be aware that surgical reconstruction isn't nearly as simple an operation as a tubal ligation, and the chances of conception are very slim. Sterilization should only be considered as a final method of contraception.

Hysterectomy—The Most Effective Sterilization?

Several physicians advocate hysterectomy as a means of final sterilization. Women occasionally experience irregular bleeding after a tubal ligation; this might be due to the operation interfering with the blood supply to the ovaries. To avoid this, many gynecologists recommend hysterectomy as sterilization because it avoids later complications. For women with uterine abnormalities, irregular bleeding, or vaginal prolapse who have completed their families, hysterectomies might possibly be considered as a means of sterilization. This most drastic form of sterilization should be limited to rare, clearly indicated instances.

When Should Sterilization Be Considered?

All factors considered, one basic element remains: Only a woman who has completed her childbearing, or a woman for whom pregnancy and childbearing would be dangerous, should undergo sterilization. Women in their early twenties with unwanted pregnancies shouldn't hastily decide to have their tubes tied because they are temporarily angry at the entire male population. Likewise, young women with one or two children would be wise to use a form of birth control until they are older and certain they have completed their families. There are few emotional side effects to sterilization in the case of the thirty-five-year-old career woman, whereas there are many when dealing with the occasional young woman who never wants to see another man in her life. When the anger ebbs and she returns three years later with a prospective husband, she faces the uncertain prospect of reversibility. A woman should not only think twice, but perhaps three times before she consents to sterilization.

Which Type of Sterilization Should a Woman Choose?

The simplest form of tubal sterilization is the Band-Aid procedure —tubal sterilization via laparoscopy. This procedure requires only one or two days of hospitalization, and the incision can usually be made inside the navel so that no scar is visible. Whether a silastic ring or a hemoclip is used is left to the discretion of the physician. A laparoscopy cannot be performed if you have had previous extensive abdominal surgery or if you are very obese. A laparotomy is then suggested.

What Does Tubal Sterilization Cost?

Among private physicians, fees vary from doctor to doctor. If you have good health insurance, it might pay a portion of this fee. It would be wise to discuss the fee with the doctor or his secretary before the surgery. The hospital fee is usually covered by health insurance. If you go to clinics, the operation is often completely covered. Patients with Medicaid usually get the entire procedure covered through the Medicaid. However, check locally, since this also varies from place to place.

MALE STERILIZATION

Vasectomy, or sterilization of the male, is not *castration*. Castration is a removal of the testes, and the connotations surrounding it in former days prevented the growth of popularity of vasectomy, which is a completely different procedure. Anything that remotely resembled tampering with the male organs was in the past avoided. As the unwarranted fears relating to vasectomy were dispelled, it affected more men on a worldwide basis. In spite of the fact that vasectomy is much less complex than tubal ligation, tubal ligation was for years the preferred method of sterilization. Recently, however, the popularity of vasectomy has increased rapidly.

In Asia, for example, vasectomies have exceeded tubal ligations in number. Between 1968 and 1972, six million vasectomies were performed in India. The rates are equally staggering in Pakistan,

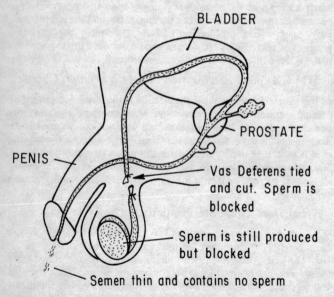

Fig. 10–5:   A vasectomy. The vas deferens (the tube which leads the sperm from the testes to the prostate gland) has been tied and cut. This blocks the sperm, which continue to be produced in the testes.

Nepal, and Bangladesh. In fact, the numbers have been increasing in many Third World countries, most notably in Latin America.

The concept of vasectomy was initiated in 1885 by Felix Guyon of France, who concluded that blocking off the *vas deferens* (the two tubes which carry semen) caused an atrophy of the prostate. At the beginning of this century, vasectomy was performed for eugenic reasons on criminals, the mentally ill, and those with hereditary diseases. It became popular in Asia in the 1950s, as it tried to replace ineffectual birth-control practices.

Even in the United States and Europe, vasectomy has seeped into the consciousness of the male population. As oral contraceptives received adverse publicity, and as feminism stirred feelings of male responsibility, the figures took on a startling change. In 1969, a quarter of a million men in the United States had vasectomies. In 1970, it was three quarters of a million, a two hundred percent jump!

Procedure of Vasectomy

The operation is simple enough and, in most cases, is done by a urologist in his office. As there are many different techniques, a specialist may perform a specific type of sterilization.

In most cases, the patient is given a local anesthetic, injected into the skin of his washed scrotum. Although an occasionally squeamish man may ask for a general anesthetic, it is not recommended. The pain is minimal and he can usually be released minutes after the surgery.

After the scrotum is numb, a small incision is made and the *vas deferens* are pulled out. Clips are placed on the two ends and a small piece is excised. Depending on the skill of the physician, a suture may be used instead of a clip. For those so trained, *electrocautery* or *electrocoagulation* of the vas can be performed.

A small gauze bandage is then placed on the scrotal incision and held by an athletic supporter, or *scrotal suspensory*. The patient need stay off his feet only the first day.

The follow-up to this simple operation is as important as the surgery itself. The patient should not engage in sexual intercourse for at least a week. The pressure can prevent the vas from healing.

Secondly, the patient must know that he is not sterile for at least six weeks. All the residual sperm and products of ejaculation must be expelled before complete sterilization is effected. The stored sperm may take from one to several months to leave the body. Postoperative semen tests are recommended. These tests normally begin at the sixth week and end when two consecutive sperm counts are found negative.

Again, there are contraindications to sterilization, although they are much less severe for the man than for the woman. Local infections and blood disorders are the primary ones, but even previous hernia surgery can be a hindrance to the operation, depending on its severity.

Problems with Vasectomy

Those who undergo vasectomies should be warned of possible postoperative side effects. Most, such as discomfort and swelling, are common and go away in a week or so. Certain infections and hematomas can develop, and are treated accordingly.

Epididymitis (swelling and tenderness near the testes) has occurred in less than one percent of all vasectomies. It is treated with heat and/or a suspensory.

Sperm granuloma, an inflammatory response to the leakage of sperm, is another post-op problem. Again, it is usually not severe enough to be harmful, but if it does cause problems, the sperm can be drained surgically. *Granuloma* occurs in 0.1 to 3.0 percent of all vasectomies.

Sperm antibodies can be produced to destroy the sperm retained in the male's body following vasectomy. It is theorized that these sperm antibodies may interact with fats circulating in the bloodstream, resulting in the formation of plaque on blood vessel walls and other cardiovascular problems. However, this has only been confirmed in monkeys.

Reversibility

Again we approach the subject of reversibility, and again the prospect is not favorable. There are three major methods of reversal of vasectomy being researched. Only one is past the point of experimentation. This process is called *vas anastomosis* (also *vasovasotomy*). This is a surgical reconstruction of the vas. The vasovasotomy is a lengthy surgery which must be performed by a specially skilled surgeon employing microsurgical techniques. To date, it has been fairly successful, but not many physicians are familiar with this difficult operation.

There are two other methods of reversal which are still in the experimentation stage: (1) storage of the semen, and (2) vas-occlusive devices. Neither of these methods is yet accepted. The vas-occlusive (blocking) clips and silicone rings have been used only on monkeys. As for semen storage, this is not really reversibility; it is artificial insemination. A man about to decide whether he should be sterilized should know that vasovasotomy is his only chance of reversal. The word *chance* should be stressed.

Physical Factors

As vasectomy becomes more prominent the world over, certain physiological questions have been asked.

First is the question of the alteration in the male hormone count. The *spermatogenesis* (production of sperm) continues unchanged soon after the operation. There is no FSH or LH change whatsoever. There is, however, an increase in testosterone, which is produced in the testicles. If anything, this is a positive factor, as it is thought to increase desire.

Another controversy is the issue of sperm antibodies. It is true that one third to one half of all vasectomied men develop antibodies to sperm. This is an immunity established within the body which inhibits sperm activity. The condition is known in fertile men, but is more common in infertile ones.

Does Vasectomy Lead to Heart Disease?

The sperm antibody which follows vasectomy may be involved in the development of atherosclerosis. In a very well-controlled and well-conducted study by Drs. Nancy Alexander and Thomas Clarkson ten monkeys were fed a high cholesterol diet for six months. Five of the monkeys were then vasectomized and all were maintained on the high cholesterol for another six months. At the end of this time a significant increase in atherosclerosis was shown in the vasectomized monkeys as compared to the similarly treated control group. Although the number of animals in this initial test sample was small and the amount of cholesterol employed about twice as high as that in the average American diet, the results were consistent and significant. This study has been expanded and the results confirmed. At the present time it might be advisable for a man with a heart condition, history of high blood cholesterol, or atherosclerosis to reconsider vasectomy very carefully until the final results of long-term testing are available. If a man is already vasectomized, it might be advisable for him to avoid excess dietary cholesterol.

Psychological Factors

There is a psychological factor that remains in many men—fear. The fact that a doctor takes steel instruments, scissors, and hypodermic needles to his genitals can overwhelm many a timorous man. Yet a healthy man should be able to allay any fears with proper counseling. After all, there is certainly a bright side to being sterile.

First, in the hands of a skilled surgeon, the failure rate almost does not exist. The pregnancy rate is 0 to 0.15 percent. The recanalization of the vas is as unlikely as honesty in politics. It is, in fact, this release from anxiety which enhances the sex lives of a majority of vasecto-mized men.

In the United States alone, sterile men have a twenty percent higher frequency rate of sexual intercourse. Without the bother of birth control, the possible financial burden, and the increase of testoster-one, the sterile man has become more sexually active.

The only noticeable sexual change is that the semen is somewhat thinner. This is because the semen is coming only from the gland and the prostate. Indeed, when a man decides whether or not he should undergo a vasectomy, the emotional and financial relief should far outweigh some remotely possible physical change. However, men with serious neuroses or sexual maladjustments are not advised to submit themselves to the surgery. The psychological ramifications can be much more harmful than the physiological ones.

Recommendation

Vasectomy should not be performed so that a man can be more promiscuous. It should be an act of respect. Still, in Western culture, pride often stands in the way. Some men fearful of losing their masculinity would rather have their wives undergo the more compli-cated surgery than have a vasectomy in ten minutes. This is chauvinistic. For a couple healthy in mind and attitude, the vasectomy seems to be the preferred method of sterilization.

What Is the Cost of Vasectomy?

Done by a private physician, the complete cost (with interview, operation, and sperm count after the procedure) should be about $150 to $200. These prices are, of course, individual. Medicaid or private health-insurance companies might cover part or all of these expenses.

Further Information

If you want more information about voluntary sterilization and vasectomies in particular, contact your nearest Planned Parenthood affiliate (you can find it in your telephone directory) or one of the regional offices listed below:

Great Lakes: Illinois, Indiana, Michigan, Ohio, West Virginia, Wisconsin: 2625 Butterfield Road, Oak Brook, Illinois 60521 (312)986-9270

North Atlantic: Connecticut, Delaware, District of Columbia, (Maine), Maryland, Massachusetts, New Hampshire, New Jersey, New York, Pennsylvania, Rhode Island, Vermont: 810 7th Avenue, New York, New York 10019 (212)541-7800.

Southeast: Alabama, Florida, Georgia, Kentucky, (Mississippi), North Carolina, South Carolina, Tennessee, Virginia: 3030 Peachtree Road N.W., Rooms 301–303, Atlanta, Georgia 30305 (404)233-7117.

Central: Arkansas, Iowa, Kansas, (Louisiana), Missouri, Nebraska, New Mexico, Oklahoma, Texas: 2829 West Northwest Hwy, Dallas, Texas 75220 (214)350-8664.

Western: Alaska, Arizona, California, Colorado, Hawaii, Idaho, Montana, Nevada, (N. Dakota) or (S. Dakota), Utah, Washington, Wyoming: 785 Market Street, San Francisco, California 94103 (415)777-1217

*Parenthesized states indicates Planned Parenthood is not physically represented there.

The United States national voluntary agency for sterilization information is:

Association for Voluntary Sterilization
708 Third Avenue
New York, N. Y. 10017 (212)986-3880

chapter 11

ABORTION

The moral issue of abortion has been argued elsewhere, and it is not the purpose of this book either to condemn or condone. Our purpose is simply to present the medical facts. Abortion is now legal, and every year many women have their pregnancies interrupted. Whether or not you feel you have the right to terminate a pregnancy, you definitely have the right to know precisely what an abortion procedure entails.

Before legalized abortions were common, it was an everyday occurrence for women to arrive in hospital emergency rooms with serious hemorrhaging and infection from illegal backroom abortions. Many women died, and many more became sterile. Those who made it through physically unscathed were often emotionally devastated, stigmatized by the thought of having been through an underworld operation. Many kept the experience secret, fearing censure and the disdain of their family and friends.

Abortion has now become an accepted fact of life. Women can feel secure about having the procedure performed under sanitary conditions with modern techniques, and they can often share their fears and reservations with their friends without suffering embarrassment or social ostracism. Moreover, physicians are no longer forced to stand by and watch a woman die because of legal restraints.

Not only have abortion techniques improved tremendously in the past decade, but attitudes have changed so much that psychological and emotional counseling on abortion are now available in many places. This fulfills an urgent need. Thankfully, women have finally seized control of their own bodies.

HISTORY OF MODERN ABORTION

Abortions are categorized by the length of pregnancy. Pregnancies are broken up into trimesters. The first trimester lasts up to the twelfth week after the first day of the last menstruation, or the tenth week after conception.

Abortions were most commonly performed during the first trimester and the general method was a dilation and curettage (D&C). First the cervix was opened with instruments of increasing size until it would permit the passage of a curette, or spoon-shaped instrument (or catheter or coat hangers in the case of some illegal abortions). Then, bit by bit, the fetus, the placenta, and the membranes—the products of conception—were scraped away. This procedure was lengthy, and the uterine walls, which are soft during pregnancy, would often be punctured. Extensive bleeding often occurred. Sometimes the cervix was torn during the procedure. Occasionally too much tissue was scraped from the uterus, causing scar tissue that led to infertility. Even in the few legal abortions that were performed by this method, complications were frequent. Illegal abortions almost always led at least to minor problems.

The Chinese were the first to abandon this procedure. In the late 1950s, they introduced the *vacuum aspirator*. By the following decade, the vacuum technique had spread to Europe, England, and finally to the United States. By dilating the cervix to a lesser extent and by shortening the procedure considerably without actually scraping the uterine walls, vacuum aspiration transformed abortion into a relatively safe operation.

After the twelfth week of pregnancy and until about the twenty-fourth week, a *midtrimester abortion* is performed. Instead of mechanically aspirating the products of conception, this abortion is induced by mimicking a natural miscarriage. Over the years, various solutions have been used as catalysts. One of the first such methods involved *intraamniotic injection of a saline solution* into the sac of fluid surrounding the fetus. This was described in 1934 by a Bucharest physician. Later researchers developed a fifty percent glucose solution. However, this proved too congenial a medium for infection, even when administered with antibiotics, and the procedure was abandoned. Other solutions, such as a mixture of formaline and urea, were subsequently used. Some of these solutions were even found to be effective when injected between the fetal membrane and the uterus, without ever penetrating the amniotic sac.

The use of saline gained widespread acceptance in the 1940s, until reports from Japan and England showed a high incidence of infection, uterine hemorrhaging, and occasionally brain hemorrhaging. Saline is still used today, but in limited, safe doses and only under strict supervision. It has, in many places, been replaced by the prostaglandins.

Following the Second World War, Swedish researchers succeeded in isolating a substance called prostaglandin from the prostate gland and the semen. This substance causes uterine contractions, and in 1970, reports from Sweden and Uganda confirmed that it could be used successfully to induce *midtrimester abortion*. Unfortunately, this type of abortion was accompanied by nausea, vomiting, and diarrhea. The drug was administered in many different manners until it was found that intraamniotic injection alleviated severity of the side effects and provoked uterine contractions strong enough to cause expulsion.

THE FIRST SIGNS OF PREGNANCY

If conception occurs, the pituitary secretes a hormone called HCG (human chorionic gonadotrophin), which stimulates the corpus luteum, or yellow body, in the ovary to produce progesterone. Progesterone, in turn, prepares the uterus to receive the fertilized egg. Four weeks after conception, or six weeks after the last period, most HCG production is replaced by the placenta, an organ whose sole purpose is to provide nourishment to the fetus. HCG is excreted in the urine and levels of HCG in the urine can be measured in the laboratory. This laboratory measurement of urinary HCG is the most commonly employed pregnancy test and takes from four to eight hours to complete. These tests can be performed in a doctor's office with a diagnostic kit, but the levels of HCG in the urine must be very high for a positive reaction; the laboratory test is more sensitive. A positive reaction in either of these tests means that you are pregnant, but the opposite is not true. It is possible to have a negative pregnancy test, particularly in the first three to five weeks after conception, yet still be pregnant. Pregnancy tests should be repeated every week until there is either a positive sign of pregnancy or the most positive sign of nonpregnancy—menstruation.

A urinary pregnancy test is usually not positive until two weeks after the first missed period, six weeks from the last menstrual period, and four weeks from the time of conception. In order to have the ability to detect pregnancy *with accuracy* soon after conception, researchers at Cornell University Medical Center in New York have developed an ultrasensitive receptor assay for HCG which gives a positive reading as early as two weeks after conception, even before the first missed period. The levels of HCG in the blood are tested with this technique, and while at the present time there are no widespread facilities beyond the original research institution for application of this test, it should be generally available in the not-too-distant future.

One of the first visible signs of pregnancy is enlargement of the breasts and deepening in color of the areola surrounding the nipple. A physician can check the uterus for signs of softening, but uterine enlargement is usually not detectable until six or seven weeks after a missed period. Nausea, a bloated feeling, and breast tenderness are often the first signs noted by a patient. Persistent elevation of the Basal Body Temperature is another indication of pregnancy. If all these signs are monitored and pregnancy is detected early enough, abortion can be relatively simple. The earlier the abortion is performed, the fewer are the complications that can be anticipated.

MENSTRUAL EXTRACTION, OR MINIABORTION

The quickest, easiest, and safest method of abortion is the so-called *menstrual extraction* developed by a California physician in an effort to minimize the psychological trauma of abortion. The procedure was initially performed on women who had missed a period, yet showed negative pregnancy tests. It was felt, though, that if a woman did not know she was pregnant, the abortion procedure would have a better chance of psychological acceptance. Thus the name—menstrual extraction, which is the simple removal of the endometrium which would normally be expelled during menstruation. Some feminist leaders even advocated replacing the normal form of six-day menstruation with this operative procedure, which lasts only a few minutes. Extensive studies, though, have indicated that this procedure should not be performed on nonpregnant women, since there are dangers of infections and excessive bleeding. Because of this, the term *menstrual extraction* is now considered a misnomer and the technique is called a *miniabortion*. It is the recommended procedure only if a pregnancy test is positive and a woman is less than 7 weeks from her last menstruation.

A miniabortion is performed either in a clinic or in a doctor's office. The procedure is not without discomfort, chiefly because of the need for mechanical cervical dilatation (opening of the cervix by instruments). This problem can be overcome with the use of prostaglandin suppositories.

The ability of prostaglandins to soften or "prime" the cervix prior to the procedure and thus reduce the trauma of miniabortion is promising, but still under investigation. Until results are conclusive, and prostaglandin is available for this purpose, a woman is advised to take either a tranquilizer or a mild painkiller thirty minutes prior to the procedure (the doctor should always be advised as to the pharmacological agent that has been taken). The woman is placed on an examining table with her legs in the stirrups, a position similar to that used in the normal pelvic examination. A manual internal examination is performed to determine the size and position of the uterus. A speculum is then inserted into the vagina to provide the physician with good visualization of the cervix. The vagina is swabbed with an antiseptic solution. A local anesthetic of Novocaine is injected with a very fine needle at three points on the cervix—the top and on either side. The cervix is then held with a special type of forceps, called a tenaculum. A thin, flexible, plastic tube five to seven millimeters in diameter is inserted through the cervix into the uterus. With most patients, the cervix does not have to be dilated to permit insertion of the plastic tube; this minimizes cervical damage. The plastic tube is attached to a suction apparatus. Through mild suction, the lining of the uterine wall, complete with the products of conception, is gently removed within one or two minutes. On occasion, the tube is removed and cleared, then reinserted to make certain that removal is complete. Since the procedure can be associated with strong uterine cramps, nausea, and a feeling of sweating and faintness, the woman should not be moved from the examining table for fifteen to thirty minutes. It is advisable for a woman undergoing this procedure to be accompanied by a friend or relative to help her return home safely.

There are many advantages to this procedure. It is fast, relatively simple, can be performed without the need for general anesthesia, and the cost of a hospital stay is eliminated. A woman should not have intercourse or use a tampon for three to four weeks after the procedure to avoid complication or infection. Bleeding after the procedure should stop within one to two weeks. If it continues, you should return to your doctor for evaluation. Normal menstruation usually occurs four to eight weeks after the procedure.

FIRST-TRIMESTER SUCTION ABORTION

Today, a suction abortion, or curettage, is the technique of choice for interruption of pregnancy between the seventh to the twelfth week after the last menstrual period.

The art of suction abortions has progressed significantly in recent years. When suction or vacuum abortions were first developed, many of the pumps did not exert sufficient power, and in several instances complications occurred. Since the liberalization of abortion laws around the world, more attention has been given to the development of safe abortion apparatus, and the procedure has become more sophisticated. Still, complications do occasionally occur, and it is important to go to an experienced, competent physician to minimize these risks. If you want an abortion but are unsure where to go, a Planned Parenthood clinic or referral center in the city nearest you should give you reliable information.

Suction abortion can be performed up to the twelfth week of amenorrhea, or the tenth week after conception. After that time, the fetus is too large and severe bleeding may occur if a suction abortion is attempted. A good chance also exists that the physician may tear the cervix to accommodate such a large fetus.

Suction abortion can be performed either under local or general anesthesia. Most abortion clinics prefer local anesthesia because the patient can go home much sooner after the procedure. Hospital abortions are usually performed under general anesthesia, since the hospitals feel that this procedure, although it is more expensive, should be available to women who do not wish to be conscious during the abortion. Even at hospitals, though, one will usually be admitted in the morning and go home the same evening. A patient placed under a general anesthetic will experience no pain during the abortion.

Technique of First-Trimester Suction Abortion

The technique of suction abortion is outlined as follows: If the patient is undergoing local anesthesia, she will usually receive an intramuscular injection of one of the various painkillers such as codeine or Demerol. The patient is then placed on the operating table with her legs in the stirrups. An internal examination is performed to determine the size and the position of the uterus. The vagina is then washed with an antiseptic solution and a local anesthetic is injected into the cervix to numb the nerves. If a patient is having this procedure performed under general anesthesia, she initially receives an intramuscular injection of Atropine one hour prior to the procedure. This decreases the mucous secretion of the lungs in preparation for the later administration of general anesthesia. An intravenous infusion is then started. The anesthesia is usually initiated with intravenous injection of sodium pentathol through the intravenous infusion. The sodium pentathol puts the patient to sleep and then a general inhalation anesthetic, such as nitrous oxide, is administered

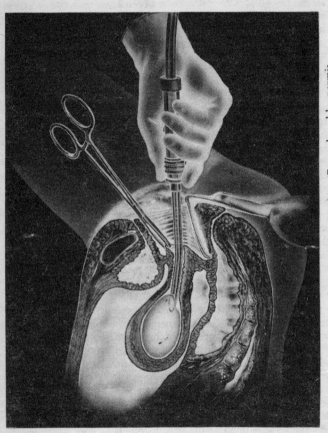

Fig. 11-1: Technique of suction abortion. (Reproduced by permission of the Berkeley Bio-Engineering, Inc., San Leandro, California.)

through a mask during the operation. Once the patient is completely asleep, she is examined and her vagina is washed with an antiseptic. From this point, the procedure for patients under local and general anesthesia is identical.

The cervix is held by a tenaculum and then dilated slowly by the insertion of a progression of cervical dilators, each one somewhat larger than the last. The cervix is stretched until the opening allows the insertion of a suction tip *(vacurette)*. These tips have diameters ranging from 8 to 12 millimeters and, as a rule, a patient is aborted with a tip that is one size larger than the week of gestation; that is, if a patient is eight weeks from her last menstrual period, the physician will employ a nine-millimeter suction tip. As the vacurette tip is inserted into the uterus, it is attached to a suction apparatus via a flexible tube. This vacuum aspirator can either be an electrical or a mechanical pump, and it indicates the amount of vacuum suction it produces (see picture). The suction should go up to at least 60 centimeters of water pressure to evacuate completely the products of conception. The suction from the pump gently loosens the fetal tissue from the uterine wall and aspirates it through the suction to contract the uterus, thus decreasing the blood loss. With local anesthesia in a clinic, an injection of *ergotrate* is used to contract the uterus; this can cause nausea and vomiting.

If the abortion is performed under general anesthesia in a hospital, the patient is usually fully awake and ready to go home four to five hours following the operation. With a local-anesthesia abortion, the patient can go home after about two hours, but may feel a little faint and should be accompanied by a friend or relative.

Suction abortion under local anesthesia is not without discomfort, so it might be advisable to take a tranquilizer beforehand, if the clinic or the doctor permits it. The pain usually subsides during the first hour following the procedure.

A woman experiences contractions the first few days after the abortion as the uterus returns to normal. Bleeding usually occurs for up to two weeks following the procedure. In order to minimize the pain, a woman should take it easy the first few days after the abortion to give the uterus a rest and to decrease bleeding. If the bleeding is heavy or if a temperature develops after the operation, the clinic or doctor should be contacted immediately.

Blood type should be checked before any suction abortion. If a woman is more than six weeks pregnant and her blood type is Rh-negative, she should have an injection of Rhogam, an anti-Rh-positive agent which prevents a woman from being immunized in future pregnancies (this is usually not necessary after a miniabortion). If the fetus has Rh-positive blood, and some of its blood gets into an Rh-negative bloodstream, an allergic reaction results causing subsequent pregnancies perhaps to abort spontaneously or result in death of the fetus. Rhogam prevents this from occurring.

A woman should be aware that the cervix will take three to four weeks to close up following a suction abortion. Because it is dilated, the uterus is particularly susceptible to infection, so during this period women should refrain from inserting tampons into the vagina or engaging in intercourse. Any object pushed into the vagina at this time might push bacteria from the vulva into the uterus. She may shower, but not bathe.

Since ovulation might occur two to three weeks after an abortion, birth control should be planned immediately. If the pill is the chosen method of birth control, the cycle should begin a few days after the abortion. If a woman opts for an IUD, it can be inserted while she is still anesthetized from the abortion. Regular menstrual periods usually occur four to eight weeks following an abortion.

ABORTION IN THE GRAY ZONE

The so-called gray zone is that period of time between the twelfth and the sixteenth week after the last menstrual period. During this interval, the fetus is too large for an ordinary suction abortion and there is too little amniotic fluid (the fluid which fills the sac surrounding the fetus) to allow an intraamniotic injection for a midtrimester abortion. This means that women who discover that they are pregnant after three months, or for some reason put off their decision to have an abortion until that time, must wait an additional month until they enter the time of the midtrimester, when abortion is feasible. Psychologically, this can be an extremely long month.

Recent research, however, has developed new techniques for "gray zone" abortions. These abortions are accomplished by means of prostaglandins, drugs which cause uterine contractions and abortion, or by a surgical procedure called D&E, Dilatation and Evacuation.

The half-life of natural *prostaglandin* in the circulation is less than thirty seconds, which means the body inactivates the drug in about half a minute. Therefore, vaginal prostaglandin E2 suppositories are ideal for administration, because the prostaglandin is released slowly when the suppository is placed in the vagina. The suppositories are held in the vagina by a diaphragm that is altered by having a portion of the center removed. A physician may then determine when the abortion has occurred. Without the diaphragm, the prostaglandin tends to leak out, requiring more repeated suppository insertions, perhaps every two hours. With the diaphragm, suppositories must still be inserted repeatedly, but only every three or four hours. Expulsion of the products of conception usually occurs within ten to fifteen hours after insertion of the first suppository. Side effects such as nausea and diarrhea can be somewhat alleviated with prophylactic drugs.

Another form of prostaglandin has been developed which can induce abortion in the "gray zone"—a synthetic prostaglandin called 15(S)-15-methyl prostaglandin F2 alpha. This drug is injected intramuscularly every two to three hours and results in expulsion of the products of conception in about fourteen hours. This analog seems to relax the cervix as it stimulates the uterus, thus reducing the pain associated with abortion.

These two forms of "gray zone" abortions—vaginal administration of prostaglandin E2 suppositories and intramuscular injections of 15(S)-15-methyl prostaglandin F2 alpha—may also prove useful as midtrimester techniques. Often, traditional midtrimester abortions with intraamniotic instillation of saline cause excessive bleeding or are difficult to perform. Research continues into the development of the prostaglandin for abortion induction. These methods for gray zone abortions have been approved by the Food and Drug Administration.

Dilatation and evacuation (D&E) is a procedure for surgical interruption of pregnancy beyond twelve weeks of gestation. D&E is gaining increased popularity in certain medical centers, but it can be a potential source of danger in inexperienced hands. The D&E technique is similar to the one previously described for surgical interruption of first trimester pregnancy, but there are some important differences. First, D&E usually requires general anesthesia. Second, successful D&E necessitates an increased degree of cervical dilatation to permit complete removal of the products of conception at this advanced stage of pregnancy. If this dilatation is forced with mechanical instruments, problems such as cervical damage and laceration can arise. Attempts at minimizing this possible hazard involve the use of laminaria tents, made of dried seaweed, inserted in the cervical canal; the laminaria cause gradual dilatation of the cervix by swelling as they absorb fluid. Prostaglandin suppositories, administered a few hours prior to surgery, may also produce the desired cervical expansion. Once the cervix is dilated, either by priming or forced mechanical dilatation, the products of conception are removed by a combination of suction and forceps and the surgery is concluded with sharp curettage.

The advantages of the procedure are that it is rapid, relatively pain free, and requires only a single-day hospital stay. The possible problems encountered with D&E include cervical injury, laceration, uterine perforation, and heavy bleeding. It should be pointed out that the safety of the D&E largely depends upon the skill and the experience of the physician. Even the most experienced and skillful physician, however, will encounter increasing difficulty with D&E in advanced gestation. If a woman desires D&E for termination of pregnancy, she should consult her gynecologist as soon as the conclusive decision to abort is reached.

There is usually some bleeding and mild cramping for one or two weeks following the gray zone abortion. The same instructions as for midtrimester abortions should be followed after this procedure.

MIDTRIMESTER ABORTION

Midtrimester abortion, or the interruption of pregnancy from the sixteenth to the twenty-fourth week of gestation, is the most difficult and complicated of all the abortion techniques. Although pregnancy may be legally interrupted up to the twenty-fourth week from the last menstrual period, many hospitals and clinics will not perform the procedure after the twentieth week unless the woman's health is in danger or there are indications of a malformed fetus. These restrictions are observed in some institutions in order to avoid any possibility of delivering a fetus with signs of life, a circumstance which proves very disturbing to both the woman having the abortion and the professional staff attending her. Women should be aware of the difficulties related to midtrimester abortion. Because of the difficulties, if a woman is considering pregnancy interruption, she should have it interrupted as soon as it is known she is pregnant.

Pregnancy can be interrupted between the sixteenth and the twenty-fourth week of gestation by intraamniotic instillation of either saline or prostaglandin, or by hysterotomy.

Intraamniotic Instillation

An intraamniotic instillation of either saline or prostaglandin causes abortion by stimulating the uterus to contractions similar to those of labor, and the products of conception are expelled, mimicking a natural miscarriage. Abortions of this type are considered major procedures and should only be performed in hospitals on an inpatient basis so that the woman can be carefully watched throughout the entire procedure. In this way, if any complications occur, they can be immediately and adequately handled by a competent professional staff. A woman undergoing this type of abortion must expect a hospital stay of one and a half to three days in an uncomplicated procedure.

A woman must fast for at least six hours prior to her admission to the hospital. On admission, a blood specimen is obtained for typing and cross-matching, so that blood replacement is immediately available if the woman has bleeding complications. An intravenous infusion is then started.

The woman is then taken to either an operating or treatment room and is asked to lie on her back on the treatment table. The procedure is initiated by a careful washing of the lower abdominal region with an antiseptic solution; there is no need for shaving of the abdomen. A sterile drape is placed over the lower part of the body and the area from the pubis to just below the navel is left exposed. The physician performs the operation wearing a mask and sterile operating gloves to eliminate the risk of infection. The physician palpates the abdomen to determine the position of the uterus and the appropriate area for the injection. A local anesthetic such as Novocaine is injected into the area where the needle will be inserted. Once this area is anesthetized, the procedure, an *amniocentesis,* is performed. In general, *amniocentesis* is the puncturing through the abdominal wall of the amniotic sac, the sac of fluid which surrounds the fetus, by a fine needle and the aspiration or withdrawal of some of the amniotic fluid. This procedure is performed for a variety of reasons, such as determining the genetic makeup of the infant for chromosomal studies, determining fetal abnormalities and fetal lung maturity at term, and finally for the initiation of abortion by intraamniotic instillation of drugs.

If saline is used to induce the abortion, an 18-gauge, 3½-inch-long spinal needle is inserted through the abdominal wall and into the amniotic sac. Between 50 and 200 cubic centimeters of amniotic fluid are withdrawn via a syringe attached to the needle. Approximately 200 cubic centimeters, or approximately seven fluid ounces, of a 20 percent saline solution are slowly injected through the needle by a syringe into the amniotic fluid.

Some medical centers instill (slowly inject) a combination consisting of 80 grams urea plus 10 to 20 milligrams prostaglandin in a fluid volume of 200 to 300 cubic centimeters. This "cocktail" has been found to be more effective than an instillation of saline alone.

If, on the other hand, prostaglandin alone is used, only a very small amount of amniotic fluid is withdrawn. This is simply to determine the correct positioning of the needle. Eight milliliters, containing forty milligrams of prostaglandin F2 alpha are slowly injected into the amniotic sac. The needle is then removed and the site of the amniocentesis covered with a sterile dressing. If it is done by an experienced physician, amniocentesis is a rapid and relatively painless procedure.

The woman's blood pressure and pulse rate are then measured. If the readings are within normal limits, she is returned to her room and requested to remain in bed for one hour. After this time, the woman may be allowed to walk around for as long as she wishes. A clear liquid diet is provided until the expulsion of the fetus. For the first few hours after the amniocentesis, a woman should experience only a minimal amount of pain. As time passes, abdominal cramps of increasing strength develop, similar to cramps experienced with the onset of menstrual flow. The cramps, or contractions of the uterus, cause a softening of the cervical muscle in preparation for the dilation required for the expulsion of the products of conception. As cervical dilation occurs, the pain associated with cramps increases to a peak. This happens immediately prior to the expulsion of the fetus, and the cervix is the most stretched at this point. In women who have not previously delivered a child, the pain associated with this type of abortion is somewhat stronger than in women who have had children.

During the early part of the abortion, a woman may receive a tranquilizer such as Valium to help relax her over the abortion period. As pain and cramping increase, something stronger, such as Demerol, is required. However, if an injection of Demerol is administered too early, it stops the uterine contractions and prolongs the abortion. Demerol should not, therefore, be given before the cervix begins to dilate. As contractions become stronger, a woman feels more comfortable in a sitting position than in a supine position. As the woman begins to feel strong rectal pressure, often an indication that passage of the fetus is imminent, she may be asked to sit on a bedpan (to facilitate the passage of the abortus) and asked to use voluntary abdominal exertion. When the abortion takes place, the patient usually remains in her hospital bed and is aided by the nursing staff. Only rarely is she transferred to an operating or delivery room.

The time from the intraamniotic instillation of either saline or

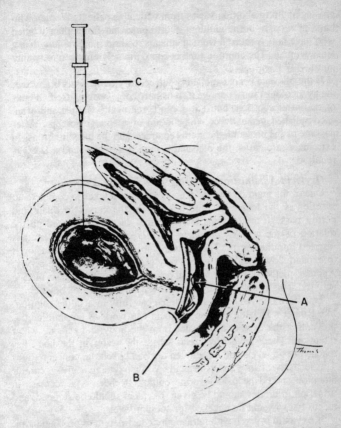

Fig. 11–2: Midtrimester abortions are usually performed by in-traamniotic instillation of either a hypertonic saline solution or prostaglandin. During amniocentesis, the needle is inserted through the abdominal wall into the uterus and amniotic fluid is aspirated with a syringe, as shown in C. The hypertonic saline or the prostaglandin is then injected and the needle withdrawn.

Vaginal suppositories, as shown in B, containing prostaglandins have been administered for induction of midtrimester abortion and a number of various techniques are under investigation. Some investigators also insert a diaphragm, as shown in A, to prevent the leakage of the suppositories.

prostaglandin to abortion varies from patient to patient. Women who have previously borne children abort somewhat faster than women who have not. A relaxed woman appears to abort more rapidly than a tense woman. The abortion time is approximately eighteen to twenty hours.

If the placenta is not expelled spontaneously as the fetus is aborted, the gynecologist must remove it. It usually comes out by itself an hour or two after abortion, but if it doesn't, removal is simple and often accomplished manually or with the aid of a sponge forceps. After passage of the placenta, the uterus contracts and the bleeding stops. In extremely rare cases, the placenta is hard to remove, and a D&C is required.

Oxytocin Administration during Midtrimester Abortion

One of the main factors influencing the time it takes to complete an abortion is the length of time it takes for the cervix to dilate and permit passage of the fetus and placenta. In order to speed up the dilation of the cervix, *laminaria digitala* (dried seaweed steam) is inserted into the cervix. The laminaria absorbs body fluid, causing it to expand slowly and to create a very gradual dilation of the cervix. Another method of decreasing abortion time is to increase uterine activity. This is achieved by the intravenous infusion of oxytocin.

This hormone must be administered carefully in a saline solution, like Ringer's lactate, because oxytocin can work as an antidiuretic, preventing the excretion of water from the body and causing water retention. There have been cases where the water in the body has reached toxic levels and has diluted the bodily sodium concentration. This leads to seizures and even death. When oxytocin is given, careful attention should be paid to urine output. If there is a decrease in urination, diuretics should be given, oxytocin should be stopped, and electrolytes should be checked for sodium levels.

If oxytocin is given with intraamniotic instillation of prostaglandin, it may cause overly violent contractions which rupture the cervix. However, if the oxytocin is not administered for six hours following amniocentesis, there are few problems. After instillation of saline solution, there should be a two-hour interval before administration of oxytocin.

What to Expect following a Midtrimester Intraamniotic Abortion

The patient may leave the hospital six to ten hours after the abortion. For two weeks following a midtrimester abortion, there will be bleeding and the passing of a few large clots. The patient should try to remain relatively inactive. Because the cervix is dilated, no foreign objects should be introduced into the vagina or infection may be pushed into the uterus. This means no tampons and no sexual intercourse. A woman may shower, but not bathe during this time. After four weeks, the patient should have a follow-up examination. If the uterus has healed and the cervix has closed, normal sex life may resume.

Birth control should begin as soon as possible. If a woman elects to use the pill, she should begin taking it a few days after the abortion.

If heavy bleeding or a sign of infection occurs after a woman has left the hospital, she should immediately contact the clinic or doctor who did the abortion. If neither can be reached, she should go immediately to the nearest hospital emergency room. Women should expect a very heavy flow during the first menstrual period following abortion.

Since midtrimester abortion is actually induced labor, the endocrine mechanism of the body is fooled into producing milk. Women should expect milk secretion for several weeks after abortion. Nothing can be done about this, but a tight breast binder or bra helps decrease tenderness. Breast movement stimulates milk production, as does applied heat.

If a midtrimester abortion is performed by an experienced physician in a good hospital, the procedure resembles a miscarriage and no physical harm should result to the uterus. The ability to conceive and have children will not be affected. In fact, it might even be easier to conceive since the cervix has been opened.

Hysterotomy

Hysterotomy is an operative abortion, a procedure almost identical to a Caesarean section, in which the products of conception are surgically removed. This is considered a major operative procedure requiring a hospital stay of six to eight days. After a hysterotomy, a woman will have a scar on her abdomen. More importantly, she will also have a scar in her uterus. In the future, she will have to be delivered by Caesarean section. Because of this, hysterotomy is seldom employed.

The operation is usually performed under general anesthesia, but can be done with spinal anesthesia. When the woman is asleep, the abdomen is shaved and sterilized. The patient is draped sterilely and an abdominal incision is made, either transverse (from side to side) or up and down. When the abdomen is open, an incision is made in the lower part of the uterus. The amniotic sac containing the products of conception is carefully freed from the inner uterine wall and removed via the incision. The uterus and the abdomen are then surgically closed.

The patient is given a postoperative intravenous infusion for two days. She is then slowly given clear liquids. Finally, during the last part of the hospital stay, she is allowed to have solid foods. If the woman's recovery is uncomplicated, she is usually discharged on the seventh postoperative day.

A patient undergoing a hysterotomy must expect a longer period of recuperation than if her pregnancy is terminated by intraamniotic instillation of either saline or prostaglandin. Complete healing does not occur for four to six weeks following surgery, and during this period, a woman should not have intercourse, lift any heavy objects, or even return to work.

Hysterotomy is associated with the highest complication rate of any type of abortion and should only be performed in a very limited number of indicated cases, such as in cases of uterine abnormalities.

Mental Health and Late Abortions

Besides the medical complications, late or midtrimester abortions have also been associated with more pronounced psychological difficulties. The late abortion is usually a rather painful procedure—it is actually a drug-induced miscarriage—but psychological trauma is often a greater problem for women who undergo this type of abortion. Many hospitals recognize this and have set up counseling centers to deal with the depression which often accompanies midtrimester abortions. Because the fetus is so far advanced, many women have religious conflicts. Unmarried women may allow a pregnancy to continue too long in the hope of marrying the child's father and are emotionally devastated when he refuses. Still others refuse to face the possibility that they are pregnant, sometimes indicating a weak grip on reality and the potential to break down.

The psychological depression that can occur after late abortion may be very severe, sometimes suicidal. Some women are so depressed that they require hospitalization. This should be recognized by the family and parents, who should help any woman as much as possible after any abortion. Women should know that this depression will disappear and if the abortion was performed in a recognized clinic or a good hospital, there should be no difficulty in conceiving and carrying a child in the future. It is important to note that many women emerge from an abortion experience unscarred and with a healthy attitude toward contraception.

If you need psychological counseling and don't know where to get it, your nearest Planned Parenthood center should be able to help. There should be a Planned Parenthood office in your state, but if you don't know how to contact it, call the main office in New York City at (212)541-7800. Counseling and referral for abortion can also be obtained in many cities from the Clergy Consultation Service, an organization of women and men of all religions who recognize the difficulty a woman experiences when she has an unwanted pregnancy. This organization is also able to refer you to the best abortion facility or the best counseling. Their main office is also in New York City, and they can be reached at (212)254-6230.

CHOOSING THE METHOD OF ABORTION

When a woman is pregnant and does not wish to maintain the pregnancy, it is important for her to decide on interruption as early as possible. The miniabortion and the early, first-trimester curettage are the least complicated procedures, in both the medical and psychological senses. As a general rule, the later an abortion is performed, the higher the complication rate. Statistics collected from 1972 to 1975 in the United States indicated that the death rate associated with suction abortion was 1.6 per 100,000 abortions; the death rate related to intraamniotic instillation of saline was 22.9 per 100,000 abortions; and the death rate for hysterotomies was 45.0 per 100,000. Prostaglandin was approved by the Food and Drug Administration in 1973, and initial studies indicate that it is even safer than saline. Labor and full-term delivery are associated with a death rate of approximately 20 per 100,000; thus it is evident that early abortion is even safer than full-term delivery.

When performed by experienced physicians, intraamniotic instillation of prostaglandin is the safest form of abortion from the sixteenth to the twentieth weeks of gestation. However, because of the possibility of the fetus being aborted with some signs of life in an abortion performed after twenty weeks, the majority of physicians induce abortion with saline in these later gestations.

Recent research indicates that intraamniotic instillation of saline results in damage to the placenta and fetal death, as well as causing an expansion in the volume of the uterus. It is hypothesized that instillation leads to the release of prostaglandin; it is the prostaglandins which cause uterine contractions, which result in the expulsion of the products of conception.

ABORTION IN THE FUTURE

In the future, with more sex education and counseling, women will better understand their bodies and be better able to detect the signs of pregnancy early. It is hoped that pregnancy testing facilities or home pregnancy kits for detection of early pregnancies will be readily available to every woman to determine if she is pregnant without fear of recrimination. If a pregnancy is confirmed and cannot be maintained, it should be interrupted in the earliest stage, when there is the greatest margin of safety and a lesser chance of permanent damage to the body.

Research is being conducted with the administration of different types of prostaglandins for the induction of very early first-trimester abortions. It may be that, in time, prostaglandins will replace many types of mechanical abortions or suction techniques. Prostaglandin causes uterine activity, which results in the expulsion of the products of conception. In the future, this type of prostaglandin may even be used to induce a period if a woman is a few days late.

chapter 12

INFERTILITY

Infertility—the inability of a couple to conceive—is, for many people, a completely irrelevant concern, since most young couples are preoccupied with preventing conception and many even live in constant fear of unwanted pregnancy. In fact, the most remote thought in a young woman's mind is that she might be barren. Probably as a result of our upbringing and cultural conditioning, we tend to expect our bodies to perform on demand, and for this reason, many couples become hysterical if they do not conceive within the first months of trying.

Our social attitudes and values are undergoing profound changes at present. Many women now postpone childbearing until their late twenties, early thirties, or even later years, waiting until they have fulfilled career ambitions as well as other personal goals. Because of this, more and more women are coming to realize that it is increasingly difficult to get pregnant as they get older. This is caused by many factors, not the least of which is the fact that women and men can develop various medical conditions in the intervening years which make conception more difficult and which may even cause sterility.

The realization that a couple might be sterile often comes as a shock and can cause tremendous psychological distress. This is particularly true of couples who have postponed childbearing in order to achieve certain career goals and a degree of financial security. When such couples are faced with the realization that they might remain childless, their dreams can be completely shattered.

The word *infertility* has a nightmarish ring of finality. The thought of it cuts straight to our genetic core, for it is our biological heritage, to say nothing of our societal expectation, to reproduce. That is how our species survives and progresses. Yet, far from being a permanent condition, infertility is often the result of a relatively minor psychological, physical, or chemical problem. It is a condition which can be reversed. Rather than being a permanent curse, infertility is often a matter of poor timing, nervousness, or hormonal imbalance. In this chapter, infertility is defined as the inability of a couple to conceive after *one year* of coitus without contraception. About ten percent of all married couples fit this description.

Partly as a response to the great number of unwanted pregnancies in our society, many people believe it is easy to conceive. Actually, it is rather difficult to conceive. Women are fertile for only two to three days each month, while sperm survives in the uterus for only two to three days. Therefore, conception usually occurs only during a period of three to five days each month. If the timing is off, it can take months for a woman to become pregnant. Patience is often a successful self-help fertility program, but if patience fails after one year, it is time to consult a fertility specialist.

CAUSES OF INFERTILITY

The process of fertilization is so complicated that any minor disorder can prevent it. First, an egg must be released from the woman's ovaries. This egg must be able to move freely into the fallopian tube, which in turn must be normal and unobstructed all the way into the uterus. While this occurs, hormonal changes should open the mouth of the cervix during ovulation to make a channel for the sperm. The sperm, assuming the man is able to produce healthy, motile (fast-swimming) sperm, must then reach the egg alive and penetrate it. Then the fertilized egg must move into the uterus and embed itself in the uterine wall, at which time it should be under the influence of the correct hormonal conditions.

This complex process can break down from a wide variety of causes originating in either the woman or the man, or both (as, for example, when the woman develops an allergic reaction to the man's sperm).

Female infertility can be caused by emotional stress, radical weight changes, thyroid dysfunction, vaginitis, mycoplasma (microorganisms in the cervix or the vagina), amenorrhea (cessation of menstruation), ovarian cysts, endometriosis, pelvic tumors, cervical stenosis (narrowing of the cervix), or synechia (scar tissue in the uterus).

Male infertility can result from excessive drinking, stress, urinary infections, or hormonal disturbance. It can also be caused by permanent damage done by mumps, venereal disease, or physical trauma to the genitalia. Most often, however, male infertility stems from the presence of varicose veins in the testes or congenital malformations. Occasionally, it occurs without apparent cause.

These causes are discussed at greater length later, but there is one additional problem that deserves mention here: the fear of infertility. Sometimes a couple assumes that they are infertile because they have been unable to conceive after several months of trying. This assumption becomes an emotional stress that, in itself, is enough to prevent normal conception. Such couples often conceive soon after seeing a fertility specialist, even if he prescribes no treatment.

Finally, many women believe that a tilted uterus prevents pregnancy. This is a myth. Recent studies have shown that the angle of the uterus has no influence on fertility. Some doctors still perform surgery to move the uterus forward by tightening the uterine ligaments, but any subsequent improved fertility is to be attributed to psychological rather than physiological factors. This procedure is now performed only if the uterus is tilted back so far that the veins are obstructed, causing abdominal pain.

JOGGING AND INFERTILITY

Too much strenuous exercise, such as excessive jogging, can interfere with ovulation and menstruation. The physical demands involved in these activities can result in a signal to the brain to inhibit the release of *gonadotrophins*, the regulators of the cycle. Ovulation and menstruation are thus inhibited as a form of defense mechanism: If the amount of blood lost through menses is minimized, a woman's blood count is elevated and the extra oxygen required by the physical strain is available to the working muscles. If a woman who indulges in competitive or long-distance running experiences difficulty in conceiving, she would be wise to cut down on the amount and intensity of her physical exercise. Excessive physical exertion can have similar antifertility effects in men. If a male athlete finds that his sperm count is depressed, he would similarly be well advised to reduce his physical activity.

WHAT TO DO BEFORE CONSULTING A SPECIALIST

Since conception is such a complicated process, there is no reason to suspect a fertility problem until at least a year of intercourse without the use of contraceptive measures has elapsed. In the case of women taking the pill, a longer period may be necessary from the time she stops taking the pill, since it may take a few months for normal ovulation to resume.

On the other hand, older couples might consider seeing a specialist after about six months of unsuccessful attempts at conception, since the mechanism of ovulation in the woman deteriorates with age and the amount and motility of sperm begins to decrease in men as early as the mid-twenties. Thus the older a couple is, the more difficult it becomes to conceive, and the greater the likelihood of infertility for such couples.

During this trial period, intercourse should be carefully timed to fall within the few fertile days each month when the woman is most likely to conceive. These days usually fall about fourteen days prior to the onset of the next menstrual period, no matter what the length of the menstrual cycle. Because of this, the couple should have intercourse daily from between seventeen to eleven days prior to the onset of the woman's next menstrual period. Chances of conceiving before ovulation are greater than after ovulation.

After coitus, the man should withdraw his penis from the woman's vagina so that the sperm will not dilute on the shaft of the penis. Pillows placed beneath the woman's buttocks give the sperm a much-appreciated downhill swim. Any jelly or Vaseline used during intercourse may harm sperm, so saliva is recommended if a lubricant is necessary.

Emotional stress can disrupt both male and female hormonal balance, so periods of relaxation, like vacations, are good times to conceive. The man should be careful not to drink too much or become exhausted from too much sightseeing. He might even want to take vitamin supplements.

A good example of stress-related infertility is the case of a woman who held a hectic professional position—one that made her extremely nervous. This, coupled with her anxiety concerning her inability to conceive, was making her infertile. Her physician, who found nothing abnormal during a physical examination, suggested she take a glass or two of wine each evening to help her relax, and one evening at a party, she had intercourse standing up in the garden and conceived.

If, after relaxing, eating properly, cutting down on excess drinking, taking regular exercise, timing intercourse, and following the optimum coital procedure for conception, a couple has not conceived after one year, it is then time to seek professional help. It is important to find a fertility specialist, not just any gynecologist. Even though most gynecologists claim to have some expertise in treating infertility, this does not qualify them as fertility specialists. The head of the department of obstetrics and gynecology at any major medical center should be able to refer a couple to a competent fertility specialist.

FREQUENCY OF SEX

During the investigation of the frequency of sex, it is important to understand the relationship between the partners and the amount of sex experienced. It is important to know that orgasm has no influence on the ability of a woman to conceive. Orgasm is merely satisfying and pleasurable for the partners, but conception can occur even without it, as, for example, during artificial insemination, where there is no sexual pleasure at all. During the investigation of a couple's sex habits, it is not so much a question of how often they have sex as it is the understanding of having sex on the right days. In this area, the physician should help a woman calculate the days when she is most likely to be fertile, since this time of maximum fertility amounts to only a few days each month. There are different beliefs as to how often intercourse should take place during the woman's fertile days. Some physicians believe that couples should have intercourse only once every other day in order to build up the semen and break down the acid-base difference between the sperm and the mucous plug. On the other hand, if sperm are too old, they tire easily and have less motility. Therefore, it is probably advisable during a woman's fertile days for a couple to have intercourse every day. It is also important, during those days, that the man is well rested, takes vitamins, and does not drink too much.

DIAGNOSING FERTILITY PROBLEMS

Infertility Workup

The first step in determining the cause of infertility is a comprehensive medical history and a physiological examination. You should be absolutely candid with your doctor. Remember, it is his responsibility to keep your medical history confidential, even from your husband. Your doctor should know about any previous pregnancies, miscarriages, or abortions (especially illegal ones) which you may have had, because these indicate that you do ovulate, at least occasionally, and this information could also point to possible fallopian complications resulting from infection or scar tissue. If you have conceived before but your partner has not, the problem could be his, not yours.

A menstrual history is vital to a proper understanding of the nature of infertility. If regular periods occur every twenty-eight days, ovulation is highly probable, so the problem must be elsewhere. Irregular menstrual bleeding, sometimes spanning eight weeks between periods, might indicate a problem such as Stein-Leventhal syndrome, in which the ovaries are enlarged and have a thicker capsule, making ovulation difficult or impossible.

An erratic menstrual history may also indicate hormonal imbalance, especially when accompanied by increased hair growth on the face and arms. This can often be solved with hormone injections or fertility drugs.

The release of hormones is radically affected by anxiety. Two key hormones, the releasing hormones FSH-RH and LH-RH, are produced in the hypothalamus area of the brain and stimulate the production of FSH and LH, both of which are released by the pituitary gland. Anxiety affects the hypothalamus and, in turn, affects the release of these hormones, resulting in sterility. For example, a group of women college students who were under a great deal of stress were found not to release these hormones at all, and therefore developed amenorrhea. However, as soon as they went home to their parents for a vacation and were relaxed, they released these hormones again, and normal menstruation resumed. FSH and LH are responsible for stimulating the ovaries to produce estrogen and progesterone, and without them, abnormal menstrual periods result. It is important to include any psychological or emotional stress in your history so your doctor can consider these factors in his diagnosis.

At this point, it is worth noting that approximately 25 percent of all infertility problems are caused by male infertility. This is due either to the fact that the man does not produce enough sperm or that his sperm are abnormal in size or shape. For example, some men produce sperm with two heads, two tails, and various other abnormalities. Often a man produces enough sperm, but if their motility (i.e., swimming speed) is too slow, this can cause sterility in the man, even if his sperm are normal in shape and size.

Since such a high percentage of infertility is caused by male infertility, it is important for a man to undergo a complete physical examination, including a sperm analysis, in order to determine if a couple's infertility problem is related to any physical abnormalities in his reproductive system. In this way, if the problem lies with the man, the wife can be spared the time, inconvenience, discomfort, and expense of extensive tests when, in fact, it is her partner who is infertile.

Of course, certain diseases in a woman's past may have caused damage to the ovaries or fallopian tubes. Venereal diseases are particularly dangerous, so a woman should not be shy about reporting them to her doctor. He is there to help cure infertility problems, not to pass any kind of moral judgment.

If there is any thyroid dysfunction in your family, you should be tested. Actually, you should have this done anyway. Thyroid function is very closely associated with ovulation, and many infertile women who complain of fatigue show a low level of thyroid function in blood tests. A thyroid pill often cures both the fatigue and the infertility.

The loss or gain of as little as five pounds can also throw off a woman's menstrual cycle. Therefore, if you have been dieting or if you have recently gained weight, be sure to include this information in your medical history. A return to normal weight generally causes your menstrual cycle to return to its normal pattern.

Any physical examination prior to diagnosing the cause of infertility should be thorough. Your eyes should be normal, your neck should be without thyroid gland enlargements, your heart and lungs should be functioning normally, and your blood pressure should be normal. Any problems in these areas could mean trouble, from thyroid dysfunction to kidney problems. For instance, if your blood pressure is high, you could be suffering from chronic hypertension. This is sometimes caused by kidney abnormalities, which in turn often cause infertility. A urine sample can isolate many of these problems, and at the same time, it can be checked for possible diabetes.

A pelvic examination often reveals startling problems, such as a total congenital absence of the uterus or fallopian tubes. A speculum inspection of the cervix should be performed to be sure that it is open. The hymen should also be examined to make certain that it is not intact. A bimanual examination, with two fingers in the vagina and the other hand on the abdomen, reveals any uterine tumors. You must relax completely for this examination to be successful, although this is often more easily said than done.

Basal Body Temperature

One essential indicator which the doctor will want to evaluate is your basal body temperature (BBT). This is usually taken orally, although some physicians prefer it be taken rectally. BBT takes a month to measure, so you should have taken your BBT for one month before visiting your doctor. This not only saves time, it also gives

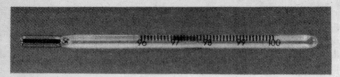

Fig. 12–1: Ovulation Thermometer. This is a special type of thermometer, since it is only able to measure temperatures between 96° and 100°F.

your doctor the advantage of additional data for his initial diagnosis of your fertility problem.

BBT is obtained by taking your temperature every morning, beginning on the first day of your period, as soon as you awaken and before you get out of bed. It is important that the basal body temperature be taken before you smoke a cigarette, brush your teeth, drink coffee, make love, or do anything else, since the slightest activity affects BBT. After a month of plotting your BBT on a graph, you know exactly when, or if, you ovulated.

Immediately after menstruation, the ovaries are stimulated by the hormone FSH to produce an egg. During the growth period of the egg, the BBT remains relatively low and stable, but at the time of ovulation, there is a small *decrease* in the BBT, followed by a sharp increase (see Fig. 5–2).

As the egg makes its way into the uterus, the scar tissue in the ovaries, where the egg was expelled, turns into the so-called yellow body, or corpus luteum. This yellow body starts to produce progesterone, which reduces the contractions of the uterus and tubes, thereby simplifying conception. This increase in progesterone also increases body temperature, which remains high until immediately prior to menstruation. If your BBT shows an early drop at this point, you probably have a luteal problem, caused by insufficient production of progesterone. While it is possible to conceive with this condition, the contractions of the uterus might increase, squeezing the egg out of the womb and resulting in miscarriage. Treatment is therefore recommended if you have a luteal problem.

If the BBT does not decrease before the anticipated time of your next menstrual period, you might be pregnant. BBT is the cheapest and easiest pregnancy test. If you have reason to believe you are pregnant, continue charting your BBT for another two weeks just to be sure, at which time a pregnancy test can be done.

The Cervical Factor

The cervix is more than a passive barrier to be negotiated by the sperm; it is an active organ whose functioning is essential to conception. Studies show that cervical problems are responsible for between 30 and 50 percent of all female infertility.

The cervix changes shape throughout the menstrual cycle. For instance, it opens and shortens to let blood pass from the uterus during the menstrual period. It is during this phase that vaginal infections can be sucked into the tubes by the pumplike contractions of the uterus, resulting in *salpingitis* (inflammation of the fallopian tubes), or even into the abdominal cavity, resulting in *peritonitis* (inflammation of the peritoneum, the smooth, transparent membrane that lines the abdominal cavity). After menstruation, the cervix usually points backward and closes to an opening of only about one millimeter.

At the time of ovulation, the cervix usually opens to about three millimeters. It softens and points forward in order to catch the sperm.

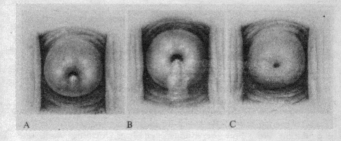

Fig. 12–2: A close-up view of changes in the cervix throughout the menstrual cycle. (A) A few days after menstruation has ceased, the cervical canal is closed and the cervix points backwards. (B) The cervix, during ovulation, moves forward, and the cervical canal opens to approximately 3 mm in diameter to facilitate sperm transport. The cervical mucus is clear, watery, and slimy, which makes sperm adhere more easily to the cervix. (C) The cervical opening closes again during the luteal phase and will again point somewhat backward. The cervical mucus has almost disappeared. (Reproduced by permission from *Progress in Infertility;* 1968; Little, Brown and Company, Inc.; Boston, Massachusetts.)

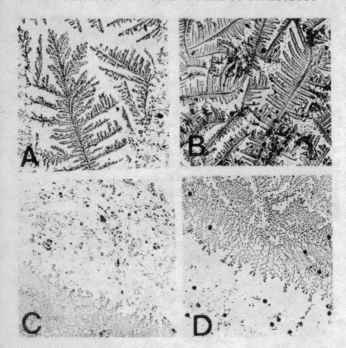

Fig. 12-3: Fern pattern of the cervical mucus. This illustration shows how the dried mucus, as it appears under a microscope, changes throughout the menstrual cycle. (A) The fern pattern a few days after menstruation. (B) A well-developed fern pattern at the time of ovulation. Note how the mucus crystallizes, forming small, fine channels in which the sperm can travel. (C) The fern pattern is broken up in the mid-luteal phase, days 20–24 of the menstrual cycle. Sperm cannot pass through this mucus. (D) Poorly developed fern pattern in a patient with a vaginal infection, which could be contributing to her infertility problem.. (Reproduced by permission from *Progress in Infertility;* 1968; Little, Brown and Company, Inc.; Boston, Massachusetts.)

The cervical secretions become thinner, like saliva, to aid the sperm's passage through the fine channels of the mucous plug at the mouth of the cervix. Many women describe this change as "becoming wetter."

This wetness also increases sexual sensations, remotely resembling the mechanisms of *estrus* ("in heat") in other species. After ovulation, the mucus thickens. Women who practice the rhythm method of birth control call this their "dry" or "safe" period. What is vital to understand here is that all of these changes are governed by estrogen levels.

Your doctor can ascertain a great deal from mucus samples. The mucus should stretch up to ten centimeters and be long and slimy. This enables the mucus to draw the sperm into the cervix and lead it on into the uterus and tubes. If there is no change in the amount of mucus and its ability to stretch (also called *Spinnbarkeit*), there may be no ovulation.

The Postcoital Test

Dr. Papanicolaou, who discovered the Pap-smear test for cancer, found that cervical mucus, when dried, forms distinctive patterns which change as the mucus changes. When a woman is fertile, these patterns, during ovulation, resemble in shape a fern or palm leaves, opening channels through which the sperm can swim freely. This pattern is important in evaluating the estrogen and hormone levels. When the mucus thickens, after ovulation, the "leaves" appear to bunch up and the channels are closed off, acting like miniature diaphragms to prevent the entrance of sperm.

A visit to the doctor as soon as possible after intercourse, preferably within two to three hours, enables him to extract samples of sperm and mucus to determine whether the sperm is able to move through the fern patterns. This test is also valuable for finding out if the sperm can survive in the mucus, since many women are allergic to sperm, and this reaction causes the sperm to die in the mucous plug.

The Influence of Vaginal Infections on Fertility

The effect of vaginitis on fertility is hard to evaluate, but there is little doubt that increased discharge lowers sperm concentrations by diluting semen. Trichomonas in the vagina is likely to cause an increased pH in the vagina, and this elevation of the pH could interfere with sperm survival. Whether the elevated pH permitted the vaginal infection to develop or whether it is secondary to the discharge produced is uncertain. Vaginal moniliasis does not increase the vaginal pH. However, clinical vaginitis of both types may diminish fertility because the resulting discharge impedes sperm migration and dilutes the sperm concentration. It is, therefore, important to understand that infertility can be caused by infections of the vagina, and the physician should examine you for both monilia and trichomonas, as well as for cervicitis. If any of these conditions are present, they should be treated, as they could be the only factors causing infertility.

Mycoplasma

Mycoplasma is a condition wherein microorganisms are found in the cervix and vagina. Some studies have recently shown that this condition *could* influence fertility by decreasing sperm motility and/or survival; however, other studies deny the importance of these findings. Treatment with tetracycline (250 milligrams, taken four times a day for ten days) should be sufficient to kill the infection. It might also kill other infections present, and therefore increase fertility. However, when a woman is treated with a broad-spectrum antibiotic such as tetracycline, the balance in the vagina between yeast and bacteria is often altered, thereby causing a yeast infection, which, in turn, causes infertility. Therefore, if you are treated with antibiotics, you should always be treated at the same time with an antiyeast medication such as mycostatin suppositories or any other antiyeast cream or jelly, to maintain the proper balance between yeast and bacteria in the vagina.

Tubal Insufflation (The Rubin Test)

The Rubin Test, in which the fallopian tubes are inflated with carbon dioxide, can determine if at least one of the tubes is open. Unfortunately, this test cannot distinguish between bilateral and unilateral blockage, nor can it determine the existence of a partial blockage of one or both of the fallopian tubes. For this reason, the Rubin Test is considered to be obsolete by many modern fertility specialists. On the other hand, the advantage of the Rubin Test is that it can be performed in the doctor's office, but other tests must be performed concurrently in order for it to have any credibility. During this procedure, if the fallopian tubes are clear, gas (carbon dioxide) escapes into the abdomen, and there is no high pressure. The escaping gas can be heard with a stethoscope, and when the woman sits up, she feels a pain in her shoulders, because the gas has irritated the thoracic diaphragm, thereby stimulating the phrenic nerve.

Hysterosalpingogram

Rather than resort to the Rubin Test, most modern gynecologists

Normal Hysterosalpingogram

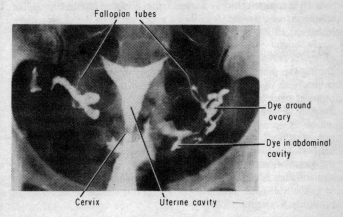

Fig. 12–4: X-ray picture of a *hysterosalpingogram,* which shows a normal uterine cavity and normal and open fallopian tubes. The dye flows freely out through the tubes on both sides and surrounds the ovaries.

and fertility specialists prefer the *hysterosalpingogram,* an X-ray of the uterus and the fallopian tubes. In modern hospitals and clinics, where extensive infertility studies are performed, X-ray facilities have been set up specifically for this test.

First, the patient lies on a gynecological table. A special forceps (a tenaculum) holds the cervix, while a tubelike instrument connects a syringe to the cervix. A water-soluble dye is then injected with the syringe into the uterine cavity, flushing through the tubes. This dye, as it shows up on an X-ray film or a fluoroscope, reveals any abnormalities of the uterus or the tubes. Often the dye flushes out obstructions in the tubes, and if no other problems are influencing the woman's infertility, the pregnancy rate increases 40 to 50 percent within four months of this test. The hysterosalpingogram can be painful, so a Valium or an aspirin tablet might be taken beforehand. Aside from identifying obstructions, a hysterosalpingogram can also indicate cervical stenosis and/or synechia (scar tissue inside the uterus).

Endometrial Biopsy

In an endometrial biopsy a small spoon is placed through the vagina and cervix into the uterus to take a specimen from the endometrium (see Fig. 16–2). As has been described before, the lining of the uterus, or endometrium, changes and becomes thicker toward the end of the menstrual cycle, making it ready for implantation of the egg. During the menstrual period, the endometrium is expelled due to contractions of the uterus. A biopsy from the uterine lining determines if ovulation has occurred. The best time for the biopsy is the first day of menstruation, because when the uterus starts contracting, the cervix opens and it is easier to insert the biopsy instrument. This test is painful, but less so if it is performed during the time of menstrual bleeding. A good pathologist grades the biopsy by studying the vascularity and structure of the tissue, thereby determining if ovulation has occurred and if implantation was possible. Endometrial biopsy is still considered a good test, and it should be a part of an infertility workup.

Laparoscopy

If, after a hysterosalpingogram or a Rubin Test, your doctor suspects pelvic adhesions, he should perform a laparoscopy (waiting three to four months after the hysterosalpingogram to see if conception occurs in the interim). This is a fairly simple procedure, usually performed in a hospital under general anesthesia because it causes severe pain when the abdomen is distended with four liters of carbon dioxide. A periscope is inserted through the navel to give the doctor a complete view of the pelvic organs. The periscope is the same instrument used for tubal cauterization or ligation during voluntary sterilization (see illustration in Chapter 10, Voluntary Sterilization).

Small adhesions and obstructions are treated through the laparoscopy. Sometimes a problem requires more extensive surgery, such as a *laparotomy* with a *tuboplasty* (see Tuboplasty, below), and the patient should be prepared for this eventuality so that the doctor can proceed while she is still under anesthesia. Laparoscopy is also used to evaluate pelvic tumors or endometriotic masses. Several women have become pregnant after this operation, even when no cause of infertility was found. This could be due either to psychological factors or to the fact that the operation perhaps stimulated the ovaries to normal functioning.

Culposcopy

As in a laparoscopy, a periscope is inserted into the abdomen during colpotomy. Instead of being inserted through the navel, the periscope is introduced through the vagina for this procedure (see Fig. 16–7). Today, culposcopy has been largely replaced by laparoscopy, because a culposcopy can push into adhesions and cause even further damage. At the same time, the procedure is uncomfortable for the patient, since she must be in a knee-chest position under local anesthesia (see Fig. 16–6). Most physicians today have abandoned the culposcopy.

Tuboplasty (See also Microsurgery)

If laparoscopy reveals abnormalities such as adhesions or tubal occlusions of the fimbriated ends, an exploratory laparotomy (an operation in which the abdomen is surgically opened) must be performed to correct the condition. Occlusion, or blockage of the tubes, is often caused by gonorrheal infections. Other severe pelvic infections, such as those following a septic abortion or infections after delivery, also cause this closure. During the laparotomy, a dye is usually injected into the uterus so the physician can see if the tubes are open. If there are pelvic adhesions, a careful dissection and surgery must be performed, perhaps using an operative microscope, and the doctor has to be very careful in freeing the adhesions of the ovary and tubes. The rougher the physician is during this procedure, the more is the chance of subsequent adhesions.

If tubal surgery is performed, this is called *tuboplasty*. Tuboplasty calls for delicate surgery with fine instruments (microsurgery). If there are adhesions on the outer part of the tubes, they should be gently freed and the fimbriated ends opened and folded up like a flower. For conception to occur, the tubes and ovaries should be able to move freely in relation to each other. Freed adhesions could recur, and an attempt should be made to prevent this. It has also been found that if steroid hormones are injected into the abdominal cavity and the patient is treated with steroids, antibiotics, and tranquilizers after the operation, chances of recurrent adhesions are lessened.

If there is severe tubal occlusion, several modifications of tuboplasty can be done. However, it has been found that the more successful the doctor is in restoring the natural anatomy of the tubes, the higher are the chances for conception to occur afterward.

If the obstruction in the fallopian tube is closer to the uterus, one can bring the tubes closer to the uterus by reimplanting the tubes into the uterus.

If the fimbriated end is amputated due to severe adhesions or damage after infection, the chance of conception is small. Therefore, the most important task of tuboplasty is to restore the fimbriated ends of the tubes, free adhesions, and prevent the recurrence of adhesions by administering steroids, tranquilizers, and antibiotics immediately following the procedure. The ovaries and fallopian tubes are highly fragile organs, so the chance of conception after this procedure is often as low as 30 percent, depending on the extent of damage the infection has done to the pelvic organs.

Microsurgery

Microsurgery may be deemed a new approach to infertility surgery, for it is *restorative* surgery with the goal of returning delicate reproductive structures to their normal anatomical state and allowing them to function naturally. Microsurgery takes advantage of high optical magnification to permit visualization of minute tubes and vessels, and surgical suture finer than human hair to repair and restore these structures and a surgical philosophy aimed toward the most gentle and meticulous treatment of body tissues. The hands of the fully trained and experienced microsurgeon can produce near miracles in achieving or restoring fertility in both women and men. If the source of a fertility problem can be surgically corrected, microsurgery should be considered if it is applicable. There is a *caveat*, though, for not every surgeon who uses microsurgical instruments is a microsurgeon. The training for microsurgery is arduous and lengthy, but the results of this training can produce great benefits for patients. A microsurgeon must, therefore, be thoroughly investigated and carefully chosen.

Cervical Stenosis

Cervical stenosis is a narrowing of the cervix, leading to painful menstruation (dysmenorrhea). In some cases, this has been linked to a psychosomatic condition in which the fear of bleeding causes a woman to tighten her cervix to such a degree that sperm cannot enter. This condition is usually corrected with a dilatation and curettage (D&C). Following childbirth, it corrects itself.

Asherman's Syndrome—Synechia Uteri

Synechia are scars inside the uterus (Asherman's syndrome). These scars usually result from scraping the uterine walls too aggressively during abortion or for control of bleeding after delivery. Today, with modern abortion techniques, synechia are becoming less frequent.

If a D&C is not successful in freeing adhesions from synechia, a laparotomy may be necessary. After synechia are freed, IUDs effectively prevent new adhesions from forming. Birth-control pills or estrogen and progesterone therapy aid in building up the lining of the uterus.

Immunological Factors—Can a Woman Be Allergic to Her Husband's Sperm?

The human body can be allergic to anything, especially to any foreign body. To a woman, nothing could be more foreign than sperm. The simplest way to evaluate whether a woman is allergic to her partner's sperm is to perform the postcoital test, as previously described. If an allergic reaction is found, there is no known cure for this cause of infertility, but if the allergy-causing factor (i.e., the sperm) is removed, the reaction subsides somewhat. A man whose partner is allergic to his sperm should refrain from ejaculating into the vagina for several months, perhaps by using a condom, and thereafter he should use the condom at all times except during the woman's most fertile days of the month. This has resulted in many pregnancies. If the condom technique doesn't work, artificial insemination with a donor sperm may be necessary.

Endometriosis as a Cause of Infertility

Pelvic endometriosis is a condition in which endometriotic masses are spread in the pelvis. The exact cause of endometriosis is not known, but it usually develops in highly strung women who have severe menstrual cramps. The menstrual blood is pushed out through the tubes to the pelvic cavity during menstruation, where it stays like normal tissue and is under the influence of the hormones which stimulate its growth. Endometriosis can grow all over the pelvic organs and block the tubes and ovaries, thereby causing infertility. Usually if tumors of this nature are found, the patient should undergo laparoscopy or exploratory laparotomy to determine the location of the tumors.

The usual treatment involves surgical removal of the endometriosis. However, this usually grows back and can, therefore, cause persistent infertility. Recently a new synthetic hormone called danazol (Danocrine) was developed, which blocks the release of LH and

FSH, thereby causing amenorrhea. This hormone has proven effective in melting away all endometriosis and in many cases has restored normal fertility. This new hormone has helped many women who, after six months of treatment with danazol, returned to normal fertility and successfully conceived. Danazol has recently been released by the Food and Drug Administration for general use. The usual dosage is 400 to 800 milligrams daily for six months, which is usually sufficient for the majority of women who have endometriosis. Of course, some women need a more prolonged period of treatment with danazol in order to obtain the desired result.

TREATMENT OF FEMALE INFERTILITY

Infertility Caused by Pelvic Tumors or Adhesions

If the factor causing infertility in the female is tumors in the pelvis, the woman should be evaluated for an exact diagnosis. A laparoscopy, using a periscope inserted through the navel, enables the physician to examine the pelvic organs. If there are adhesions or growths around the tubes or ovaries, tuboplasty should be performed. Ovarian tumors should be very carefully evaluated and removed if they are causing infertility.

Infertility Caused by Congenital Abnormalities

If infertility is linked to unusual physical conditions such as double vaginas, uteri, or the absence of the uterus altogether, there is usually little, if anything, your doctor can do to remedy the situation. In the case of double uteri, pregnancy is possible, but the miscarriage rate is high, and premature deliveries are common. If the problem is merely a septum (a dividing wall or membrane) in the middle of the uterus, it can be removed surgically (by the Strassman operation) and the uterus can be reconstructed to reduce the chance of miscarriage. Other forms of uterine abnormalities will not be discussed here, since they are relatively rare and treatment for them is complex.

Evaluation of Amenorrhea

Amenorrhea (the absence of menstrual bleeding) is caused by any number of factors, but it always results in infertility. When a woman does not menstruate, it is because the lining of the uterus has not built up normally since the hormonal changes essential for ovulation have not occurred.

Amenorrhea can be caused by prolonged use of birth-control pills. After a certain time, the pill takes over the hormone functions of the body and, because it maintains a steady level of estrogen and progesterone, there is no stimulation to cause the buildup of the uterine lining. Once a woman stops taking the pill, it may take several months before menstruation resumes. If, after several months, menstruation does not resume, estrogen treatment followed by the administration of progesterone may bring it back.

Emotional stress can also be responsible for amenorrhea, as it affects the hypothalamus, which controls the release of FSH and LH from the pituitary gland. When this release does not occur, a woman will not bleed. This condition is sometimes called *anorexia nervosa*. Women who suffer from this condition often refuse to eat, thereby becoming increasingly thinner. This throws their hormonal balance even further off. Eventually such women break down physically and must be hospitalized. Treatment for anorexia nervosa must be of a psychological nature, and it may be a prolonged process. When the woman's weight, along with her eating habits, returns to normal, the rest of her body processes usually follow suit, and menstruation recurs.

A pituitary tumor can also cause amenorrhea. This will show up on a skull X-ray and must be removed surgically.

Hormone assays should be made to ensure that the ovaries and the adrenal glands are not overproducing the male hormone androgen. Overproduction of this hormone can also cause menstruation to stop. If an infertility problem stems from the adrenal glands, there is probably overstimulation of or a tumor in the adrenal glands. This condition requires surgery. If, on the other hand, activity in the adrenal glands seems to be normal but the level of androgen is high and thus prevents ovulation, there is a rare possibility that a masculinizing ovarian tumor is responsible. The ovaries may have several types of tumors, some producing female hormones, others producing male hormones. The recent development of sensitive methods for checking testosterone level in the blood aids in this diagnosis.

Sometimes the ovarian capsule becomes thickened. As the thickening grows, it becomes increasingly difficult for ovulation to occur and cysts form. This is called Stein-Leventhal syndrome, or polycystic ovaries, and causes irregular or absent bleeding. The problem is treated surgically by removing a wedge of the ovary so it returns to normal size. Pregnancy occurs more easily after this procedure. The new fertility hormones have also proven effective in the treatment of Stein-Leventhal syndrome.

Alkaline Douches as a Treatment for Infertility

An alkaline environment is extremely important to sperm survival, motility, and ability to penetrate the cervical mucus. For this reason, it might be beneficial for a woman to take an alkaline douche prior to intercourse during ovulation. One tablespoon of sodium bicarbonate (baking soda) added to one quart of warm water will suffice for this purpose. Precoital use of this solution might be particularly beneficial for women whose cervical mucus is less than normally alkaline. After use of an alkaline douche prior to intercourse, postcoital tests often reveal an improvement over the previous condition by showing a greater percentage of actively motile sperm in the cervical mucus. Some physicians even recommend adding a small amount of glucose to the alkaline-douche solution, since this helps create an environment in which sperm have an increased chance for survival.

Fertility Drugs

If you are not ovulating (BBT is the easiest way to determine this), then your doctor may prescribe fertility drugs. One of the most successful of these drugs, and the most benign, is *clomiphene citrate* (Clomid). This drug has made many barren women fertile. No one knows exactly how it works, but it may reduce the amount of circulating estrogen, and some women do experience "hot flashes" when taking Clomid. Once the Clomid is stopped, estrogen production rebounds, and it may be this "flood" of estrogen that stimulates and releases eggs from the ovaries. One tablet a day should be taken from the fifth day of the menstrual period. If this proves unsuccessful, the dosage can be raised to four or five tablets daily. Clomid does not generally cause multiple births, but it can.

Some doctors follow Clomid with an injection of HCG (human chorionic gonadotrophin). Your doctor should treat you with progesterone tablets or suppositories to decrease uterine contractions that can squeeze out the egg. Clomid may also improve the luteal phase merely by normalizing ovulation.

The fertility drug which sometimes causes the much-publicized multiple births is *Pergonal*. This drug is only indicated in rare cases and is generally prescribed for women who do not respond to Clomid. Pergonal is a mixture of LH and FSH collected from the urine of older women. The reason the urine of older women is used is that the secretion of these hormones from the pituitary gland is much higher after menopause. Most Pergonal is produced in Italy, where it is often collected from the urine of elderly nuns.

Pergonal is administered by injection. Your doctor then checks urine, blood, or cervical mucus for estrogen. When the estrogen reaches a certain level, an injection of HCG is administered. This should cause ovulation, but since the levels of FSH and LH are unusually high, several eggs might be released at the same time, causing multiple birth. A specialist experienced with Pergonal knows how to watch the hormone levels carefully, thus decreasing the chance of multiple birth. Still, Pergonal, which is very expensive, should be a last resort.

MALE INFERTILITY WORKUP

The production of sperm is a delicately balanced process, one that can be toppled by anything from too little exercise to too much alcohol. If sperm analysis reveals that the sperm is not sufficiently motile, that is, that it does not move fast enough, vitamin B complex or perhaps extra caffeine may be all that is required.

More often the cause of infertility is related to a hormonal imbalance. The man should have his thyroid function and pituitary production of gonadotrophin checked to be sure they are fulfilling their roles in the production of sperm. A urologist can best evaluate both these functions, as well as abnormalities such as diabetes and hypertension as they relate to infertility. Most hormonal imbalances are successfully treated with hormone drugs, whether the imbalances are caused by tension or by disease.

A partially understood cause of male infertility is varicose veins in the scrotum. Surgical removal of these varicose veins has been proven to increase tremendously the amount of normal sperm which a man produces. The prevailing theory is that the great number of veins in the scrotum raise its temperature to the point where the testes are adversely affected. Temperature control is essential to normal sperm production, and this is why in warm weather, the testicles hang low, away from body heat; but in cold weather, they draw up into the body. The temperature of the scrotum should be somewhat lower than normal body temperature.

A complete physical examination should determine the condition of the penis and the testicles. Many unexpected congenital abnormalities, such as the absence of the vas deferens (the tube which transports semen from the testes through the penis) may be discovered. Undescended testicles that have been squeezed and damaged at a young age can also be detected.

A sperm analysis must be done by a specialist. Semen is often collected at the laboratory (the man is asked to masturbate in a private room) so the sperm is fresh. For sperm to be considered healthy and capable of causing pregnancy, the ejaculate should be at least 4 cubic centimeters and should contain a minimum of 20 million sperm per cubic centimeter. The normal sperm count is about 90 million per cubic centimeter. At least 40 percent should have good motility and 60 percent should have no serious defects, such as double or abnormal head structures. The first sperm sample might appear to have a low count, since the man will probably experience anxiety the first time he goes to a urologist. The role which many men are raised to play often makes it difficult for them to admit to having reproductive problems —infertility is easily translated by cultural bias into weakness, or a less than manly condition. Thus, more than one visit might be necessary before the man feels sufficiently at ease with the doctor to render a normal sample.

Environmental factors such as excessively high temperatures, poor eating habits, severe fever, allergies, or the excessive consumption of alcohol or tobacco can also lower a man's sperm count.

In today's high-pressure world, with sexual roles under constant scrutiny, it is not unusual for a man to suffer from infertility. Though the causes are sometimes physical, the problem is usually of a psychological nature, and professional help should be sought. If the problem is physical, hormone treatment or surgery often remedy the condition.

TREATMENT OF MALE INFERTILITY

If a man's sperm count is found to be low, a specialist should evaluate the man's physical problems. For example, if the level of thyroid function is low, treatment with thyroid tablets often restores fertility. If the gonadotrophin level is low, treatment with FSH and LH is indicated. Clomiphene citrate (Clomid), the fertility tablet for women, is also sometimes effective in treating male infertility by raising the sperm count to a normal level. A testicular biopsy is indicated to determine if the testes have normal sperm production. A few other conditions are surgically or hormonally treated, but the majority of male infertility is caused by permanent damage, such as that resulting from mumps or accidents.

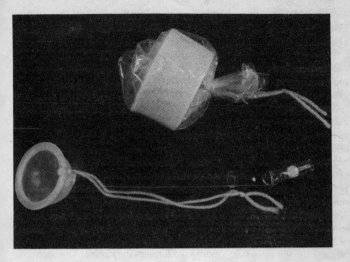

Fig. 12–5: This picture shows a vaginal sponge and a cervical cup, both used during artificial insemination. The vaginal sponge is covered with a plastic shield so it will not absorb the semen.

Men who undergo vasectomy should understand that this operation is generally not reversible and that their sterility is permanent, although isolated cases of restoring fertility through reconstruction of the vas deferens have been reported.

Unfortunately, the majority of male infertility problems cannot be treated. However, if a man is able to produce sperm, but the count and/or motility is low, the couple might consider artificial insemination.

ARTIFICIAL INSEMINATION

Twenty-five percent of all infertility problems, as previously stated, are attributable to the man. In the past, many couples have turned to adoption as an alternative to conception, but with the decrease in unwanted pregnancies due to modern birth-control techniques and legalized abortion, it is becoming increasingly difficult to find an adoptable child. Contemporary couples with infertility problems often solve their problem through artificial insemination.

The term *artificial* insemination is unfortunate. There is nothing really artificial about it. Perhaps *therapeutic* insemination would be a more accurate term. The procedure is timed to coincide with the woman's ovulation. If she has a regular twenty-eight-day menstrual cycle, insemination should be performed as many as three times between the tenth and the fourteenth days of the cycle. First, the doctor should check the fern pattern of the cervical mucus to ensure that the sperm will be able to penetrate it. Then the sperm should be checked, whether the husband's or a donor's is used. When brought to the doctor, the semen should be transported in a small bottle. The bottle should be kept warm (slightly below body temperature) or the sperm may die. Sperm are injected directly onto the cervix by the doctor in the hope they will move more quickly into the uterus and tubes. Insemination directly into the uterus is extremely painful and not particularly successful. A sponge is placed in the vagina to prevent the sperm from running out, and the woman's hips should be elevated slightly for fifteen to twenty minutes.

Alternatively, a cervical cup can be used. This apparatus fits over the cervix and has a tube running out through the vagina. The sperm is injected through the tube to the cervix. Uterine contractions create enough suction to hold the cup on the cervix, and a small valve prevents the sperm from escaping. The tubing is then folded into the vagina. Still, the woman should elevate her pelvis and remain on the table for fifteen to twenty minutes. After twenty-four hours, the woman removes the cup simply by pulling it out. There will be mucus and perhaps a little blood in the cup after removal, but this is normal.

The difficulty of artificial insemination is not in the procedure itself; rather, it lies in arriving at the decision to resort to this procedure. Most men find the idea threatening to their egos, especially if donor semen is used. Sometimes if the husband's sperm count is low but not necessarily useless, the doctor may mix the husband's sperm with the donor's. Although this might create an allergic reaction, just the possibility that the successful sperm was the husband's can work psychological wonders.

Many couples worry about who their donor will be, having read horror stories about blood donors recruited from Skid Row. Sperm donors are carefully screened and are matched as closely as possible to the prospective father. Hair color, eye color, race, and religion—all of these factors are taken into consideration when matching a sperm donor to the prospective father. Most sperm donors are medical students and generally an intelligent group of men.

One obvious advantage of artificial insemination over adoption is that the woman carries the child and the couple is involved in its birth. An understanding between the parents that no blame should be assessed for the original infertility is essential; it could just as easily have been the woman's problem as the man's. Sometimes professional counseling helps a couple understand that an artificially inseminated child is still their own child, a whole child, born of their love.

If the man is not infertile but has some inheritable disease—for instance, certain central nervous system diseases—or if he and the woman have incompatible Rh factors in their blood which may have already caused spontaneous abortion or stillbirths, the couple should consider artificial insemination with donor sperm. This greatly increases the possibility of a normal birth.

If artificial insemination is correctly performed by a specialist, conception should occur within a few months, although this is a generalization and not a firm rule. It may take years. The rate of success with artificial insemination is around 70 percent.

Is Artificial Insemination with the Husband's Sperm Worth the Effort?

Many people feel the entire procedure of artificial insemination is not worth the time and effort that it requires. Such couples often ask if it is not possible to achieve the same results at home with concentrated effort, by having intercourse during a woman's most fertile days and by using all optimum conditions for intercourse such as elevating the woman's buttocks by placing pillows under the pelvic area. It is true that this home method helps somewhat, especially when the man withdraws his penis from the woman's vagina shortly after ejaculation to prevent the dilution of the sperm on the shaft of the penis. However, if, after six months of trying at home, a couple still has not conceived, it is definitely a good idea to consult a doctor about artificial insemination.

Frozen Semen

In the past fifteen years, insemination with frozen semen has made progress. Today approximately one thousand babies have been born who were conceived with frozen, stored semen. Only about one percent of these have evidenced any abnormalities (as compared to six percent of the general population). The rate of successful impregnation with frozen sperm is only fifty percent. It is, however, a very

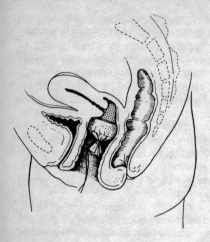

Fig. 12-7: Artificial insemination in which a vaginal sponge is placed high in the vagina to prevent the sperm, which are seen around the cervix, from leaking out.

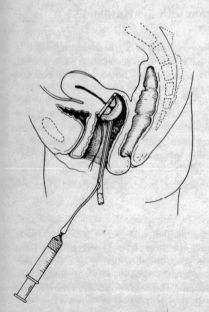

Fig. 12-6: This picture shows the cervical cup placed around the cervix and the semen being injected into the cup through plastic tubing. The little round plastic ball in the tubing pushes down to the cervical cup to prevent the leakage of sperm.

practical method of donor insemination, since sperm banks have a large selection of donors, meeting almost all imaginable male genetic characteristics. The frozen sperm can easily be stored in the doctor's office for several days, and this makes insemination possible on weekends and in the evening. In this way, a working woman does not have to interrupt her office hours in order to visit her doctor's office.

The procedure for artificial insemination with frozen sperm is slightly different from that with fresh sperm, in that frozen sperm is actually allowed to thaw in the vagina. Motility is reduced more than 50 percent in some cases, so insemination is tried every month until impregnation occurs. The average length of time for a woman to become pregnant using this method is about eight months.

Should a Man Store His Semen Prior to Vasectomy?

Whether a man should store his sperm in a sperm bank prior to vasectomy has been increasingly discussed. Thus far, very few men have made use of this possibility. Even though this prospect appears attractive to some men, particularly to men who feel it might still be important to them, at some future time, to reproduce, it should be clearly pointed out that this procedure is still relatively new, and scientists do not know exactly how many years the sperm can be stored. It is known that sperm loses its motility, and the percentage of this loss is increased in direct proportion to the length of time during which the sperm remains frozen. As previously stated, the chance of conception with frozen sperm is only about 50 percent. Furthermore, there is no guarantee that a power failure might not occur one day, resulting in the destruction of all sperm stored in a given sperm bank. All of these factors should be taken into consideration before a man elects to undergo voluntary sterilization. In view of all this, it seems more reasonable to postpone vasectomy until a man has completely fulfilled his desire for reproduction.

Surrogate Mothers—Artificial Insemination and Donor Uterus

In any discussion of artificial insemination, one usually considers the case of the fertile female partnered with the infertile male; however, over the past few years, there has been discussion concerning artificial insemination of the husband's sperm into another woman who would act as surrogate mother, carrying the child until delivery and then surrendering it for adoption to the child's genetic father and his wife. This concept has even been explored in a recent movie, *The Babymaker;* however, in this case, the father impregnated the surrogate mother naturally. Such a procedure would undoubtedly cause a number of psychological problems, and family conflicts are certainly not suggested as a solution to fertility problems.

Nonetheless, one case has recently been publicized in which the husband was fertile and his wife infertile, and adoption was difficult. The husband placed an ad in a newspaper stating that he was married to an infertile woman and wanted to have a baby through artificial insemination with a woman whose background was similar to his wife's. There were more than 160 responses to this ad, and even though the man was willing to pay a good deal of money for this donor uterus, he found many women willing to carry the child just for payment of the doctor and hospital fees. The husband gave his sperm to a physician, and a woman submitted to artificial insemination. The woman delivered and the father adopted his child. The two parents never met. Although there are very few reports of this kind, artificial insemination with a donor uterus is considered another way to help the childless family and at the same time ensure that some of the family's genes are transmitted to the child.

TEST-TUBE BABIES

"Test-tube baby" was the term used to describe Louise Brown, the first live-born child to be conceived outside the mother's body in 1978. The term is a misnomer as it suggests the baby actually develops and grows outside the body. The proper term is *"in vitro* fertilization" since the mother's ovum (egg) is fertilized by the father's sperm *in vitro,* that is, in glass outside the woman's body. The full procedure is complex and requires the skills of several medical disciplines. The pioneering work in this field was done by Drs. Robert M. Edwards and Patrick Steptoe.

A woman whose infertility is based in tubal disorders such as damaged, blocked or missing fallopian tubes, who is healthy, with no ovulatory difficulties, and has a fertile partner, would be a candidate for *in vitro* fertilization.

When the fallopian tubes are blocked or missing, it is impossible for the normal pathway of conception to occur. What happens in nature must be replicated with great skill in the laboratory in an effort to bypass the tubes by artificially performing their vital functions. This is achieved in three basic steps.

Phase 1—Obtaining the Egg

The mother's egg or ovum must be obtained at the precise time of ovulation when it is about to be extruded from the ovary. At this time, the egg is mature and can be fertilized. The time of ovulation must be precisely determined by a battery of hormone tests. The operation to obtain the egg is called laparoscopy (see Chapter 16). Once the egg is collected, it is placed in a glass dish (therefore the term *in vitro,* in glass) containing blood serum and nutrients.

Phase 2—Fertilizing the Egg

Once the ripe egg has been obtained it must be fertilized. The husband's sperm is added to the dish containing the egg along with certain chemicals which permit the capacitation of the sperm, the ability of the sperm to fertilize the egg. The egg and sperm are placed in an incubator at body temperature in the hope that fertilization and cell division will occur. Great care must be taken to keep everything as free from contamination as possible. If the egg is fertilized, it will be ready for reimplantation within two and one-half days.

Phase 3—Reimplanting the Egg in the Uterus

The timing of the reimplantation of the fertilized egg must be again extremely precise. The zygote, two and one-half days after fertilization, is introduced into the uterine cavity by means of a slender tube passed through the cervix. If the zygote is at the right stage of development for implantation, and the mother's uterus is at the proper stage for reception, the fertilized egg will attach to the uterine wall and normal development will begin.

The Future of *In Vitro* Fertilization

The birth of Louise Brown in England in 1978 proved that "test-tube" fertilization is possible and raised expectations in women for whom pregnancy had been impossible. The birth of other children and even a set of twins conceived outside the womb has been reported (in Australia). The Norfolk General Hospital, Norfolk, Virginia, has established a clinic to provide for *in vitro* fertilization in this country. There have been many attempts to achieve a single successful conception that have ended in failure, however. The success-to-failure rate has been estimated at one pregnancy for every one hundred attempts. However, a number of ethical problems have been raised. Will women in the future be able to hire surrogate mothers to carry their children? Whose baby would it be? These problems will only arise if *in vitro* fertilization becomes widespread. Since the technique requires exquisite skill and care, it will most likely be limited to the strictest indications.

chapter 13

UTERINE ABNORMALITIES

DEFINITION AND DESCRIPTION OF THE UTERUS

The uterus is a muscular organ whose sole function is to house the fetus during its growth and development. To this end, the interior of the uterus goes through monthly variations to prepare for conception.

The uterine wall is composed primarily of smooth muscle cells. These cells are lined by fibrous (connective) tissue and vascular tissue. The fibrous tissue supports the muscle cells, while the vascular tissue supplies blood and other energy-giving components to these cells through blood vessels.

As a muscular organ, the uterus has contractions or cramps continuing for the entire monthly cycle, even throughout pregnancy and delivery. Those cramps are much stronger at the time of menstruation, but they are evident throughout the month, even if they are not felt by the woman. The pain at menstruation is caused by the dilatation (opening) of the cervix. This dilatation permits the passage of the endometrium (the lining of the uterus), which is squeezed out of the uterus during menstruation.

CONGENITAL MALFORMATION

During the first three months of female fetal development, the beginning of the brain system, the intestines, and the urogenital systems are formed. The uterus (As well as the kidneys, the vagina, and the bladder) is developed from tissue originating on each side of the body, the so-called Müller's and Wolffian ducts. As these ducts fuse together in the midline, the uterus is formed. The urogenitalia sinus, located in the lower part of the abdomen, joins with the newly formed uterus to create the vagina.

During this intrauterine life, an occasional developmental abnor-

331 UTERINE ABNORMALITIES

mality can occur. This is commonly precipitated by certain infections or viruses in the first three months of pregnancy or by any condition which might prevent the complete fusion of this tissue in the midline. In severe instances, a girl baby can be born with neither a vagina nor a uterus or with other severe malformations of the reproductive and urinary tracts. Sometimes the uterus will be only partially fused, and a child will be born with a double uterus. There are many variations of this, all of them dependent upon the degree to which this fusion has occurred.

Such abnormalities often cause no symptoms and thus go largely undetected until they accidentally are discovered, either because a girl does not start menstruating or experiences trouble which leads to a complete gynecological examination. If malformations are suspected, they can be confirmed by special tests or procedures such as *hysterosalpingogram, laparoscopy,* or *hysteroscopy.*

Imperforated Hymen

During fetal development, the Müller's and the Wolffian ducts meet the urogenital sinus and form the hymen, a mucous membrane located approximately half an inch inside the opening of the vagina.

The hymen is closed to varying degrees in different women. In certain cases, there is very little hymen located on the wall of the vagina. In other cases, the hymen almost completely closes the vagina and makes penetration extremely difficult. If the hymen is completely closed (imperforated hymen), a problem would develop when the woman starts menstruation—the blood will collect behind the hymen period after period and cause severe pain, eventually requiring surgical intervention *(hymenectomy).*

An intact hymen has long been considered a symbol, if not absolute proof, of virginity. In fact, it is not. Some hymens are so undeveloped that they are apparent only to a doctor as a *fragment* of tissue on the wall of the vagina. Intercourse can occur without breaking the hymen and so can conception.

If the hymen is so tight that intercourse is impossible, even after several attempts, you should see a doctor. He might have to perform a hymenectomy, a surgical procedure in which the hymen is cut open at several places and then sutured so that it remains open. After this procedure, a woman might have to use vaginal dilators if she does not have regular sex to keep the hymen open. This condition, however, in no way affects a woman's ability to become pregnant.

DEVELOPMENT OF FEMALE GENITAL ORGANS

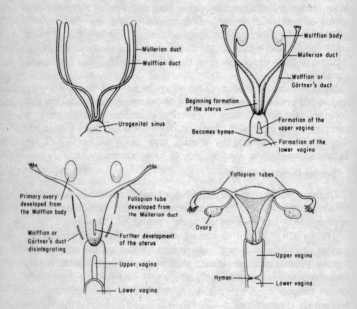

Absence of the Vagina or Uterus

Some women are born without a vagina or a uterus. Although this can occur separately, usually the absence of a vagina means the absence of a uterus, also. However, the ovaries are often intact, so normal development of sex characteristics occurs.

Women often do not realize this type of problem until they attempt intercourse and discover that there is no real opening, or until they consult a gynecologist about absence of menstruation.

This condition is not genetically derived; rather, it is a developmental abnormality occurring in the fetus often as the result of some disease or drugs taken by the mother during pregnancy.

If a woman has no vagina, which might be discovered through self-examination, the physician should test her chromosomes to determine if they are normal. He should also perform a laparoscopy (with a periscope inserted through the navel) to determine if the uterus

Fig. 13–1: Development of Female Genital Organs. The genitalia start to develop during third to the fourth week of fetal life. Primitive cells fuse to become the Wolffian or Gaertner's duct about the fifth week after conception. The Müllerian duct starts to develop at about the sixth week of fetal life, about the same time as the urogenital sinus. *(See upper left drawing.)* The upper part of the Müllerian ducts develops into the fallopian tubes while the lower portion fuse together and form a uterus at about eight weeks after conception. *(See upper right drawing.)* The upper portion of the Wolffian duct develops into the Wolffian body which eventually becomes the ovary in a female (it would be a testicle in a male). The urogenital sinus likewise develops into the vagina.

The lower left drawing shows the stage of development approximately eleven to twelve weeks after fertilization. The development of the Fallopian tubes and the uterus has become clear. The Wolffian body has formed into a primary ovary, which will subsequently move downward. In the male fetus, this gonad moves all the way into the scrotum. The lower portion of the Wolffian or Gaertner's duct disintegrates in a female fetus. In a male, it develops into the *vas deferens* (the tubes carrying the sperm from the testes to the urethra).

The vagina lengthens and the vaginal opening becomes apparent. The hymen will be located between the developing of the upper and the lower vagina. If this normal progression is disturbed during the second to fourth month of fetal life, an abnormal uterus or vagina can result. Such disruption can be caused by drugs taken by the mother, or by various types of infections, as well as by radiation from X-rays. By the sixteenth week of fetal life, the female genitalia have their characteristic appearance, but development continues until birth. The lower right picture illustrates this final stage of development.

and ovaries are present and normal. If the uterus and ovaries are both present, which is rare in these cases, a surgical vagina can be constructed with the same plastic surgery techniques used in male to female sex-change operations. In this operation, a tunnel is created, then covered with a skin graft obtained from the inside of the thigh. The finished product has all the characteristics of a real vagina, from touch to smell. Since the skin graft is placed directly on nerve tissue, sensation is not impaired and frequency of orgasm is absolutely normal. This procedure can be performed even when the uterus and ovaries are missing, but in that instance, conception is not possible.

Double Vagina and Uterus

During the first three months of fetal intrauterine life, developing tissues from either side of the abdomen might not join properly. In some rare cases of female fetuses, two vaginas and two uteri may result. Quite often, each vagina is connected quite cleanly to one cervix, one uterus, and one fallopian tube, and the woman will exhibit no abnormal symptoms. A double vagina is usually divided by a membrane that is pushed to one side or the other by a penetrating penis, so it feels normal to both the man and the woman. Conception can occur in either uterus.

Problems occur, however, when the fetus begins to stretch the uterus. Since one sac of a double uterus cannot stretch as far as a normal uterus, premature birth or miscarriage is frequent. Surgery is not always necessary to remedy this condition, but if pregnancy occurs, the obstetrician should pay special attention to prevent complications.

What Problems Occur with Uterine Abnormalities

As seen in the illustration, there are various types of uterine malformations caused by incomplete fusion of the two parts of the uterus during the first three months of embryonic development. Any variation can occur, from a complete separation of the womb with a double uterus (uterine *didelphys*) or a double vagina to only a small uterine septum (a membranous partition within the uterus). Occasionally, only one side of the uterus develops, a condition known as *uterus unicornis*.

A woman with a double uterus can conceive. The only problem usually is miscarriage or premature delivery. Still, no corrective surgery is indicated.

If there is an incomplete septum in the middle of the uterus, pregnancy can also occur without problems, although there is a higher incidence of miscarriage. If a woman miscarries too often, a *hysterosalpingogram,* an X-ray of the uterus in which the septum or the abnormality can be clearly seen, should be ordered. If the septum is causing miscarriage, corrective surgery should be performed. This entails a Strassman's procedure, in which the septum is removed and the uterus is repaired. After this operation, women can usually carry children with no further problems.

A woman with a unicornis (or "one horn") uterus usually experiences no problem in conceiving if her cervix is open and a normal fallopian tube and ovary are present.

Many women have variations of uterine abnormalities without ever knowing about them, since they experience normal menstrual bleeding and childbearing. These conditions need to be evaluated—by a physician or by X-ray—only if problems occur.

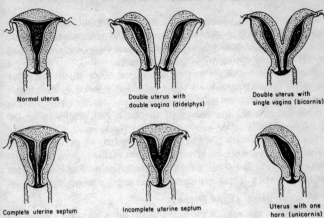

Fig. 13–2: Some congenital uterine abnormalities. In the top row to the left is a normal uterus. In the middle is both a double uterus, a double cervix and two vaginas. To the right is a double uterus with only one cervix and one vagina. In the lower row to the left is a uterus with a complete uterine septum. In the middle, is an example of a uterus with a small septum. To the right, is an example of a one-sided uterus; the other side did develop in this particular case.

Tilted Uterus

Normally the uterus is positioned forward, against the bladder. In infancy, the uterus lays backward a bit, but it shifts forward as it develops. However, in about 20 percent of all women, the developing ligaments holding the uterus forward loosen, and the uterus tilts back against the rectum. This syndrome is called *tilted uterus*.

Until recently, there was a widespread belief that a tilted uterus caused, among other things, infertility. Today, unless a tilted uterus causes pain or physical problems, it is usually left untreated. It is now considered to be a genetic condition, like freckles or a big nose.

There is a second type of tilted uterus that is not congenital, but is acquired usually from pelvic inflammation or endometriosis resulting in adhesions which pull the uterus backward. This is often painful and associated with infertility.

Acquired tilted uterus can also occur after childbirth, since delivery stretches the uterine ligaments and these ligaments subsequently relax after birth. With each delivery, the ligaments become weaker and looser, allowing the uterus to lean back more.

The most common symptom associated with tilted uterus is backache. This is probably a result of blood trapped in the uterus, causing the uterus to become enlarged and tender. This uterine tenderness inflames the nerves of the back and results in severe backache. This is called *pelvic congestive syndrome*.

Many women with tilted uteri also complain of pelvic pressure stemming from the pressure the uterus exerts on the rectum. Constipation generally follows, and there is abdominal pain often mistaken for inflamed ovaries. These symptoms increase prior to menstruation.

Treatment of Tilted Uterus

Treatment depends on the severity of the symptoms. When no symptoms are present, no treatment is necessary. If the symptoms are minor, some doctors simply prescribe an exercise regimen, stressing exercises in the knee-chest position to allow the uterus to fall forward and empty any congested blood.

Another alternative to surgery is the insertion of a *pessary,* a device which acts like a crutch to hold the uterus forward.

If your gynecologist suggests surgery, you should solicit a second opinion from another doctor. Surgery is sometimes required, but more often it is abused. The surgery is not dangerous; it is often merely unnecessary. The operation basically entails tightening the ligaments which pull the uterus forward.

FIBROID TUMORS OF THE UTERUS

The word *tumor* is shocking to everyone. If a doctor suddenly looks up after completing a pelvic examination and says, "You have a tumor of the uterus," most women will immediately begin planning their own funeral arrangements. It is a common fear, one that is possibly devastating to the psychological well-being of every patient.

It should be clear from the start that having a tumor *does not necessarily mean cancer*. A tumor is merely an enlargement or growth. That growth can be either benign or malignant. A benign tumor is noncancerous; only malignant tumors are cancerous. In the vast majority of cases (approximately 99 percent), a fibroid tumor is benign or noncancerous. This statistic should calm women's natural fears about fibroid tumors, but it should not divert attention away from other possibly serious ramifications of a fibroid tumor.

Definition and Origin of Fibroid Tumors

A fibroid tumor of the uterus, also called a *myoma* or a *leiomyoma,* is caused by abnormal growth of cells within the uterine wall (the *myometrium*). There are contrasting theories concerning the type of cells in the uterine wall that develop into fibroid tumors.

One theory is that fibroid tumors arise from primitive cells which normally develop into muscle cells, fibrous cells, or blood vessels. For some unknown reason, this normal development of primitive cells into special cell types has not occurred. Instead, these primitive cells develop into fibroid tumors. Since there is no known reason why these cells shouldn't develop along their normal lines into special types, this apparent malfunction could be genetic in origin. This theory tends to support the undeniable fact that fibroid tumors run in the family—if your mother had fibroid tumors, you have a higher risk of developing the same condition than a woman whose mother was free of fibroid tumors.

A second belief holds that the myomas come from the fibrous (connective) tissue cells in the uterine wall.

Other investigators have suggested that fibroid tumors originate in the fibrous tissue or muscle cells of the blood vessels in the uterine wall.

Finally, some scientists firmly believe that myomas are developed from the smooth muscle cells of the uterine wall, since the fibroid tumors have been found, on microscopic examination, to be composed of muscular tissue. This lends credence to the Latin words *myoma* and *leiomyoma,* both of which refer to muscle. If this is true, though, the layman's term—fibroid tumor—is technically inaccurate, since it is the muscle tissue, and not fibrous tissue, which causes the tumor.

The type of cells from which fibroid tumors develop is, however, more of scientific curiosity than clinical interest. What is important is the cause behind the growth of fibroid tumors, how to prevent or minimize their growth, and how to treat them in their various stages.

General Characteristics

Myomas are the most common tumors afflicting the female organs. It has been estimated that more than 20 percent of all adult women have fibroid tumors, although the vast majority of these women exhibit no symptoms of these tumors.

The incidence of fibroids is, inexplicably, five times greater in black women than in white women. Although it is not statistically verified, the incidence of fibroids tends to be higher in East European and Jewish women than in other white women. The youngest female known to have fibroid tumors was an eleven-year-old girl. Rarely do new tumors develop after menopause, and the majority of myomas found after the change of life actually developed before the menopause. If a new tumor does develop after menopause, there is more reason to believe it is malignant.

A woman can develop a single fibroid tumor, yet development of multiple tumors is far more common.

The size of fibroid tumors varies widely, from microscopic to enormous. The largest tumor ever reported weighed over one hundred pounds.

White in color, fibroid tumors are dense in structure. They are encapsulated and form whorllike masses.

Genetic Occurrence of Myomas

There are several misconceptions among women concerning the development and growth of fibroid tumors. Most of these misconceptions arise from fear and the subsequent ignorance it produces or from a misguided sense of morality.

It should be stated at the beginning that frequency or type of intercourse, or any past traumas or accidents, have absolutely nothing to do with the development of fibroid tumors.

The reason fibroids occur is most likely genetic. The significantly higher incidence of fibroids running through specific families backs up this genetic theory. As mentioned before, the more frequent occurrence of myomas in certain races also supports this belief. Since this genetic trace seems undeniable, it is vital that a woman in one of the racial or familial categories which have a greater tendency to myomas be aware of her situation. In this instance, a woman should be more alert and have a gynecological examination twice yearly to monitor the occurrence and/or growth of fibroids. Moreover, she should understand the phenomenon of myomas and not be frightened if a doctor tells her she has a fibroid tumor of the uterus.

Hormonal Stimulation of Fibroid Tumors

A woman is probably born with the seed of a fibroid tumor in her uterine wall. Although we don't know what exactly sets off the impulse for this seed to develop into a myoma, a growing body of evidence indicates that the female hormone estrogen may be the culprit. This is supported by the observation that these tumors almost always occur between the first menstruation and menopause—the only time when women produce estrogen hormones. Furthermore, when the production of estrogen is highest—during pregnancy —fibroid tumors grow more rapidly. Concomitantly, after pregnancy —when estrogen production diminishes—fibroid tumors usually regress to a certain extent. It has also been observed that there is a rapid enlargement of myomas in cases of estrogen-producing ovarian tumors.

Birth-control pills, particularly the kind with high estrogen content, have also been found to stimulate rapid growth of fibroid tumors. For this reason, many women taking oral contraceptives develop fibroids. Of course, these women might have developed fibroid tumors in any case, and the birth-control pill might only speed the onset of myomas. Women with increased genetic tendencies to fibroid tumors should, then, probably avoid use of oral contraceptives, particularly those with high estrogen content. Women who already have diagnosed tumors should definitely not use estrogen-containing birth-control pills. If you are taking an oral contraceptive and your physician discovers a myoma, even if it is very small, you should immediately discontinue the use of the pill and find another method of contraception.

It has recently been discovered that there is an association between high-fat diets leading to obesity and an increased level of estrogen production. It seems that obesity overstimulates the body's hormone production. This, in turn, leads to a greater stimulation of fibroid tumors, as well as an increased incidence of breast cancer (which is probably also dependent on estrogen levels). This indicates another important function of diet, but it also shows that if you are one of those women with a higher tendency to myomas, you should avoid becoming overweight.

Usually the growth of fibroids is slow. If, however, you have rapidly growing myomas and this fast growth cannot be connected to the overstimulation of hormones (such as by pregnancy or use of oral contraceptives), the fibroid tumor should be *very* carefully monitored. It is this type of tumor which is most often malignant.

Types and Descriptions of Fibroid Tumors

Fibroid tumors can be found in three general locations in the uterine wall, and the location of each fibroid determines the type of tumor in question and the treatment.

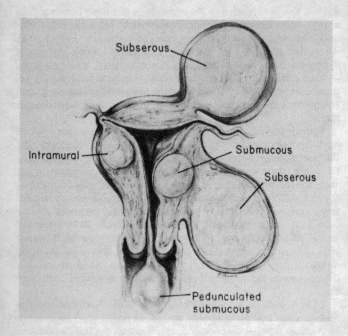

One type is the *intramural*, or *interstitial*, fibroid tumor, located in the middle of the muscular wall of the uterus. This type of tumor usually grows entirely in the wall, causes no pain, and poses no problem when it is small. If the intramural tumor is large, it will occasionally obstruct the fallopian tubes and/or the birth canal.

A fibroid can also be located in the subserosal area of the uterus, directly beneath the peritoneum (the outer lining of the uterus). This is the *subserous*, or *subperitoneal*, fibroid. These can grow anywhere on the outside of the uterus. Although they might cause some pain, they are usually not dangerous as long as they remain small. The subserous fibroids will occasionally achieve great size without causing any other symptoms, except perhaps a feeling of heaviness. If they are located in front of the uterus, they may press on the bladder and cause urinary discomfort, such as frequent or difficult urination. If they grow on the lower part of the uterus, the subserous tumors might also block the

Fig. 13–3: Three different types of fibroid tumors. On the left is an *intramural* fibroid, located *inside* the muscle wall of the uterus. As you can see, if this tumor grew to a large size, it could obstruct the passage to the fallopian tubes. On top of the uterus is a *subserous* fibroid. This tumor is *outside* the uterus and, although it is rather large as pictured here, it does not interfere with uterine function. A second *subserous* tumor can be seen in the lower right portion of the picture. Even at this relatively large size, this tumor would not generally cause any symptoms. However, in this location, on the lower aspect of the uterus, this tumor might be stimulated and grow due to the increased hormone level during pregnancy. It might grow to such an extent that it would obstruct the cervix and vagina and make natural delivery impossible. In the middle of the diagram, on the right side of the uterus, is a *submucous* fibroid, lying just underneath the endometrium (the lining of the uterus). This is protruding into the uterine cavity, pushing the endometrium in front of it. This breaks the smooth contour of the uterine cavity and can, therefore, cause bleeding. Protruding down through the cervix into the vagina, a *pedunculated* submucous can be seen. This pedunculated tumor started inside the uterus, but was expelled from the uterine canal by uterine cramps. It is still attached by its stalk to the inside of the uterine cavity and can, therefore, cause pain and bleeding. Each tumor is whorllike in substance, contrasted to the normal tissue of the uterine wall.

birth passage if they are large. This would make a natural delivery impossible. Sometimes large veins on the surface of subserous fibroids might rupture, causing severe internal hemorrhaging.

The subserous fibroids occasionally become *pedunculated*, meaning that they grow like a flower on the outside of the uterus, attached to the uterine wall by a stalklike protuberance. A pedunculated subserous myoma will also cause no problems unless it twists around its own stalk, thereby cutting down the blood supply to the tumor. This causes extreme pain and can only be treated by surgical removal of the pedunculated tumor.

A third type—the *submucous* fibroid—grows inside the uterine wall just beneath the endometrium (the lining of the uterus) and protrudes into the uterine cavity. Even though submucous myomas comprise only 5 percent of all fibroids, they are the type that instigate the most problems. Submucous fibroids will, when they enlarge, break the smooth lining of the uterus, thereby causing heavy bleeding. This bleeding can, at times, become so severe a woman might bleed to death without medical attention. She might well require emergency surgery. A submucous fibroid can also disturb pregnancy. When the placenta, or afterbirth, starts to grow inside the uterus, it might grow into the area of the myoma. This area will not have the same blood supply as the normal part of the uterus. Consequently, the placenta will not adhere adequately to this area. This might result in bleeding and miscarriage.

Some submucous fibroids might also become pedunculated as they grow larger. The uterus then regards the fibroid as a foreign body, and it attempts to expel the fibroid by contractions. Even when the uterus succeeds in expelling the pedunculated fibroid through the cervix, the myoma will still be attached, via its blood-supplying stalk, to the uterine wall. This so-called self-aborting tumor tends to become ulcerated and infected and must be surgically removed.

If you have a fibroid, make sure you know what kind it is and where it is located. Remember, fibroids vary with each person—one woman will have a subserous fibroid while her best friend or sister will have an intramural or submucous fibroid.

It is also important to know that it is not the number of fibroid tumors you have that is important. The vital fact is the size and location of the tumors.

The only type of smaller tumor you, as a patient, should be concerned about is the submucous fibroid. It is potentially the most dangerous type, since it may cause severe hemorrhaging.

Diagnosis of Fibroid Tumors

A fibroid tumor is usually diagnosed during a pelvic examination. A competent physician will most often be able to feel any abnormality in the size and shape of the uterus, particularly if the patient is relaxed during the examination. A thorough physician should, as soon as he feels even the slightest abnormality of the uterus indicating the development of a fibroid tumor, inform the patient of his diagnosis and the size and location of the fibroid.

Unfortunately, some doctors are not that good at determining the size and location of fibroid tumors. These doctors might unnecessarily frighten you by telling you that you have a large tumor that is very dangerous when, in fact, you have a small tumor that is quite harmless. No matter how much you like your doctor, if he suddenly springs this kind of diagnosis on you—a diagnosis that will scare most people—you should get a second opinion. This is especially true if you have been receiving regular examinations in which you were told you had no abnormalities.

To confirm a physician's diagnosis of a fibroid tumor, *sonography* (or *ultrasonography*) can be used. This is a newly developed technique which has become extremely popular in diagnosing both pelvic masses and the size of the fetus during pregnancy. Sonography has replaced X-ray for a variety of diagnoses, since ultrasound is completely harmless to the body. Essentially similar in principle to radar, sonography employs acoustical rather than electronic frequencies in making a diagnosis. Sonography projects a high-frequency sound into the body, and the impulses of the reflection of that sound measure the size and location of the tumor as it is shown on the sonar screen. If there is any doubt as to the location and size of your fibroid tumors, sonography might be the ideal tool to give you an exact description of your uterine tumors. Besides, it is completely painless and most hospitals have ready access to the equipment.

There might be occasional difficulty with sonography in determining whether a tumor on the side of the uterus is of ovarian or uterine origin. Ovarian tumors are far more dangerous than uterine masses. For this reason, it must be determined whether a mass is ovarian. To check this, a physician could perform a laparoscopy. This is a procedure usually done under a general anesthesia, though sometimes local anesthesia can be used. During this operation, a periscope-type instrument (a laparoscope) is inserted through the navel. By looking into the laparoscope, the doctor will have a direct view of the uterus, the fallopian tubes, and the ovaries. This allows an exact description of the size, shape, and origin of the tumor.

If there is a suspicion that you have a submucous fibroid, one of the best methods of diagnosing this condition is an X-ray of the uterus, called a hysterosalpingogram. With this type of X-ray, dye is injected into the uterus and a picture is taken. If a submucous fibroid tumor exists, it will distort the shape of the uterine cavity. This distortion will be readily seen on the X-ray.

A few doctors prefer to perform a D&C (dilatation and curettage) to determine the presence of a submucous fibroid tumor. During this procedure, the physician will explore the uterine cavity with a curette (a spoonlike instrument) in order to find out if the walls are smooth and regular. If the walls are irregular, a submucous tumor is most likely penetrating into the uterine cavity.

What Can You Do If You Have a Fibroid Tumor?

Most fibroid tumors cause very few problems, so if you show no symptoms whatsoever, the best thing you can do is relax and not worry about them.

However, if you have one or more fibroids with no symptoms, you should be seen by a good gynecologist two or three times a year to check the size of the fibroids. This is the only important action on your part, because you and your doctor can then determine what, if anything, is happening with the fibroid tumors.

If there is rapid growth of the fibroid tumors, it might cause suspicion. Rapid growth is one of the symptoms of malignant tumors, but is not an indisputable sign; tests may be necessary to find out if the tumor is, indeed, malignant. Sometimes you might even need an operation to remove the fibroid tumor for further analysis. This should determine whether the tumor is malignant. It should be pointed out, however, that this type of condition is extremely rare, happening in only one-half to one percent of all cases, and almost always when there is rapid growth of the fibroid tumors.

If your fibroid tumor causes hemorrhaging, you should have an examination under anesthesia and a D&C to determine the location of the fibroid. If the symptoms are severe, you should probably have an exploratory laparotomy, an operation in which the abdominal cavity and the uterus are explored.

Contraception and Fibroid Tumors

If you have a fibroid tumor, yet you experience no problems with it and can bear children, you really don't have to do anything about the condition except refrain from taking birth-control pills with high estrogen content.

You might, though, desire some form of contraception. Here a diaphragm may be the answer. Still, fibroid tumors sometimes disturb the vagina to such a degree that a diaphragm will not fit properly.

An IUD might be a perfect solution in this situation. Not only is there no hormone stimulation, the enlarged uterine cavity will make insertion of an IUD fairly easy. An IUD is not recommended when dealing with submucous fibroids, though, since it will probably cause more bleeding.

Of course, condoms and foam are other solutions to this problem and are widely used when fibroids disrupt normal contraceptive techniques.

As stated before, submucous fibroids often cause miscarriage. While certain cultures believe miscarriage is God's will and therefore a natural form of contraception, it is hardly the ideal method for today's woman. If you have a submucous fibroid where hemorrhaging and miscarriage occur, you should probably have the tumor removed.

It is important to realize that a tumor can be taken out without removing the uterus.

Fertility and Fibroid Tumors

The vast majority of women with myomas have no difficulty whatsoever in conceiving. If, though, you do have any trouble conceiving, it might be due to obstruction of the reproductive passages by fibroid tumors. Surgery might be indicated in such an instance, but because myomas related to fertility are so rare, the physician should perform a thorough testing prior to any surgery.

The doctor should take an X-ray of the uterus (a hysterosalpingo-gram). If the X-ray shows that the fibroid tumors are obstructing the fallopian tubes, there might be cause to remove the fibroids. However, the physician should first make sure your ovaries are functioning normally and that you have a normal ovulation pattern. This is done by taking daily basal body temperature (BBT), which shows an increased temperature just after ovulation. The doctor can also take a biopsy from inside your uterus to make certain you do ovulate. Sadly, many women have operations to remove fibroid tumors only to find that it is an abnormal ovulation pattern which is preventing concep-tion, not the fibroids.

The potential father is often overlooked. The doctor should examine his sperm to ensure his fertility before *you* undergo an operation to remove fibroids. Again, countless women have gone through such an operation only to find that the hopeful father does not have a healthy sperm count.

If these checks are made and it seems that the fibroid tumors are the cause of your infertility, it would probably be wise to have them removed.

Can Fibroid Tumors Be Removed without a Hysterectomy?

If the fibroid tumor is enlarged to an abnormal extent or causing symptoms, you will most likely need a *myomectomy,* an operation in which the fibroids, or myomas, are removed. This operation is performed to save the uterus (and avoid an unnecessary hysterec-tomy).

It is very important for every woman to understand that all visible fibroids can be removed from the uterus. Thereafter, a doctor will perform a plastic reconstruction of the uterus so it will heal and be like a completely normal uterus. Usually, a woman experiences normal menstruation after this reconstruction, and often maintains the ability to bear children.

When Should Fibroid Tumors Be Taken Out?

Fibroid tumors are very complex and unpredictable. Accordingly, each case has to be determined on its own merits. There are, though, some general guidelines which may help.

If the tumors are in the wall of the uterus, you will not need to have them removed unless they are extremely painful, cause infertility, or, as mentioned before, grow very rapidly.

When the fibroids are on the outside of the uterus, they can twist, causing severe pain. They should immediately be removed if this happens. Fibroids can also degenerate, meaning that if the blood supply to them decreases, they will begin to rot and cause severe pain. In this instance, the fibroids should also be removed.

During pregnancy, when the uterus starts to enlarge, the blood supply to the fibroids often increases. This causes the fibroids to grow. If these fibroids are subserous, they will generally be harmless. Many women deliver babies even though they have enormous fibroids on the outsides of their uteri. At other times, fibroids located on the lower part of the uterus can occasionally grow to such an extent that they obstruct the birth canal. Natural delivery would then be impossible and a Caesarean section would have to be performed.

Sometimes the fibroids on the outside of the uterus cause a disturbance in the uterine wall which might cause an early or premature delivery. For this reason, women with fibroids that seem to be growing during their pregnancies should take it easy during those pregnancies. Heavy lifting and energetic intercourse should be avoided in the later stages of pregnancy.

If a woman has experienced several miscarriages due to fibroid tumors, she should have an operation to remove them. She should, though, insist that her uterus be preserved and a plastic reconstruction done.

When Is a Hysterectomy Indicated?

According to the American College of Obstetricians and Gynecologists, a physician has the right to perform a hysterectomy, the surgical removal of the uterus and cervix, when the uterus grows beyond the size of a twelve-week (or three-month) pregnancy from a fibroid tumor.

Unfortunately, many physicians abandon this rule. These doctors tell the patient her uterus has reached the twelve-week point of growth when, in fact, it hasn't.

Other doctors may perform an inadequate examination, and this results in your getting a less than accurate description of a fibroid condition. Sometimes physicians tend to exaggerate the seriousness of the condition, often leading to unnecessary surgery.

Some doctors will observe the growth of fibroid tumors for a long time, then suddenly tell the patient she needs a hysterectomy. Not only is this an example of bad medicine, the sudden change in the doctor's attitude could frighten any woman.

Without a doubt, there are too many hysterectomies performed without the proper indications. Hospitals are aware of this and try their best to control the situation. Each hospital has a committee that examines all tissue removed during surgery. This is done in an attempt to prevent unnecessary operations.

Malignant Fibroid Tumors

For the layperson, a malignant fibroid tumor is always associated with cancer; the medical profession will refer to this malignancy as *myosarcoma* (or *leiomyosarcoma*) of the uterus.

A malignancy goes through various stages. Like everything else, it is better to catch a malignancy in an earlier rather than a later stage. If a fibroid tumor is removed in an early stage of malignancy, it might not have spread. In such an instance, you might be completely cured. Because of this, it is important to remove malignant tumors as soon as they are diagnosed.

The incidence of sarcomatous changes in fibroid tumors is less than 0.5 percent, so when discussing malignancies, women should not get the idea that they are inevitable or common. Low-grade malignancies can even be removed by myomectomy alone. On the other hand, a more definitive treatment consists of a total hysterectomy and bilateral *salpingo-oophorectomy* (the removal of the entire reproductive system—the uterus, fallopian tubes, and ovaries). This is an extremely rare operation, and the likelihood of it happening to you is so slight that you shouldn't be needlessly concerned about it.

How Can You Protect Yourself?

In cases where you do not fully understand your doctor's explanation about why you need a hysterectomy, or in cases where a doctor's sudden change in attitude scares you, you should get a second, or even a third, opinion.

Many patients who are told by doctors that they need a hysterectomy go to other doctors for a second opinion and find that they do not, after all, need an operation.

It is important to realize that it is *your* uterus. You probably should not trust any doctor who does not make it exactly clear why you need the operation, or a doctor who seems to be *pushing* you into an operation without sufficient cause.

Of course, it is vital to your own protection that you understand the nature of fibroid tumors. If you do, it will be very difficult for a crooked or incompetent physician to talk you into an unnecessary hysterectomy. If you have any doubts whatsoever, get a second opinion.

There are good reasons for this.

The chance of malignancy in a fibroid tumor is extremely small. Usually a fibroid causes no harm, even if it has reached the size of a three-month pregnancy, the size at which your doctor can legally operate.

Also, if you are in your late forties, as you get closer to menopause, your hormone level will decrease. There will, therefore, be less stimulus of female hormones to the fibroids. At this point, the fibroids usually decrease in size and often disappear. Certainly, if this is the case with you, a hysterectomy would be unnecessary unless there were severe symptoms, even if the tumor was, again, of the three-month-pregnancy size. Of course, if the tumor does not shrink by itself after menopause, it might be advisable to have an operation.

At times, a fibroid tumor is mistaken for an ovarian tumor. The two often grow in the same region, and many excellent physicians have trouble distinguishing between them. If there is even the slightest chance that you have an ovarian tumor, an operation (maybe just a laparoscopy) must be performed, at the very least for diagnostic reasons. An ovarian tumor is much more serious than a fibroid tumor. The possibility of cancer is higher and it should be considered a dangerous condition. Still, if you have doubts, you should seek a second opinion before submitting to an operation.

Hysterectomy versus Myomectomy

If you are in your mid-thirties and have fibroid tumors which start to grow rapidly, your doctor might be right when recommending a hysterectomy. Still, if you have no problem with fertility and no heavy bleeding or abdominal pain, a hysterectomy might be unnecessary. Under those circumstances, a myomectomy might be indicated, and you should ask your doctor to take out the fibroid tumors but to leave your uterus intact. If your doctor refuses to do this, you should definitely get a second opinion.

It must be remembered that in the majority of cases, if the uterus is no more than four months' pregnancy in size and there are no symptoms, a myomectomy will accomplish the proper aims. You will then be left with a normally functioning uterus and, as long as the fallopian tubes are not damaged and you still have normal ovulation, you should be able to bear children.

However, if you have a uterus that is more than three months pregnancy in size, and you have decided not to have any more children, you might *want* a hysterectomy. With a hysterectomy, you will be sterile, but you will still have normal hormone production as long as the ovaries are not removed.

If the uterus is extremely large, say four or five months' pregnancy in size, the uterus probably should be removed, because it might otherwise cause too much pressure and heaviness on the adjacent internal organs. For instance, a uterus of this size could push the bladder, which would either make urination difficult or too frequent.

Unless you want a hysterectomy, and many women do, you should always fight to keep your uterus. It is, after all, *your* body and no one can force you to have any operation that you don't want. A myomectomy often accomplishes the exact aim of a hysterectomy, but without the result of permanent sterility.

Of course, if symptoms of heavy bleeding and pain are excessive, a hysterectomy is probably in order. But when faced with an operation of this importance, especially if you don't want it, you should *always* get a second opinion. Unfortunately, there are always a few incompetent physicians in the medical profession, and you should watch out for them. Getting a second opinion protects both you and your doctor, so no good doctor will object.

Warning!

In the past few years, there has been much publicity about unnecessary hysterectomies. Unfortunately, too much of this publicity is true. There are irresponsible, incompetent, and greedy people in every profession, and medicine is no exception.

It is important for you to understand that doctors make a great deal of money through hysterectomies. Some unscrupulous physicians could give patients high-estrogen birth-control pills just to speed the growth of fibroids.

Other doctors follow the progress of the fibroids while preparing you for a hysterectomy. Sometimes they wait as long as three or four years; by that time they have your trust. Then the day comes to scare you and they announce that the tumors have started to grow rapidly and you should have a hysterectomy, either immediately or in the near future.

At that point, you should get a second opinion. Remember, if the second doctor confirms the diagnosis of the first, it is a compliment to your original doctor.

It is vital that you realize that only *you* can decide if you should have a hysterectomy. Not that you should be your own doctor, but you should understand your body completely and have thorough biannual examinations. If your doctor does not make your condition clear to you, you should ask him to draw a sketch to further clarify the problem. Bring your husband or boyfriend, or even a close woman friend, and get a thorough explanation.

Once you have established the reliability of your doctor, and once you completely understand your condition, then you can make an intelligent decision with a clear conscience.

Sex and Hysterectomies

There are some very damaging myths concerning sexual enjoyment after hysterectomies. Some cultures, mostly black and Hispanic, believe a woman loses her sexual value and allure once this operation has been performed. This is a mostly male-dominated belief, probably springing from some misguided sense of *machismo*, and is sheer nonsense. This sort of stupid judgment has even caused many intelligent women to hide from their sex partners the fact that they have had hysterectomies.

Without a doubt, the removal of the uterus has little to do with sexual pleasure for either the woman or the man. During intercourse, the penis enters the vagina, not the uterus. The uterus is connected to the vagina by the cervix, and no penis can penetrate the cervix and enter the uterus. It stands to reason, then, that removal of your uterus will not interfere *in any way*, except perhaps psychologically, with your sex life.

PROLAPSE OF THE UTERUS

Prolapse of the uterus is a condition in which the muscles and ligaments holding the uterus weaken, causing the uterus to sag into

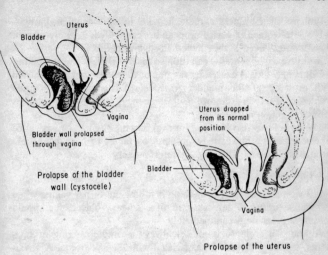

Fig. 13–4: Different types of uterine prolapse. Left, an example of a *cystocele,* where the bladder wall has prolapsed out through the vagina. A case like this can usually only be treated by surgery. Right, an example of a prolapsed uterus in which the uterus has dropped from its normal position and the cervix is almost at the level of the vulva. This almost eliminates the vagina, and the uterus, furthermore, pulls on both the bladder and the bowel. This can often be treated by a pessary.

the vagina. This, in turn, shortens the vagina and sometimes pulls the bladder backward. Prolapse of the uterus is generally found in older women. It is more prevalent in women who have borne children, yet the condition is seen in women who have never been pregnant.

Prolapse of the uterus was seen much more often in the past, when women had several children and were often in labor for days. This was particularly true if the childbirth was difficult and a traumatic delivery of a very large child caused extensive tearing of the vagina and uterus. This condition is less frequent today, largely because many women limit their families to one to two children. Deliveries today are carried out under much supervision and Caesarean section is done if the delivery is judged too traumatic.

Prolapse of the uterus is more frequent in white women, particularly white women of East European background. It is rarely seen in black women, even if they have had several children.

In severe cases, a uterus can drop so far that it feels like something is falling out. This is caused by sagging of the uterus and is associated with prolapse of the bladder *(cystocele)*. This condition causes problems of urinary control and frequency, and usually requires corrective surgery.

The bowel can also *herniate* (or sag) into the vagina. This is called a *rectocele*. The bowel may prolapse so far as to even be visible through the vagina. This, too, requires surgery.

Diagnosis of Prolapse

If a woman feels as if something is falling out of her vagina when she walks, urinates, defecates, or lifts a heavy object, she should consult a gynecologist immediately.

Although a prolapse is almost always a simple sagging of ligaments, cancer is sometimes associated with this syndrome. A physician should take X-rays to ensure that the kidneys, bladder, and rectum are intact. A *cystoscopy* should be performed to double-check the bladder for similar symptoms. Several other tests may be necessary to narrow down the diagnosis.

Treatment of Prolapse

A uterine prolapse is often treated with a pessary—a ring inserted into the vagina which keeps the uterus in the anatomically correct position. The difficulty with a pessary is that it needs to be removed for cleaning at least every two to four weeks. Furthermore, it causes a persistent vaginal irritation and discharge and it often erodes through the vaginal mucosa and causes an ulcer. Many women have no difficulty and are very happy with a pessary; however, others complain that it interferes with sexual intercourse.

If surgery is necessary, a hysterectomy is often performed through the vagina, and the muscles and ligaments surrounding the bladder are tightened. If a rectocele is present, it will be pushed back into position, and the hernia repaired.

Hysterectomy is not absolutely necessary in many cases, but since prolapse usually occurs in older women, removal of the uterus should not affect the woman in any way. This surgery is rather difficult and should be done only by gynecologists well trained in vaginal operations. If the surgery is not done perfectly, the bladder might

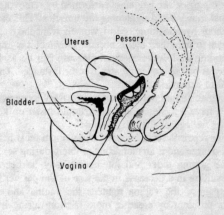

Fig. 13–5: A corrected uterine prolapse. The uterus has been moved back into its normal anatomical position and is held in place by a pessary.

prolapse again, or the surgery could leave symptoms such as inability to control urination. Difficulty of intercourse can also occur if the surgeon makes the vagina too tight.

During the operation, the gynecologist should pass a catheter from the abdomen to the bladder so the urine can drain into a bag, giving the vagina a chance for proper healing. Some surgeons place a catheter into the bladder via the urethra; this is no longer recommended since it causes discomfort and can result in infection. It is important to go only to the best hospital for this procedure, a hospital with competent anesthesiologists; since this procedure is usually performed on older women, anesthesia itself can cause serious problems. The hospital stay for this type of operation will usually be between six and ten days.

Posterior Repair of a "Too Large" Vagina —Increased Sex Life

The same operation that is usually performed for uterine prolapse can be done for women who do not have a complete prolapse but feel that childbirth and age have caused relaxation of the muscles which keep the vagina tight. These women feel their vaginas are getting too loose, and usually they lose some sexual pleasure.

Posterior repair of the vagina is performed by removing a portion of the vaginal mucosa and tightening the muscles. This can be done with or without hysterectomy. Most women want the vagina tightened, but want to keep their uterus because they feel it is important for sexual functioning. However, sexual pleasure can be as great after hysterectomy as before—even greater in some instances. The uterus is not essential to achieving orgasm.

Still, a woman should not have an unnecessary hysterectomy. If a woman does have a hysterectomy, she should *insist* on keeping her ovaries under the age of fifty, if possible.

A posterior repair is recommended if a woman feels her vagina is becoming too large and is an increasing problem during sex. Her mate may also be getting older and intercourse may be becoming less frequent, resulting in a decrease in the size of the partner's penis. A posterior repair of the vagina tightens the vagina and sometimes relieves this problem by creating more friction during intercourse. Since it is done through the vagina, there are no scars on the abdomen, and the operation has often increased sexual pleasure.

ENDOMETRIOSIS—THE CAREER WOMAN'S DISEASE

Normally, the *endometrium*, or uterine lining, becomes thick and spongy during ovulation to accommodate a fertilized egg. If conception does not occur, the excess endometrium is expelled during menstruation.

Endometriosis is a condition in which some of this endometrial buildup backs up through the fallopian tubes and into the pelvic cavity. Endometrial tissue is then mostly found on the ovaries, in back of the uterus, or on the bowel, but it has been known to spread throughout the body to the eyes, the lungs, and even the brain.

Although the exact mechanism for its spread is unknown, one of the most accepted theories was developed by Dr. Sampson in 1921. As the endomctrial tissue backs into the pelvic cavity, he postulated, it implants and then reacts to hormonal changes just as it would in the uterus. Thus the tissue grows every month, but it is not expelled during menstruation. This growth causes problems as it spreads, creating adhesions (which can cause infertility) and pelvic pain. It might also spread through the body in the same manner as tumors.

Women who develop endometriosis are often tense, well-educated and prone to stress and menstrual cramps. Because of this profile, it is thought that endometriosis is caused by tension. Tension tightens the cervix to the extent that menstrual blood cannot get through. This, in itself, would force some of the menstrual wastes back into the fallopian tubes and into the abdomen.

Women with prior histories of *hysterotomy* (a procedure like a Caesarean section performed for late abortion, through an abdominal incision) often develop endometriosis in the abdominal scar.

The first symptom of endometriosis is increased pelvic pain prior to menstruation. This is often misdiagnosed as tilted uterus, polycystic ovaries, or pelvic infection, but a careful examination should reveal an irregular pelvic mass behind the uterus or on the ovaries that characterizes the disease. This mass becomes more tender when progesterone and estrogen levels rise prior to menstruation. It can also create an adhesion between the uterus and the bowel, causing painful bowel movements. *Peristalsis* (waves of involuntary contractions of the bowel) can also cause pain in this condition. Similar adhesions between the ovaries and fallopian tubes can cause infertility.

It is thought that seven to eight million women in the United States suffer from this condition, but only ten to fifteen percent of the cases are diagnosed. If a woman suspects that she has endometriosis, she should make her physician aware of this suspicion, and fully detail her symptoms.

Treatment of Endometriosis

One of the best cures for endometriosis is, simply, childbearing. This halts ovulation for nine months, during which the endometriosis is not stimulated. Subsequently, delivery opens the cervix, causing less painful and more efficient menstruation.

Often surgery is necessary to determine whether the lump behind the uterus is, indeed, endometriosis, and not cancer. During surgery, the physician will remove most of the tissue, but because of the considerable spread of this condition, he cannot remove it all. Relapse is, therefore, common. Because of this, many women will have to undergo repeated surgery. For this condition, surgery is as much a diagnostic tool as it is a treatment.

Birth-control pills have been used against endometriosis, although this use of oral contraceptives has not received Food and Drug Administration approval. Some doctors have found that long-acting progesterone injections alleviate the symptoms, but *the most promising drug treatment for endometriosis is danazol (Danocrine).* Danazol is the only drug approved by the Food and Drug Administration for treatment of this condition. It is closely related to the male hormone testosterone and inhibits the release of LH and FSH, therefore preventing ovulation. Danazol also prevents cyclic variation in estrogen and progesterone levels, so no stimulation of the endometrium or the endometriotic tissue can occur. The body subsequently absorbs the inactivated endometriotic tissue as if it were dead tissue. Many women who have had fertility problems stemming from endometriosis have been able to conceive after danazol treatment. This drug seems to be a real breakthrough for treatment of endometriosis, and women should be placed on danazol as soon as the diagnosis is made to prevent the spread of this condition. Women should also take danazol after surgery to make certain that the tissue that was not removed during surgery is completely eroded. The suggested treatment is 400 to 800 milligrams of Danocrine daily for at least six months, depending on the extent of the disease. Many physicians today start patients on 600 milligrams daily and vary the dose depending on patient response.

Danazol acts as a contraceptive during the treatment and has also been found effective in the treatment of *chronic cystic mastitis*, a very painful condition in which the breasts become cystic and painful. Women suffering from this condition can benefit from a Danocrine treatment of 200 to 400 milligrams daily. This treatment also results in amenorrhea, becoming a safe and effective means of contraception. Unfortunately, danazol is rather expensive, but it is well worth the expense. Perhaps a discount drugstore can offer a bargain. In any event, the majority of Danocrine users will find that this expense will be reimbursed by their medical insurance.

ADENOMYOSIS

Adenomyosis is a condition in which the endometrium, or the uterine lining, invades the myometrium, the uterine muscle fibers, causing an enlarged uterus and severe pain prior to menstruation. Abnormal uterine bleeding usually occurs. Most cases occur in women in their forties, but adenomyosis has been seen in fourteen-year-old girls. Most women, though, develop adenomyosis after childbearing; its occurrence before childbearing can lead to infertility problems.

There is some controversy over treatment of adenomyosis. It is sometimes treated with hormones, but hormone treatments have not proven successful all the time. Many physicians advocate hysterectomy. This seems to be the safest solution unless a woman is approaching menopause or can live with the symptoms. After the change of life, the symptoms of adenomyosis generally disappear on their own.

chapter 14

OVARIAN ABNORMALITIES

Ovarian abnormalities are cysts or tumors of the ovaries. These abnormalities can be divided into benign, or noncancerous, and malignant, or cancerous. The words *cyst* and *tumor* are used synonymously by most physicians. A cyst means a fluid-filled enlargement and a tumor just means a growth or an enlargement. The word tumor, therefore, does not necessarily mean that the growth is malignant. If a physician finds an enlargement or a cyst on an ovary during a pelvic examination, there is no way he can determine immediately if the finding is malignant or benign.

The ovaries are very delicate and important organs. They store the potential eggs (oogonia) throughout a woman's life, and develop one each month into a mature egg or ovum. The ovaries also produce hormones such as estrogen and progesterone, which develop and maintain a woman's secondary sexual characteristics. These hormones prepare the uterus for pregnancy and regulate the menstrual cycle. The ovaries are very active organs undergoing constant internal changes. All these functions interrelate like biochemical clockwork, and a delicate balance is necessary for a woman's body to work correctly. If this mechanism is disturbed or fails to work correctly one month, ovulation might not occur and a cyst could develop.

The most common ovarian abnormalities are cysts. These fluid-filled growths that often enlarge the ovaries can be either benign or malignant. Most malignant ovarian cysts occur after menopause, though they may begin growing during the reproductive years. A cyst that does not disappear spontaneously may be malignant and should be removed surgically.

BENIGN OVARIAN CYSTS

By far the most frequent ovarian cysts are nonmalignant, particularly if they develop before menopause. The most common of these are called *functional cysts,* because they develop from tissue that functions, that actively changes every month with ovulation. These cysts are often larger than the ovary itself, though rarely more than three inches in diameter. If they are any larger, they are highly suspect in terms of malignancy and should be evaluated. Functional cysts can be divided into three types: *follicular cysts, corpus luteum* (or *lutein*) *cysts,* and *Stein-Leventhal cysts* (or *polycystic ovarian cysts*).

Follicular Cysts

Every woman is born with follicles, one of which develops into a Graafian follicle every month, producing an egg. This process depends on a fine chain of hormonal reactions. If, for some reason, there is a weak or missing link in this chain, the Graafian follicle, instead of producing an egg, becomes a follicular cyst. Sometimes these cysts grow to the size of lemons.

Symptoms of follicular cysts are mild. Women may experience a feeling of fullness or heaviness, and there may be a dull ache in the side, but these symptoms subside as the cyst disappears. Usually the fluid is reabsorbed by the ovarian tissue, and after a month or two, the cyst shrinks away.

Follicular cysts can rupture spontaneously, causing internal or abdominal bleeding. There can even be cramps causing such severe pain that hospitalization is required. However, this type of bleeding generally stops by itself, and the lesion heals. Follicular cysts can also be ruptured during rough intercourse or a blow to the abdomen. These cysts have very thin walls, so care must be taken not to bump into anything that may break the cyst. Intercourse should be very gentle or avoided.

If the cyst does not disappear spontaneously within a few months, your physician may prescribe birth-control pills to depress the hormone level that may be stimulating the cyst. If this doesn't work, an exploratory laparotomy should be conducted and the cyst excised and examined for signs of malignancy.

Corpus Luteum Cysts

After the Graafian follicle ruptures to release a mature egg, a yellow body, or *corpus luteum,* forms within the ovary and begins to secrete progesterone. If there is bleeding into this corpus luteum, a cyst may form, filled by the blood. If the fluid is made up predominantly of blood, it is called a *corpus luteum hematoma.* The blood elements are usually reabsorbed gradually and replaced by a clear fluid. The cyst is then called a *corpus luteum cyst*. These cysts are rarely larger than three inches in diameter.

Because this type of cyst develops in the corpus luteum, which exists only after ovulation, corpus luteum cysts occur only in women during the reproductive years.

The symptoms are usually minor: a slight delay in menstruation, persistent or scant bleeding. Pain in one side can occur, giving symptoms resembling those of a tubal pregnancy. Immediate surgery is rarely necessary. If your physician is not secure in his diagnosis, it can be confirmed by a laparoscopy, a "Band-Aid" operation, where a periscope device is inserted through the navel to inspect the ovaries, the uterus, and the fallopian tubes.

As with a follicular cyst, corpus luteum cysts can rupture easily, so intercourse must be gentle and heavy lifting avoided. If one ruptures, severe internal hemorrhaging may make surgery necessary. If not, the cyst usually disappears in a few months.

Stein-Leventhal Disease—Polycystic Ovarian Syndrome

In 1928, Dr. Irving Stein described a list of characteristics he found in a certain group of patients who had come to him with infertility problems. These women had most or all of the same symptoms: irregular menstrual bleeding *(oligomenorrhea)*, often with months between periods; abnormal hair growth *(hirsutism)* on the face, arms, and legs; enlarged clitoris; and obesity. Years later, Dr. Leventhal conducted a hormone analysis on this type of patient and identified such patients as a special group. He subsequently called the syndrome *Stein-Leventhal disease,* or *polycystic ovarian syndrome*. This condition is characterized by enlarged ovaries caused by small cysts. The surface of the ovaries becomes hard and glistening white, probably too hard for the egg to break through, causing a new cyst to develop every month. If ovulation does not occur, infertility results.

No reason is known for the development of Stein-Leventhal cysts, but the syndrome is thought to be genetic. Since the ovaries are enlarged, they produce more of the male hormone testosterone, which leads to hirsutism. Not only will there be abnormal hair growth on the face and limbs, but the pubic hairline will tend to extend triangularly toward the navel.

The ovaries will also produce more estrogen, increasing the chances of developing cancer of the endometrium (uterine lining) or breast cancer. Cancer of the endometrium is always signaled by abnormal bleeding, and if it is caught early, it can almost always be cured. Breast cancer treatment is significantly easier and less drastic if the cancer is found early, so monthly self-examinations are extremely important for women with Stein-Leventhal disease. When a woman with this disease reaches her mid-forties, she should have a mammogram (breast X-ray) every year or two.

Treatment of Stein-Leventhal Syndrome

Treatment of polycystic ovaries varies with the symptoms. Some women require no treatment. In fact, the higher hormone levels often give women more energy and can even increase libido.

If the woman misses her period, she may think she is pregnant. If she is not, her physician can usually induce menstruation by prescribing progesterone tablets or an injection to slough off the uterine lining and cause bleeding. However, this sometimes causes heavy bleeding with cramps and clots because the lining has built up excessively. If this happens, a D&C might be necessary.

Infertility due to Stein-Leventhal disease occurs because the woman doesn't know when she ovulates, or if she ovulates at all. Fertility drugs such as Clomid may induce ovulation. If they do not work, a wedge resection of the ovaries might be required. This is an operation in which a portion of each ovary is removed to reduce the enlarged organs to normal size. This is done during an exploratory laparotomy. No one knows exactly why this operation works, but many women are able to conceive after undergoing it.

This operation reduces the testosterone level, at least temporarily, which helps reduce hirsutism, but the ovaries may enlarge again. If the patient takes daily estrogen, or high-estrogen-containing birth-control pills, it also reduces the testosterone level, again decreasing abnormal hair growth. However, the hair already grown does not disappear; electrolysis is, therefore, necessary to remove the hair. This can be done on the face, while the hair on the legs and arms can be shaved or removed by cosmetic hair remover. Women with too much hair on the abdomen should shave. Many women do this because they do not want the hair to show outside a bathing suit.

MALIGNANT OVARIAN CYSTS

If an ovarian cyst does not disappear after three months, you should consult a gynecologist, especially if it is larger than three inches in diameter. It should be examined carefully by X-rays and sonography. If it seems suspicious, an exploratory laparotomy might be required to remove the cyst. The cyst should then be sent for pathological analysis in a laboratory to determine whether it is malignant.

There are three basic types of potentially cancerous ovarian cysts: *serous cyst adenomas, mucinous cyst adenomas,* and *dermoid cysts*. The cyst adenomas are far more common than the dermoids, and are precursors of most ovarian cancers. They usually grow considerably larger than functional ovarian cysts, but can still be benign, no matter how large they become. Malignant ovarian tumors account for approximately 15 percent of all cancers of women's reproductive organs.

Serous Cyst Adenoma

Serous cyst adenomas occur in women of any age after puberty. They are called the fifty-percent tumors because they are malignant about half of the time and they are bilateral (occurring in both ovaries) about half of the time. They can be too small to be felt during internal examination, or so large that they fill the entire abdominal cavity. If an ovarian cyst is found which does not disappear spontaneously after a few months, it should be carefully investigated—it could be a serous cyst adenoma.

Since there is such a large chance of this type of cyst being bilateral, if a surgeon finds one on an ovary, he should always cut into the other ovary to ensure that there is no abnormal growth there, too. After surgery, the patient should be checked regularly for a few years for recurrence. If, during this period, the serous cyst adenoma does not return, it might never return, although there have been reports of malignancy many years later. If a cyst adenoma occurs after menopause, both ovaries should immediately be removed, since this type of cyst can develop into a very dangerous malignancy (see Chapter 20, Cancer).

Mucinous Cyst Adenoma

Of all potentially malignant ovarian cysts, only 10 to 15 percent are mucinous cyst adenomas, and of those, only 12 to 15 percent develop into malignancies. They tend to be found in only one side, and are often very large. This group of cysts causes the largest tumors in the body. The largest ever reported weighed 328 pounds!

These cysts have thin walls filled with a thick fluid. Like all other ovarian cysts, if they do not disappear spontaneously within a few months, they should be removed, and the woman should return for regular checkups.

This type of cyst can also develop after menopause. Since it can transform into malignant tumor, it should immediately be removed. Because ovarian malignancy tends to occur after age fifty, a woman should continue to have at least one pelvic examination a year.

Dermoid Cyst

Dermoid cysts are so named because they often contain tissue similar to skin, and in fact often have hair, skinlike tissue, and teeth in them. They can contain elements that are developed from all three embryonic layers and can comprise all types of human cells. No one knows how these cysts originate. They represent between 10 and 20 percent of potentially malignant ovarian tumors. They are unilateral in three cases out of four, and the chance of a dermoid cyst becoming malignant is only *one percent*.

Occasionally these cysts contain thyroid tissue and produce thyroid hormone. This can cause a hormonal imbalance, possibly contributing to tumors of the thyroid.

Dermoid cysts are found most often in women in their twenties. They tend to weigh less than other tumors, since much of their mass is made of hair, sweat glands, skin, and other relatively light tissue. Because they are light, they "swim" inside the abdominal cavity, usually floating above the uterus. Therefore, during examination, if an ovarian cyst is higher than the uterus, it is usually a dermoid cyst. Since malignancy is rare, surgery can be postponed for several months to give the cyst a chance to disappear. If it proves to be a dermoid cyst, it will not disappear. If the cyst contains teeth, they will show up on an X-ray of the abdomen. If such a cyst is identified, surgery should be initiated to remove it.

Dermoid cysts tend to float, but they are usually attached to the ovary by a stalk. This attachment can cause them to twist, which stretches the nerves and can create extreme pain. Immediate surgery is then the only solution.

If a dermoid cyst should rupture, it can be highly dangerous, since it contains chemicals that can poison the abdomen. Even if there are no symptoms, these cysts must eventually be removed. Since they tend to be small, they can usually be removed through a bikini incision along the pubic hairline. Using that method, the scar is less visible. Future childbearing should be unaffected if the operation is performed by a competent surgeon.

RARE OVARIAN CYSTS

There are many other ovarian cysts, but their occurrence is very rare and need not be discussed in this book. Several of these cysts are hormone-producing: Some produce female hormones, others male hormones. Several of these rare ovarian tumors can become malignant, and they should be removed as soon as they are diagnosed. The behavior of these tumors is special and they should only be treated by a specialist.

chapter 15

SPECIAL TESTS

THE PAP TEST

The Pap test for early detection of cancer was described and developed by Dr. George Papanicolaou during the 1920s. The Pap test, originally limited to the early detection of uterine cancer, was acclaimed by the American Cancer Society as the most significant discovery in the field of cancer in our time. Later, Dr. Papanicolaou extended the application with his discovery of a diagnostic technique to include other areas of the body, such as the lungs, the stomach, the kidneys, and the bladder.

Dr. Papanicolaou was primarily interested in cytology, the discipline of cell studies. He discovered a special method by which he could stain cells in order to distinguish normal from abnormal cells more easily under the microscope. Using this staining technique, he was able to characterize cells taken from areas of inflammation and also to detect cells which indicated early cancer development. He could therefore describe normal cells, common abnormalities of cells, early cancer and late cancer, as well as inflammation.

This unique staining method and description of cancer was initially researched at The New York Hospital, where *smears* were taken from the vagina. These smears contained cells shed from the cervical and vaginal areas. By microscopically examining these cells using this special staining technique, it could be determined whether they were normal or abnormal. This correlated with cases of diagnosed cancer, leading to a complete description and thesis by Dr. Papanicolaou. This test is now called the *Pap smear*.

The Pap Smear for Women

Twenty years elapsed from the time of Dr. Papanicolaou's earliest description of his method of cancer detection to its complete acceptance. At that time, scientists around the world discovered that

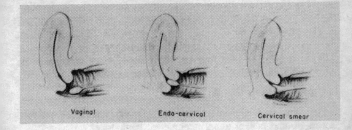

Vaginal   Endo-cervical   Cervical smear

Fig. 15–1: The Pap Test.

Dr. Papanicolaou's staining method and description of early detection of cancer were indeed correct, and that by taking smears from the vagina and cervix, one could identify early and late cancer. The Pap smear became a worldwide technique.

The technique of the Pap smear is fairly simple and involves taking at least three smears, or samples. The first smear is generally obtained from the vaginal pool—the pool of cells which, immediately prior to the examination, have collected behind the cervix. This smear contains cells discharged from the fallopian tubes and the uterus, as well as the cervix and the vagina. This is the most important smear, since abnormal cells from cancer inside the uterus, and occasionally in the ovaries, can be detected through it.

The second smear is obtained from the endocervix. This is the area at which the lining from inside the uterus and outside the cervix usually join. The physician inserts the swab into the cervix and rotates it a few times so cells from the area will be taken.

The third slide, called a *cervical swab* (cervical scraping), is obtained by a special *spadle,* which is inserted and rotated around the cervix a few times.

After a swab has been obtained, the physician transfers it onto a slide. The slides are sprayed in order to fix the cells so they will not be destroyed during transport to the laboratory. When the cells reach the laboratory, they undergo the special Papanicolaou stain. A technician or physician examines the slide under the microscope to see if the cells are normal or abnormal. If the cells are abnormal, a clear description of the cells is carried out.

Essentially, this is the Pap smear. Many physicians take only two smears, a technique believed by many laboratories to be inadequate. The more smears taken, the more cells the technician will have to look at. This gives a clearer and more distinct diagnosis. In cases in which the patient earlier experienced slight abnormalities of the cervical cells, it is wise to take four or five smears, since this gives the cytologist or the physician more material to examine.

Can Anything Go Wrong?

There are two factors of error in the Pap smear: incorrectly obtained smears or smears sent to an incompetent laboratory.

If the smears are not obtained correctly, or if the smears are not sprayed immediately, the cells within the smears can be damaged. It is then impossible to study the cells under the microscope.

If the smears are not sent to a highly sophisticated laboratory, a correct reading might not be given. To save expense, and for other reasons, some laboratories employ younger, less experienced technicians who do not have long experience in reading Pap smears. For this reason, you should ask your doctor which laboratory he uses for the smears and do some checking on your own regarding the laboratory's reputation.

What Can a Pap Smear Determine?

A Pap smear can correctly evaluate the condition of the cells. In the cervix, the cells change throughout the month, depending on the hormonal level. Since estrogen influences the vaginal and cervical cells one way and progesterone another, physicians can determine the time of the cycle from which the smears have been obtained. A Pap smear can, therefore, indicate a woman's estrogen level. This level is important to a woman about to go into menopause, since her physician is then able to determine if she needs hormone-replacement treatment. Tangentially, it is also important to women who have irregular menstrual bleeding as an aid to which treatment should be instituted.

The results of a Pap smear are classified according to the degree of cell abnormality. Class I is a completely normal smear with no abnormal cells. Class II shows mildly abnormal cells, *not* cancer. The changes can be due to a vaginal infection such as *trichomonas*, but could also be the first indication of the development of a more severe abnormality. Class II Pap tests should be repeated within three to six months. Class III indicates moderate-to-severe cervical change—not yet cancer—but a cervical biopsy is suggested to evaluate the condition more completely. Class IV indicates the presence of cancer cells; a tissue biopsy must be performed, and treatment must be instituted immediately.

The description for abnormal cells is called *dysplasia* and is further divided into *mild* and *severe dysplasia*. Cervical dysplasia is a condition in which the cells of the cervix have become abnormal. In certain instances, severe dysplasia develops into early cancer, or *carcinoma in situ*. This is an early cancer which can be completely treated. From the time the severe abnormality, or early cancer (carcinoma in situ), is discovered to the time a fully developed cancer occurs, there might be a lapse of a few years. This depends on the individual. However, as soon as the suspicion of an early cancer arises, a patient must undergo treatment. Treatment might consist of a large biopsy performed during a so-called colposcopy, or the removal of a cone-shaped portion of the cervix (see "cone biopsy," p. 378). If it is not discovered and treated, the cancer might continue into *invasive carcinoma,* which can be fatal.

The development from dysplasia into invasive carcinoma might take several years. If a woman has a Pap smear at least once a year, she can detect the condition in time to obtain a 100 percent cure and ensure survival. If a woman has had an early abnormality such as dysplasia, it is advisable to have Pap smears two or three times a year.

The Pap smear further describes infections in the cervix, guiding the physician to treatment of the particular inflammation. In a like manner, trichomonas and fungal infections can be discovered in a Pap smear.

The Pap smear is a very important test for early detection of cancer, for description and detection of infection, and for determination of hormonal levels.

The Pap Smear—How Often Should It Be Taken?

The American Cancer Society has suggested that a Pap smear every year may not be necessary. Their data seem to indicate that if a woman has had two previous negative Pap smears, she may need have the test only every three years. This approach is not without its critics, and the American College of Obstetricians and Gynecologists feels that extending the interval places the safety of the patient in jeopardy. In the U.S. 13,000 women die from cervical cancer every year; but if the condition is detected early, with a Pap smear, the cancer can be treated successfully, often in the doctor's office. A woman must make the final decision whether or not to have a Pap smear every year. The sexually active woman with several partners, however, is strongly advised to have a Pap test at yearly intervals, because of the increased likelihood of a virus being introduced. The same holds true for any sexually active woman with only one partner. Cancer of the cervix is a terrible disease and it is "better to be safe than sorry."

The Pap Smear—Not for Women Only

Despite the widely held belief that the Pap smear is used to detect cervical cancer only, the Pap test makes it possible to find and treat *many* cancers in the early, curable stages. The procedure is extensively used in both women and men to identify the cells which comprise the lining of an organ and are constantly being discarded. These exfoliated, or cast-off, cells can be removed from normal fluid and secretion, or scraped from the surface of accessible parts of the body. A small amount of this fluid or secretion is placed on glass slides, fixed, and stained so that cellular details will stand out when examined under the microscope. When malignant cells are present in a specimen, they can be identified with a high degree of accuracy.

For instance, cells are collected through sputum from areas of the respiratory tract, including the trachea, the bronchi, and the lungs. This sputum is sent to the laboratory; by detecting and examining the cells in the sputum, early or late lung cancer has been detected and many patients have been cured.

Aspiration of the stomach with a tube which collects cells from the stomach allows detection of cancer of the stomach or of the esophagus.

Cancer of the prostate gland, cancer of the kidney, and cancer of the bladder can all be detected by collecting urine and sending it to the laboratory. Although this test is used for both women and men, it has particular importance for men as one of the earliest and best methods for detecting cancer in the urinary tract.

Many *in situ cancers* (cancers still in an early stage of development which have not yet invaded the underlining tissue) have been detected cytologically by Pap smears in both women and men, as have other neoplasmas too tiny to otherwise be discovered on X-ray films.

Do Not Douche before a Pap Smear

The Pap smear taken from the vagina is a collection of cells that have been cast off from the lining of the vagina and cervix. This is a continuous process and it is, therefore, important not to douche at least twenty-four hours prior to going to the physician. In that way, the everyday vaginal flora is maintained. Douching washes away these cells and prevents the physician from obtaining enough cells for a correct analysis and diagnosis.

It is a normal human instinct to want to be clean, and everyone has been taught to be thoroughly washed before any medical examination. While this is generally appreciated, it can stand in the way of a proper examination. If you are going to the gynecologist for the detection of a vaginal infection or to have a Pap smear, do not douche before the examination. You can wash the outside of the vulva and perineum without interfering with a good Pap smear.

COLPOSCOPY—LOOKING AT THE CERVIX

Colposcopy is the examination of the cervix and the vagina through a colposcope, a binocular-stereoscopic instrument used to obtain a magnified visualization of the cervix and the vagina, enabling the physician to see clearly and diagnose any abnormality. If any abnormal tissue is present, the physician can obtain an adequate biopsy through the colposcope.

Colposcopy was developed in Germany in 1925 and is used extensively in Europe and South America to diagnose abnormalities, particularly cervical cancer. In the United States, the Pap smear replaced colposcopy, since the smear detects cells in precancerous states. Recently, however, colposcopy has been used along with the Pap smear. Any abnormality detected by a Pap smear is further investigated with the colposcope to identify the abnormality through magnification, determine its location, and obtain a better biopsy. It is even possible to remove any minor or early malignancy such as a carcinoma *in situ*.

Technique of Colposcopy

The colposcope is rather simple to use. However, it is expensive, so a hospital often has only one colposcope, or a group of physicians may have one in their office. During colposcopy, the patient lies on her back on the examining table with her legs in the stirrups. A speculum is inserted into the vagina to expose the cervix to the physician's view. The colposcope is then brought to the level of the vagina and a light source is attached so that the physician can easily see the cervix.

Various types of chemical agents can be used to improve the visibility of the cervix. A physician may apply acetic acid (which affects the cervical blood vessels) to the cervix to coagulate excessive mucus. If cervical abnormalities are present, the blood vessels form a specific pattern. The type of pattern helps determine the type of problem. Most colposcopes have cameras attached so the physician can obtain a picture and clearly demonstrate the position of the abnormality. If any abnormality exists, a biopsy can be obtained. Sometimes all the abnormal cells can be removed carefully through the colposcope.

Is Colposcopy Routine?

Some physicians who have colposcopes in their offices enthusiastically support their routine use on all patients. A Pap smear obtained by a competent physician and analyzed in a good laboratory is an adequate screening tool for most cervical abnormalities. However, if any abnormality is demonstrated by the Pap smear, it is advisable for a physician familiar with a colposcope to use this instrument as a diagnostic aid. Routine colposcopy has not been advocated except in a few institutions.

chapter 16

OPERATIONS

Surgery should be considered the last resort in the treatment of any condition, except in emergency situations such as to stop severe hemorrhage, repair lacerations and fractures, or remove an infected appendix. Surgery may be indicated in the treatment of certain cancers, although recent developments in chemotherapy and radiation therapy have proven that these methods can often replace some surgical treatments and limit the extent of surgery in other cases.

Any surgery entails a risk of complications or even death from anesthesia, infections, hemorrhaging, or misjudgment on the part of the surgeon. In gynecological surgery, there are added elements, which, though not making the procedures any more dangerous, do add to the strain of recovery. For example, removal of the ovaries causes a change in the body's hormonal balance, while removal of the uterus might have serious psychological effects.

Gynecological surgery is extremely sensitive, and it is imperative that it be performed by a specialist. That usually means a gynecologist, not a general surgeon. In the case of malignancy, the operation should be done by a gynecological oncologist.

IS SURGERY NECESSARY?

There are many reasons why too much unnecessary surgery is performed. It is partly because some physicians are not fit to practice medicine. Also, operations mean money to private physicians and training to interns and residents. Most physicians in this country are well qualified, but the Federation of State Medical Boards estimates that at least 5 percent, or 16,000 of the country's 320,000 medical doctors, are not conscientious or competent enough. Some physicians are mentally ill, and others are addicted to drugs. Some are too old and senile, while many are simply ignorant and do not care to educate themselves in modern medicine. Medical science is developing so fast that a treatment considered correct today may be outdated next year.

According to the National Center for Health Statistics, 250,000 of the 18 million Americans who underwent surgery in 1975 died either during or shortly after the operation. Many of these patients were very sick and might have died anyway, but some of the deaths could have been avoided if competent medical treatment had been available.

The main risk of surgery is general anesthesia; this is because very potent drugs are used to put a person to sleep. These drugs influence the heart, the lungs, the blood vessels, and the brain. If these drugs are not administered correctly by a well-trained anesthesiologist, they can easily result in death.

Other causes of death are postoperative blood clots, pneumonia, shock, bleeding, or infections. The incidence of these and other serious complications related to surgery varies from doctor to doctor, as well as from hospital to hospital. It is important that a person who needs surgery choose only the best doctor associated with the most competent hospital. Some smaller hospitals can be adequate if they have conscientious and competent staffs, but it is particularly important that the anesthesiologists are highly qualified.

According to a congressional subcommittee, at least 11,900 of the 250,000 surgery-related deaths in the United States in 1975 were totally avoidable, since surgery in all these cases was not indicated. Approximately 20 percent of all surgeries performed in America were, according to studies, not indicated. The rate of unnecessary surgery has not improved much since 1975. Approximately two million unnecessary operations were performed in 1978 with a loss of more than 10,000 lives and a cost of four billion dollars.

Get a Second Opinion

Dr. Eugene G. McCarthy of Cornell University Medical College in New York is presently studying the importance of second opinions before surgery. In a 1976 report, he found that 34 percent of 3,171 patients who were told they needed surgery, but voluntarily sought a second opinion, were found *not to need the operation*. In a second group, 17 percent of 1,094 patients who had mandatory second opinions were found not to need operations. Dr. McCarthy followed for three years patients who did not have surgery because of second opinions, and found that only a small percentage of these patients subsequently needed operations.

This high rate of unjustified surgery has been challenged as being nonrepresentative. Nearly 5,000 operations performed at a group of

Brooklyn and Long Island hospitals were recently evaluated and the rate of unnecessary surgery was determined to be less than 1%. However, these hospitals had stringent patient evaluation programs.

Studies have indicated that when a surgeon is paid for an operation, he is more apt to operate than if he works for a prepaid group health plan, where he is not paid extra for an operation. Furthermore, it is interesting to note that in Great Britain, where doctors are salaried, the rate of hysterectomies is 60 percent less than that in the United States.

Gynecological operations, like other operations, are performed in excess. When a woman's physician suggests an elective operation, she has the right to question the advisability of the procedure and should seek a second opinion. A woman should make sure that her physician is board eligible or certified and associated with a hospital with high standards.

Women should demand that none of their organs be removed unnecessarily. Ovaries, for example, might function until a woman is in her fifties, so should not be removed until later in life. A fibroid tumor can be removed without a hysterectomy (see myomectomy p. 386). The problem of unnecessary surgery has been recognized on a national level, and HEW is now recommending a second opinion program for surgery with its toll-free hotline, 1–800–638–6833 (in Maryland, 1–800–492–6603) to help patients find qualified consultants.

WHAT TO EXPECT AFTER SURGERY

Women who have surgery should not expect to get up immediately after the operation and drive home. After a D&C (dilatation and curettage), a patient stays in the hospital for six to twenty-four hours; older patients who require electrocardiograms or X-ray follow-up usually stay longer. For an operation that requires an exploratory laparotomy (an opening of the abdomen), a stay of six to eight days is indicated. Vaginal-surgery hospitalization may last seven to eight days. If there are urination problems, extend that to ten to twelve days. All this presupposes that there will be no complications. If any complications do arise, the hospital stay has to be extended until the problem is solved.

Regardless of what you are told, do not expect to go back to work following any major operation for three to six weeks. If you do, you are endangering normal recovery. You will be tired much of the time and will require plenty of inactivity and rest. You should be able to resume sexual intercourse after about five or six weeks. Don't be shy about asking your doctor specifically when sex will be allowed.

D&C

The most common operation of all, often called the bread and butter of gynecology, is the D&C. Though the letters stand for dilatation (opening of the cervix) and curettage (scraping the uterine wall), this operation is often jokingly referred to as a Dusting and Cleaning. The procedure is a minor one, and is carried out through the vagina so there are no scars.

There are two general reasons for a D&C: *diagnosis* and *therapy*. Many women feel that a periodic D&C cleans out potential infectious bacteria or precancerous growths. This is not true. If the uterus is normal and healthy, it cleans itself every month by menstruating. Prophylactic D&C is just asking for trouble; complications, though extremely rare, can sometimes occur. Unless your gynecologist suggests a D&C for a specific reason, don't ask for one.

For diagnostic purposes, a D&C is essentially a biopsy from the endometrium, or uterine lining. If any abnormality occurs that suggests symptoms of endometrial abnormalities, a gynecologist can, by performing a D&C, obtain enough endometrial tissue to have it analyzed in a pathology laboratory for potential malignancy.

If a minor abnormality exists in the uterus, such as a polyp, it can be removed during a D&C. This is one of the therapeutic applications of the procedure.

Indications for a D&C

The most common indication for a D&C is abnormal uterine bleeding. With younger women, many gynecologists first treat this problem with doses of progesterone to try to slough off the uterine lining and regulate accompanying abnormalities. This is especially indicated in women with high estrogen levels—for example, women with Stein-Leventhal disease—who develop too thick endometria. If drug treatment is unsuccessful, a D&C can remove the excess tissue or any abnormal growth.

In cases of a fibroid tumor breaking into the endometrium cavity (submucous fibroid), a D&C does not cure the condition, but it allows the gynecologist to diagnose the problem so that he can subsequently treat it properly. This is also true of cancer of the endometrium,

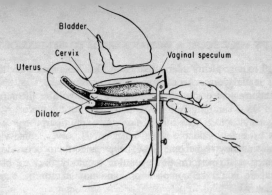

Fig. 16-1: Cervical Dilatation. Dilatation of the cervix is done in order to open the cervix so a physician is able to insert a curette during a D and C, or a suction tip in the case of a suction abortion. A speculum is inserted into the vagina to enable the physician a clear visualization of the cervix. The cervix is then dilated by using a series of dilators (special round-shaped metal instruments) with progressively increasing diameters.

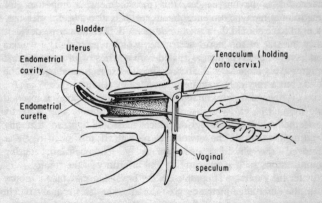

Fig. 16-2: Endometrial Curettage or Biopsy. After the cervix has been dilated, a curettage can be done. The vagina is opened by a vaginal speculum and a tenaculum (a special forceps) is placed on the lip of the cervix to stabilize the uterus. A curette is then inserted into the uterus and the physician gently scrapes the walls of the uterus in order to remove abnormal tissue, or obtain enough material for a biopsy of the lining of the uterus.

whose first sign is irregular bleeding. A D&C can save your life by giving an early diagnosis of cancer.

If abnormal bleeding is the result of a misplaced or incompatible IUD, a D&C can remove the IUD and clean out the uterus.

In general, a D&C is a simple, fairly safe, multipurpose procedure that is extremely valuable when indicated. However, some women have a tendency to become D&C-happy and try to persuade their gynecologists to perform this operation regularly. Beware of this, since there could be complications and any anesthesia entails a potential risk.

The Technique of a D&C

A D&C is usually performed under general anesthesia, although it can be done with a local anesthetic injected around the cervix. After anesthesia has been administered, the vagina is washed with an antiseptic solution and the procedure begins. The physician should first take a scraping from the interior of the cervix. This can later be compared with tissue obtained from the uterus to determine if abnormalities in the uterus have spread to the cervix. The depth of the uterus is then measured with a uterine sound. If the patient is diagnosed as having cancer, this measurement is important for determining the type of cancer treatment. It is also a useful measurement to have should the patient require an IUD (intrauterine device), since the size of the uterus determines which type of IUD a woman can have. The cervix then is dilated with a series of instruments that progressively increase in diameter. The process is gradual because the cervix has a very tight opening surrounded by strong tissue. When the cervix is opened widely enough, the *curette* (a small spoon) is inserted into the uterine cavity and scraping along the uterine wall is gently performed. The gynecologist's touch must be light so that any abnormalities inside the uterus can be felt. If too much tissue is removed, the physician can damage the endometrium, causing complications such as miscarriage and infertility in the future.

After the curettage is completed, the physician may take a biopsy from the outer edge of the cervix to send to the lab for analysis, but this is usually unnecessary since a good Pap smear renders almost the same information.

After discharge from the hospital following a D&C, a woman will usually experience slight bleeding and staining for five to seven days and on occasion up to two weeks. For the first three to four weeks following the procedure, she should avoid intercourse or the insertion of any foreign object, such as tampons, into the vagina, to prevent infection. The recovery period varies from person to person, but in general, a woman may return to work, if this does not involve physical work, in three to fourteen days.

CERVICAL BIOPSY

A biopsy, or a punch biopsy of the cervix, is a procedure by which a small piece of the cervical tissue is obtained for pathological examination in cases of suspected cervical cancer. This procedure is performed when the Pap smear is abnormal, or if an abnormal cervical lesion is seen during a pelvic examination. The cervical biopsy can be performed in the office, usually without any anesthesia since there are few nerves in the cervix. A woman usually feels only a small pinch during this procedure. This procedure can also be performed in combination with a dilatation and curettage (D&C) under general anesthesia in the hospital.

The Technique of a Cervical Biopsy

When cervical biopsy is obtained in the office, the woman is placed on the examination table with her legs in the stirrups. A speculum is

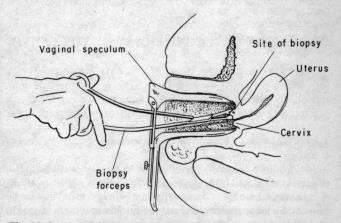

Fig. 16–3: Cervical Biopsy. Visualization of the cervix is obtained by insertion of a vaginal speculum. The biopsy is obtained with a special *biopsy forceps,* constructed so they will not damage the specimen.

inserted into the vagina, and the physician uses a special biopsy forceps. The biopsy forceps is an instrument with a sharp edge and a spoonlike opening in the middle. The physician removes from the suspicious area a small amount of tissue, which is sent for pathological examination. If the cervical biopsy is performed on the basis of an abnormal Pap smear, a physician might perform Schiller's test, which involves staining the cervix with a special iodine solution prior to obtaining the tissue. This test is based on the fact that the glycogen in the normal cells of the cervix causes them to stain dark brown when painted with potassium iodine solution. However, if there are abnormal cells indicative of a premalignant lesion, they do not stain; thus it is easier for the physician to know which area to biopsy for the most accurate diagnosis.

A biopsy of the cervix is now often performed in combination with colposcopy, allowing the physician, through the colposcope, to get a clear, magnified view of any abnormality and to take a biopsy from any suspicious area (see Colposcopy).

Women usually experience slight staining for a few days after a cervical biopsy. Intercourse should not take place for two weeks or until the tissue has healed completely. Intercourse, or even the use of a tampon, might result in bleeding or cause infection in the biopsied area. Most women experience very little or no pain following cervical biopsy.

CONIZATION OR A CONE BIOPSY OF THE CERVIX

A conization is an extended biopsy of the cervix, with removal of a cone-shaped portion of the outer cervix. This is performed when an abnormality that may be precancerous shows up on a Pap smear or a punch biopsy of the cervix. The cone biopsy removes the tissue that is most susceptible to cancer and can even remove early cervical cancer. The operation should have no effect on a woman's sex life or ability to conceive.

The operation is usually performed under general anesthesia. The patient is then placed in the stirrups and the vagina is sterilely washed. A cone-shaped biopsy is then excised from the cervix. This can be associated with heavy bleeding, and several sutures must be placed to control the bleeding. The patient remains in the hospital for a few days and is then discharged to rest at home. It is important not to have intercourse for five or six weeks, since this could break the

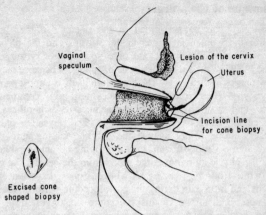

Fig. 16-4: Cone Biopsy of the Cervix. After the patient is anesthesized, the vagina is sterilely washed to prevent infection and proper visualization of the cervix is obtained by a vaginal speculum. A cone-shaped biopsy (shown to the left in the picture) is then obtained by cutting a cone-shaped portion of the outer cervix with a sharp knife. If there is any abnormality or lesion of the cervix, the physician must be sure to include that in the biopsy.

sutures and result in heavy hemorrhaging. A woman should have a Pap smear after the operation, particularly if the operation was done for removal of a precancerous lesion.

CRYOSURGERY, OR FREEZING OF THE CERVIX

Cryosurgery, or freezing, of the cervix is a relatively new technique which is used to destroy any abnormal lesion by freezing. In gynecology, this procedure is mostly used for women who have chronic cervicitis. It has also been used in the treatment of early malignant lesions, but with questionable success.

Cryosurgery and electrocauterization, or burning, are used for the same indication. The reasoning behind both techniques is that both procedures kill abnormal cells. In cervicitis, where there has been a prolonged infection and cellular damage, the physician wishes to destroy the abnormal cells. This gives newer and healthier cells the opportunity to form and replace the old damaged cells.

Technique of Cryosurgery

Cryosurgery can be performed in the doctor's office. In this procedure, the woman is placed in the stirrups and the physician visualizes the cervix with the aid of a speculum. Cryosurgery is performed without the aid of anesthesia or analgesia because there are very few nerves in the cervix. The procedure itself is almost painless.

Many types of cryosurgery machines are now commercially available, and most physicians have machines in their offices. The actual freezing takes only a few seconds. The physician places a cryosurgery probe firmly against the cervix, making sure that a sufficient area is deeply frozen, thus destroying all abnormal cells.

After the physician removes the probe from the cervix, the cervix will be white from the freezing. A woman usually experiences few symptoms and little pain during the postprocedure period. A woman should not be disturbed if this procedure is suggested in well-indicated cases, where symptoms dictate that intervention is required.

What to Expect after Cryosurgery

A woman should not expect any serious problems after cryosurgery, although it will take up to four to six weeks before all the cells destroyed by freezing are replaced by new, healthy cells. During this time, she can usually expect a profuse, watery vaginal discharge caused by the sloughing off of the damaged cells, until the normal physiological balance of the vagina is restored. She will occasionally see a slight brownish discharge, which is caused by the shedding of the old, damaged, destroyed cells. A woman should usually refrain from intercourse for at least four weeks to prevent any infection or damage to the healing cervix. At the same time, she should not wear a tampon but use a sanitary napkin. She should see her physician four to six weeks after the procedure to make sure proper healing has occurred.

Cryosurgery is recommended in *indicated cases* if performed by physicians who are competent with the procedure.

ELECTROCAUTERIZATION OF THE CERVIX

Electrocauterization, or burning, is a procedure performed to destroy abnormal cells of the cervix due to chronic cervicitis.

This procedure has been performed for many years to destroy the infected and abnormal cells, giving new, healthy cells a chance to form, eventually changing all the cells on the surface of the cervix.

Technique of Electrocauterization

Electrocauterization is usually performed in a doctor's office and can be done without anesthesia or analgesia. The woman is placed on a gynecological table and a speculum is inserted into the vagina to visualize the cervix. The physician then carefully places a small probe on the area of the cervix to be cauterized. The amount of heat applied via the probe is easily controlled by a foot pedal. The cauterization causes an actual burning of the superficial layers of cells. This usually takes a few minutes; when the physician is satisfied that all damaged cells are destroyed, the procedure is over. Cauterization is usually associated with very little pain. In fact, the majority of women feel nothing during the operation.

What to Expect after Electrocauterization of the Cervix

After cauterization of the cervix, it usually takes four to six weeks before the destroyed cells are replaced by new, healthy cells. In the interim, a woman can anticipate a watery discharge and an occasional brownish discharge as the old cells are sloughed from the vagina. The insertion of any foreign object into the vagina might introduce new bacteria and cause another infection; therefore it is advisable not to have intercourse, to douche, or to use a tampon for four to six weeks. A physician should be seen approximately six weeks after the procedure to ensure that proper healing has occurred.

HYSTERECTOMY

The most common major gynecological operation is hysterectomy, or removal of the uterus through either the abdomen or the vagina. There are two basic types of hysterectomies about which there is considerable confusion among many women: *total hysterectomy* and *supracervical hysterectomy*. The confusion stems from the misconception that a total hysterectomy includes the removal of the ovaries. In fact, a total hysterectomy simply means that both the uterus and the cervix are removed. Removal of the ovaries, the fallopian tubes, and the uterus is called a total hysterectomy with a bilateral salpingo-oophorectomy.

Supracervical hysterectomies are now not done very often. Years ago the cervix was not removed because it was a more difficult procedure and many physicians were not that well trained. The difficulties encountered in removal of the cervix are caused by its

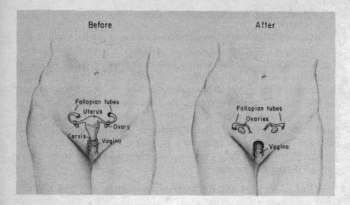

Fig. 16–5: Total Hysterectomy. A total hysterectomy is the removal of the uterus and the cervix, but *not* the ovaries or the fallopian tubes. The illustration demonstrates the anatomical position of the female genitalia before and after a total hysterectomy. When the uterus and the cervix is removed by a hysterectomy, a woman still has the same depth of the vagina and the operation should not interfere with sexual intercourse.

proximity to the bladder and the uterus. It can also cause severe bleeding. Today, however, with modern surgical techniques and better training, it is no longer considered dangerous or difficult to remove the cervix, and since this area is particularly cancer prone, most gynecologists feel the cervix should be removed with the uterus.

Many women have reservations about hysterectomies because they feel their female sexual characteristics will somehow be affected. Men, too, often feel a woman is desexed after hysterectomy. Nothing could be further from the truth. Masters and Johnson have shown that women have no orgasmic loss after hysterectomy. In some instances, the hysterectomy may even enhance sex, since the woman no longer has to worry about becoming pregnant. This does not, however, justify a hysterectomy.

Unnecessary Hysterectomies

Some physicians push women into unnecessary hysterectomies simply to earn fees. However, most unnecessary hysterectomies are performed for a less mercenary, but no less tragic, reason: namely, ignorance and incompetence on the part of the physician. Some physicians simply haven't kept up with the modern techniques or knowledge that render many hysterectomies unnecessary. They are not necessarily negligent, for there is more to keep up with in medicine than is possible for any one physician. That is the reason so many doctors specialize. Women should, therefore, make sure that their gynecologists are trained and are specialists in gynecology. A gynecologist should participate in postgraduate training and meetings to become familiar with the latest developments in the field. Some general practitioners and general surgeons call themselves gynecologists, but are not qualified. Some of these physicians, particularly general surgeons, have had minimal gynecological training and practice and tend to perform too many gynecologic operations, often not in accordance with the rules of the American College of Obstetricians and Gynecologists.

If your doctor suggests a hysterectomy and you have any reason to question this suggestion, especially if the doctor is not a gynecologist, you should seek a second opinion. Every woman has a right to this, particularly since so many unnecessary hysterectomies are performed. Every woman has the right to doubt her doctor, even if he is a trained and competent gynecologist. If you are still in doubt after a second opinion, a third opinion could solve the matter.

Unnecessary hysterectomies risk more than a woman's uterus; they can mean her life. This is one of the reasons the problem has received so much attention in the media. Of the 787,000 hysterectomies performed in the United States in 1975, 1,700 of the patients died as a result of complications, often from anesthesia-related causes. This is all the more reason to have a hysterectomy in a modern medical center where competent medical attention can be assured from both surgeons and anesthesiologists, and where consulting specialists are available if complications should occur. There is also a "tissue committee" in such hospitals, which reviews and questions the necessity of all surgical cases. This makes it more difficult for a doctor to perform unnecessary surgery.

Of course, it is unfair to say that doctors who don't work at large medical centers are not competent. Most women have seen one gynecologist for years, respect his advice, and know from experience that he is competent. Most physicians are worthy of that trust, but that does not mean you should not be aware of your options. In 1978, *The New York Times* reported that up to 22 percent of all hysterectomies were unnecessary.

It's interesting to note that half of all physicians' wives in the United States have hysterectomies by the time they are sixty-five, compared to one third of the rest of American women. Both male and female physicians are themselves operated upon some 20 to 30 percent more than the rest of the population. All common operations are overperformed equally, but don't always blame the doctors. Sometimes a woman will push the physician to do an operation. It is estimated that there will be 3.2 million unnecessary operations of all kinds this year, resulting in some 16,000 deaths. Surgery not only carries physical threat, it often causes psychological trauma.

Surgery is also costly. It has been estimated that up to $4 billion was spent on unnecessary surgery in the United States in 1978. This money came not only from patients' pockets directly, but also from taxes and insurance (driving the rates up, costing the patient more in the future). Hysterectomies also mean money to the gynecologist. The average gynecologist performs about thirty hysterectomies yearly at a charge of between $500 and $1000 for each. This means an income of between $15,000 and $30,000 annually on hysterectomies alone.

Indications for Hysterectomy

One well-justified indication for hysterectomy is cancer or precancerous signs in the uterus. Approximately 8 percent of all hysterectomies are performed for this reason. The risk to a woman's life from cancer is too great to balance the benefits of leaving the uterus. This type of hysterectomy must be done through the abdomen rather than through the vagina, since the physician must be able to check the abdominal cavity visually for tumors, metastasis, or precancerous signs. This operation should always be performed in consultation with a cancer specialist, a gynecologist-oncologist.

Fibroid tumor is another indication for hysterectomy, but only if it is causing severe bleeding or pressing on other organs. In this case, too, abdominal hysterectomy is usually necessary, particularly if the uterus is too large to be removed through the vagina. Fibroid tumors are the most common indication for hysterectomies. However, many of these operations are unnecessary, since most fibroid tumors are asymptomatic and less than one percent ever become malignant. Most fibroid tumors start to shrink when a woman reaches menopause. According to the American College of Obstetricians and Gynecologists, a hysterectomy is indicated if the fibroid causes the uterus to enlarge beyond the size of a twelve-week pregnancy. Yet some physicians tell their patients that a fibroid is larger than it actually is, thus scaring women into having hysterectomies. Tissue committees find that many fibroids removed are of less than twelve-week size. Hysterectomies for fibroid tumors account for approximately 30 percent of all hysterectomies (see Fibroid Tumors).

It is often possible to carry out a myomectomy instead of a hysterectomy. This is recommended if further childbearing is desired, or if a woman does not want to lose her uterus. In the past, this has often been left up to the physician's discretion, but a woman has the right to a second opinion if she has any doubts, or if the doctor seems to be pushing a hysterectomy.

Hysterectomy is sometimes the only solution for chronic vaginal bleeding. If repeated D&Cs and hormone therapy prove unsuccessful, the uterus may have to be removed, especially if no further childbearing is desired. In these cases, vaginal hysterectomies are often possible. Chronic vaginal bleeding is the indication in about 10 percent of hysterectomies.

Endometriosis often causes such intense pain that if treatment with drugs such as danazol does not solve the problem, hysterectomy is often required, particularly if the woman does not want to have any more children. Abdominal hysterectomy is usually the only possibility, since the physician must check the spread of endometriosis into the abdominal cavity. Also, there are generally many adhesions, making a vaginal hysterectomy very difficult.

Approximately 25 percent of all hysterectomies are done because of prolapsed uteri or dropped wombs. This operation is usually done through the vagina in combination with an A&P repair (see Anterior & Posterior Repair, page 391).

There are many other indications for hysterectomy, including severe menstrual cramps or chronic pelvic congestion, but these occur less frequently than those outlined above and vary so much from case to case that discussion here would serve no purpose.

Occasionally hysterectomy has been considered a means of sterilization, and about 9 percent of all hysterectomies are performed for this reason. If a woman has completed her family and seeks sterilization, a hysterectomy, rather than a tubal ligation, ensures not only against future pregnancy, but eliminates the possibility of uterine problems (including uterine cancer). A hysterectomy for sterilization is often performed in conjunction with an A&P repair, an operation which tightens the vaginal muscles that become loose after several childbirths. An A&P repair can often rejuvenate a couple's sex life, since the woman's vagina will be tighter and more responsive. A simple vaginal hysterectomy is usually performed for sterilization. However, women must realize that a hysterectomy is major surgery —a much longer, more involved, and more dangerous procedure than a tubal ligation, and one with many more possibilities for complications. The pros and cons of this procedure must be discussed fully with your gynecologist.

Some hysterectomies are performed for the convenience of the patient or because of the misjudgment of the physician. Some women in their twenties ask for hysterectomies because they are convinced they do not want children and do not want to be bothered with menstruation. Some women request hysterectomies since they have heard that this procedure can improve their sex lives. Obviously these are not proper indications for hysterectomy. Any of these operations involves a change of life. A woman should never let any physician remove any organs except in well-indicated cases.

Surgical Technique of Hysterectomy

A hysterectomy can be done either through the abdomen or through the vagina. These operations are usually done under general anesthesia, but they can be done under spinal anesthesia.

The abdominal route is usually employed, since a vaginal hysterectomy can only be employed in simple and easy cases. The abdominal operation can be done either through a low, horizontal incision—a Pfannenstiel incision—or with a so-called bikini cut. This incision is made underneath the hairline and is not visible. If a larger view is needed during the surgery or if the operation is done because of cancer, a vertical incision between the pubis bone and the navel is performed. If the operation is less complicated, you should ask your physician to perform a bikini cut since the scar heals more strongly and is hardly visible.

A vaginal hysterectomy is usually done as a sterilization procedure or if the uterus is not too large. Hospitalization after a hysterectomy is about a week, but a woman cannot usually return to work until four to six weeks later. Sex can be resumed six to seven weeks after the operation.

MYOMECTOMY

A myomectomy is an operation in which a fibroid tumor is removed from the uterus without a hysterectomy. This is usually done through the abdomen. If a woman who has fibroid tumors wants to have children in the future or does not want the uterus removed, she should not have a hysterectomy; she should have a myomectomy.

During a myomectomy, each fibroid tumor is removed separately from the wall of the uterus and the incision in the uterus is then closed surgically by sutures. Afterward the uterus heals normally, relieving such previous symptoms as abnormal bleeding, pain, or pressure on the bladder that are typical of fibroid tumors. If this operation is done by a competent gynecologist, the uterus will look like a perfectly normal uterus a few months later. Women can often conceive after this procedure, even if they have not been able to conceive before, as long as the fallopian tubes and the ovaries are normal.

During myomectomy, the gynecologist should remove all fibroids (more than fifty have occasionally been removed). However, it is possible to miss very tiny fibroids that have just started to develop in the uterine walls, and the condition may return. However, if childbearing is desired, the recurrence may not be for several years, giving an interim during which a healthy child can be born. In some cases it is impossible to remove the fibroid tumors because of their location or their size, and hysterectomy would be the only possible treatment. The choice is a personal one, but a younger woman is usually happier with a myomectomy.

OOPHORECTOMY

Oophorectomy is an operative procedure by which one (unilateral oophorectomy) or both (bilateral oophorectomy) ovaries are surgically removed. The indications for unilateral oophorectomy are very few; they include precancerous ovarian cysts, twisted ovarian cysts, ovarian pregnancy, ovarian abscess, and damage to an ovary due to conditions such as severe endometriosis. Bilateral oophorectomy is performed if any of the above conditions has affected both ovaries. The vast majority of bilateral oophorectomies are performed in combination with total abdominal hysterectomy, and the main indication for this procedure is cancer of the ovaries.

Should Healthy Ovaries Be Removed?

The majority of oophorectomies are performed prophylactically as a routine part of a hysterectomy. The rationale behind removing the ovaries at the time of the removal of the uterus is to eliminate them as possible sources of cancer. Some physicians feel that once the uterus is removed, the major function of the ovaries, the production of eggs for possible fertilization and pregnancy, has been eliminated and they should, therefore, be removed. However, these doctors do not seem to appreciate fully the enormous shock to a woman's entire system that is produced by surgically inducing menopause at the age of forty. Healthy ovaries in some women can function into the fifties, and artificially administered hormones can never fully compensate for the delicate balance of natural hormones produced by a woman's own ovaries.

There has been a recent controversy over the association of artificial estrogen replacement and cancer. Because of this, it seems ludicrous to remove healthy ovaries simply because they might be possible targets for cancer and then to administer artificial hormones that could render a woman more susceptible to other forms of cancer. In Europe, the number of hysterectomies performed in relation to the population is much lower than in the United States, and similarly, the number of bilateral oophorectomies of healthy, functioning ovaries is a fraction of what it is in the United States.

Prophylactic bilateral oophorectomy in women under fifty during hysterectomy is advocated by a number of physicians as a method of preventing ovarian cancer. However, a recent study has shown that in order to prevent a single death from ovarian cancer, almost 7,500 healthy, functioning ovaries would have to be removed. In other words, only 2.7 of the 10,000 yearly deaths from ovarian cancer could be prevented if prophylactic oophorectomy was performed during hysterectomy in women under the age of fifty. Bilateral oophorectomy of healthy, functioning ovaries in premenopausal women *cannot* be recommended. After menopause, when the ovaries have ceased to function, prophylactic oophorectomy during hysterectomy would be advisable.

HYMENECTOMY

The hymen is not an important anatomical part from a medical standpoint, but from a historical, cultural, and religious standpoint, it has extraordinary importance. Throughout the ages, an intact hymen has been a symbol of virginity, a sign of purity.

A hymenectomy is an operation in which the hymen is surgically opened. This operation is performed only in rare instances, when the hymen is so strong that it cannot be broken and, therefore, does not permit intercourse.

Some hymens are so thin and fragile that they can easily break during a fall in childhood or accidentally rupture during bicycling or horseback riding. Other hymens permit intercourse without breaking. Thus a woman might be a virgin, yet might not bleed during her first intercourse. If a hymen is very thick and firm, and, furthermore, if the woman is tense, as many women are when they first have intercourse, the hymen can actually prevent penetration by the penis. In cases like this, the hymen can be cut surgically and the vagina dilated until the physician can easily admit two or three fingers (size of the normal penis) into the vagina. Intercourse then becomes possible, although a lubricant like Vaseline or saliva may be necessary at first.

Most hymens are broken before or during the first intercourse. Once the hymen is broken, it never grows back. Some women who have abstained from sex for prolonged periods may feel as if their hymens have returned, but this is actually a tightening of the vagina from disuse. This condition can lead to some pain during subsequent intercourse, but additional foreplay usually solves the problem.

Re-creation of Virginity

Though the hymen will not grow back, it can be surgically repaired. Such cases have been reported among women who belong to certain orthodox religious sects. An intact hymen is often a prerequisite for marriage among certain religious groups, and marriage is often the only decent life the woman can expect. Thus, if a hymen has been broken either accidentally or through illicit sex, it becomes essential to the woman's future to have it repaired. When the hymen is subsequently ripped a second time, the woman will experience the same pain and bleeding she might have at first. This operation was supposedly done two hundred years ago on prostitutes, since they were paid more if they were virgins. Some of these women had the procedure done several hundred times.

The operation is relatively simple and entails an approximation of the loose edges of the hymen with a few superficial sutures. This can be done so that it will be impossible for a layperson to detect it.

CUL-DE-CENTESIS

This is a procedure in which a needle is placed through the vagina into the cul-de-sac (the space behind the uterus) to determine if there is any intraabdominal bleeding or infection. The operation is done if a woman has symptoms of a ruptured ovarian cyst or an ectopic pregnancy; blood is found in the abdominal cavity in both cases. If the woman has ovarian cancer, this shows up in the aspirated abdominal fluid. This operation is usually done under local anesthesia. The procedure is very helpful for a physician in order to make a diagnosis.

CULDOSCOPY

Culdoscopy, a diagnostic and therapeutic procedure, has been used in the United States since the 1940s. During this procedure, a periscope-like instrument is inserted through a small incision in the vaginal wall into the abdominal cavity, providing the physician with a view of the uterus, the fallopian tubes, and the ovaries.

Culdoscopy is rarely performed at the present time, since it has been replaced in many instances by laparoscopy. Culdoscopy is a somewhat difficult procedure, since the woman has to kneel in the so-called knee-chest position and cannot be under general anesthesia. Furthermore, the physician must insert the culdoscope somewhat blindly and might damage the pelvic organs if the patient has adhesions. This procedure is, therefore, mostly performed by physicians who have years of experience with this technique.

The Technique of Culdoscopy

Culdoscopy is usually performed in a hospital under local anesthesia. The woman is placed in the knee-chest position—kneeling, bent forward, head resting on her arms, with her chest lower than her bottom. Before the procedure, the vagina is washed sterilely. Since it is impossible to sterilize the vagina completely, some physicians are cautious about this procedure, because of the inherent risk of infection. After the vagina has been washed, a sterile drape is placed around the woman. A spinal or epidural anesthetic can then be administered or a woman can be given Demerol or other pain medication. The physician inserts a specialized speculum into the vagina to obtain an adequate visualization of the cervix and the area behind the cervix. Usually a local anesthetic is injected into the vaginal wall, and a small probe is then inserted blindly through the wall. When the position of this probe is determined, it is followed by the insertion of a larger probe containing the culdoscope. Through the culdoscope, the physician can visualize and inspect the area just behind the uterus, the ovaries, and the tubes. While a woman is

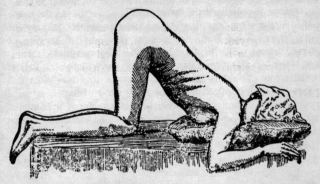

Fig. 16-6: The "Knee-Chest" Position. The "knee-chest" position has a woman resting on her knees with her body bent forward resting the chest on the table. A pillow is usually placed underneath the chest and the head is rotated to one side.

kneeling in this position, her intestines usually fall forward, lessening the chance that the bowel will obstruct the physician's view. The physician can then observe if there is any abnormality in the area.

This procedure is often performed on women with fertility problems when the physician wants to determine if both fallopian tubes and ovaries, as well as the uterus, are completely normal.

In combination with this diagnostic procedure, minor operations can also be performed with fine operating instruments inserted through the culdoscope. The most common operation is tubal sterilization. The physician can sterilize the woman by picking up the fallopian tubes and either coagulating or dissecting a piece of the tubes. Other minor operations, such as the removal of small adhesions, can be performed with fine instruments through the culdoscope.

A woman usually experiences minimal pelvic pain for a day or so after the operation. Intercourse is not advised for three or four weeks, until complete healing has occurred. She should not return to work for at least a week, or maybe two weeks, after the operation.

ANTERIOR AND POSTERIOR REPAIR

This is an operation in which the vagina is tightened by a surgical procedure; often it is called an A&P repair.

After every childbirth, the ligaments that hold the uterus in place grow weaker, especially if the infant is large and stretches the tissue greatly. At the same time, the vaginal muscles stretch, making the vagina larger. Aside from the medical problems of sagging or prolapsed uterus (see Chapter 13, Uterine Abnormalities), the increased size of the vagina can make sex less enjoyable. This is especially true of middle-aged couples. As a man grows older and engages in sex less often, his penis tends not to become as large during erection as it might have when he was younger. The combination of the smaller penis and the loosened vagina can create sexual dissatisfaction.

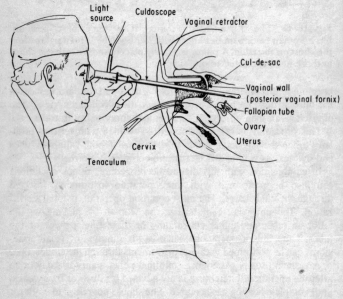

Fig. 16–7: Culdoscopy. Culdoscopy is often carried out under local anesthesia with the patient in a "knee-chest" position. The physician obtains good visualization of the cervix by vaginal retractors; the cervix is held by a tenaculum. A culdoscope is inserted in the posterior vaginal wall behind the cervix so the physician can, through this periscope type instrument, visualize the uterus, the ovaries and the fallopian tubes.

Thus, for both medical and sexual reasons, many women undergo anterior and posterior repairs. Basically, this is plastic surgery to tighten the vagina. It is often done in conjunction with a vaginal hysterectomy. An anterior vaginal plastic operation is particularly indicated if the woman has urinary difficulties. If the only complaint is that the vagina is "too loose," only a posterior repair is needed. A hysterectomy is often not indicated, and the procedure can be done quite quickly. The operation entails excision of extra vaginal tissue and tightening of the muscles, making the vagina both tighter and longer. This operation can only be recommended if there is a sexual problem stemming from a vagina that is too loose. Do not be shy about this, but discuss it with your gynecologist.

The Technique of an A&P Repair

The operation is done under general anesthesia with the patient in the stirrups. The front of the vagina is opened, and if the patient has a prolapsed uterus and has opted for a hysterectomy, the sagging uterus is readily accessible for removal. This also makes it easier for the physician to tighten the muscles. By cutting out a piece of the vaginal mucosa from both the front and the back of the vagina and tightening the muscles with sutures, the vagina becomes both tighter and longer.

After surgery, the muscles tightened around the bladder will interfere with urination for the first week or so. The urine must, therefore, be drained out. The standard treatment for this used to be a urinary (Foley) catheter placed in the bladder via the urethra; this often caused bladder infection. A new procedure in which a hollow plastic tube is placed through the abdomen via an incision into the bladder to allow urine to drain has replaced the Foley catheter. This tube does not interfere with voluntary urination, and there are fewer complications and infections.

Women should expect to remain in the hospital for seven to ten days following an A&P repair and should be extremely careful not to break the sutures loose by moving too much or even coughing violently. After release from the hospital, the patient should rest three or four weeks, being careful not to lift anything heavy. Sex can begin after complete recovery—about six to eight weeks later.

LAPAROSCOPY—THE BAND-AID PROCEDURE

The possibility of being able to observe the viscera of the human body directly through an instrument has motivated medical research for 170 years. In 1805, Dr. Bozzani constructed an apparatus in Frankfurt that used a series of mirrors and reflected candlelight to visualize the human urethra. In 1901, Dr. Kelling described a technique on dogs in which he observed the intraabdominal organs through a periscopelike instrument. In 1910, Dr. Jacobaeus of Stockholm described the first use of endoscopy in humans—he used a cystoscopelike instrument to look into the chest and abdomen. Still, it was only in the last decade that the development of fiber optics, or cold light, made it both practical and simple to develop instruments with which to peer inside the human body.

The result is the laparoscope. This instrument is quite new, but most competent gynecologists have learned its use. The laparoscope is compact, flexible, maneuverable, versatile, and extremely effective.

Indication for Laparoscopy

Laparoscopy can be performed either as a diagnostic or therapeutic procedure. The most frequent diagnostic indication for laparoscopy is to inspect the pelvic organs of women with fertility problems. In these cases, a dye is injected through the vagina and into the uterus. The dye will be passed out through the fallopian tubes if there are no obstructions. The passage of the dye can be observed through the laparoscope, and the physician can determine if the fallopian tubes are normal. The ovaries can be observed for signs of abnormality, and ovarian biopsies can be obtained to determine their functioning. Laparoscopy is also performed to determine the nature of pelvic masses or cysts. If any severe conditions that warrant immediate surgery (such as an ectopic pregnancy, a suspected malignancy, or a pelvic abscess), are discovered via the laparoscope, an exploratory laparotomy can be performed right away. The size and number of some uterine fibroid tumors can also be determined through the laparoscope, thus helping the physician in determining whether a hysterectomy or myomectomy is indicated.

The most common therapeutic use of the laparoscope is tubal sterilization. During this procedure, the fallopian tubes are picked up in the mid-portion and either coagulated or encircled by a fallopian ring. Other therapeutic indications are the cutting of small pelvic adhesions and biopsies of suspicious abnormalities.

Laparoscopy cannot be performed on extremely obese women or on women who have had previous extensive abdominal surgery, since numerous pelvic adhesions can exist and the bowel might be perforated during the insertion of the instrument.

The Technique of Laparoscopy

Laparoscopy can be carried out with either local or general anesthesia. An incision is made either in the navel or directly below it, and a small peritoneal needle is inserted into the abdomen to inflate it with four liters of carbon dioxide (CO_2) gas. The patient is tilted so her head is downward, causing the bowel to float upward toward the chest with the gas. This gives a better view of the pelvic organs (see Fig. 10–4). Because the abdomen is distended by the gas and the position of the bowel, the laparoscope has an unobstructed view of the organs. Not only does the laparoscope provide light and lens, but instruments can be introduced through it to move aside organs that block the view, or even to carry out minor surgery. Biopsies can be taken, the fallopian tubes can be grafted or cauterized (for sterilization), and dyes can be injected to see if the tubes are unobstructed. After the operation, the gas is let out and the patient usually goes home the following day. She will experience a dull pain for a week or two, but the only sign of surgery will be a small Band-Aid over the navel. That's why laparoscopy is often called the Band-Aid procedure.

HEMORRHOIDECTOMY

Hemorrhoids usually occur in women after childbirth, due to the pressure of the child restricting blood flow and causing varicose veins in the rectum. During the active phase of labor, these veins often pop up and become hemorrhoids. The problem becomes complicated if the woman suffers from constipation, and pain and infection can be extreme.

A hemorrhoidectomy to remove these veins is a relatively simple operation, usually performed by a general surgeon. Three incisions are made to remove a triangular piece of veined tissue: then the area is loosely sutured closed. The rectum is then packed, and since the patient had begun a liquid diet several days before the operation, there should be no bowel movements for a day or two to allow healing. Recovery is extremely painful, since there are extensive nerves in the rectum, and some patients are sick for several weeks. However, the benefits of the hemorrhoidectomy are easily worth a few weeks' suffering for a victim of chronic hemorrhoids.

MASTECTOMY

One of every fifteen women in the United States will develop breast cancer. Today the major therapeutic approach to this problem is mastectomy, the removal of the cancerous breast. The two major types of mastectomies are the *simple* mastectomy, the removal of the involved breast and the overlying skin, and the *radical* mastectomy, the removal of the involved breast, the overlying skin, and the muscles of the chest wall beneath the breast, as well as dissection and removal of the lymph nodes under the arm on the affected side.

History of Mastectomy

The technique of radical mastectomy for breast cancer was devised by Dr. Halsted of Johns Hopkins Medical School in Baltimore in 1882. There have been only minor changes in this procedure since then. Radical mastectomy is still the major treatment today of breast cancer in the United States, although in 1941, Dr. McWhirter, a physician of Edinburgh, proposed a so-called simple mastectomy for breast cancer. Dr. McWhirter found that there was the same five-year survival rate for simple as for radical mastectomy. Furthermore, there were fewer side effects and complications after simple mastectomy than after radical mastectomy. During a radical mastectomy, so much tissue is removed that there is a greater tendency for infection, and the tissues are stretched so much that healing is retarded. Radical mastectomy involves removal of the lymph glands in the armpit, thus there is a tendency for swelling (edema) of the arm, which can disturb the patient for a long time after surgery. Dr. McWhirter described much less swelling of the arm after simple mastectomy.

Simple mastectomy is the operation performed today for early breast cancer in Great Britain as well as the other European countries. In Germany, physicians find it difficult to secure permission for breast surgery unless a simple mastectomy is guaranteed. American physicians still prefer to perform radical mastectomies, because it is believed that a conservative attitude in the face of a killing disease is the best approach.

Breast Biopsy

If a woman is found to have an abnormal mass in the breast and there is a suspicion of malignancy, a breast biopsy must be performed. A breast biopsy can be performed either under local or general anesthesia. Some physicians prefer performing the biopsy under general anesthesia and having a diagnosis made immediately from frozen sections of the biopsy. If the mass is found to be malignant, they want to perform the mastectomy immediately because they believe the biopsy spreads the cancer. Other physicians do not hold to the theory that the biopsy stimulates the cancer. They feel that a mastectomy should not be performed on the basis of frozen sections alone, since this has led to the occasional unnecessary mastectomy. They often perform the biopsy under local anesthesia, and if the findings are malignant, the patient can at least prepare herself psychologically for the trauma of mastectomy. A breast biopsy usually consists of an incision right above the palpated tumor. The incision is usually carried out in a curved fashion so that it mimics the curve in the breast. If it is possible, the surgeon makes the incision in the edge of the areola, the pigmented area around the nipple. During this procedure, the physician excises the lump and sends it for pathological examination to determine whether it is malignant or benign. The breast is sutured up and closed, and the patient can usually go home the following day.

A needle biopsy of a breast mass is done in some institutions. A needle is placed into the mass, and part of the tumor is aspirated and sent to pathology. This can be recommended only in institutions where the pathologists are accustomed to looking at this type of biopsy, since the specimens are very small. Furthermore, if it is a negative biopsy, there is always some possibility that the surgeon did not aspirate the right area.

Radical Mastectomy

Most often in the United States, if the results of breast biopsy show a malignancy, a radical mastectomy will be performed. This procedure is performed under general anesthesia. The hair under the arm is shaved, the skin carefully washed with antiseptic solution, and the area sterilely draped. The surgeon usually has one or two assistants for this major surgery, which occasionally requires a blood transfusion. The incision for a radical mastectomy is extensive and usually has an elliptical form, starting from the middle of the chest bone around the breast to the upper edge of the armpit. The surgeon first dissects the muscles and the arteries, veins, and nerves in the armpit. The insertions of the major chest muscles under the arm, the *pectoralis major* and *minor,* are freed. The surgeon carefully dissects and removes all the fatty tissue and the lymph glands in the armpit, hoping that if the cancer has spread to those areas, this procedure will eliminate further metastasis. All the breast tissue, the skin (including the nipple), and the pectoral muscles are removed inside the incision line shown in the illustration. The rib bones are completely exposed so that one can visualize the muscles between them. The incision is then closed by sutures. Usually a physician places a drain underneath the incision, because there tends to be a formation of blood and lymph which can disturb healing. A tight bandage is placed over the incision to prevent further bleeding. The patient is usually asked not to move the arm too much the first few days, or until good healing takes place. Special exercise is then recommended. Hospitalization usually lasts at least a week. During this time, trained therapists instruct the patient as to the type of bra and clothing she can wear after the surgery. A patient is not able to work for four to six weeks after the operation, since there can be swelling of the arm and rest is required. There are very few deaths during the surgery itself. Most of the surgery-related deaths have been caused by anesthesia complications. The five-year survival rate depends on the extent of the cancer. If no cancer has spread to the lymph glands, the five-year survival rate might be close to 80 percent. If there is a sign that the cancer has spread to the lymph glands, the physician might advise radiation or cobalt therapy to kill the remaining tumor cells. A woman should only permit this procedure to be done in a hospital with competent physicians highly specialized in the treatment of breast cancer.

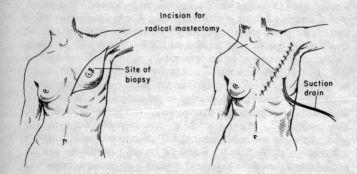

Fig. 16–8: Mastectomy. The incision line for a radical mastectomy, before and after surgery, is illustrated. In the illustration to the right, the placement of a suction drainage is shown.

A few physicians in this country perform even more radical surgery. Some physicians even prefer to remove a few ribs because they are worried that some cancer might have spread into the lymph glands between the ribs. This very radical procedure is advocated only by a few physicians.

Modified Radical Mastectomy

There has been a trend in the last few years in the United States to perform a less radical mastectomy, the so-called modified radical mastectomy. The surgeon makes essentially the same incision as with the radical mastectomy. He removes the lymph glands in the armpit but does not remove the pectoral muscles. It is very rare that cancer spreads to the pectoral muscles, so it is unnecessary to remove them, at least in early breast cancer. The scar from a modified radical mastectomy is less extensive, and breast growth is more successful after this procedure. The survival rate has been as good with the modified radical as with the radical mastectomies.

Simple Mastectomy

A simple mastectomy is an operation in which an incision encircles the breast containing the malignancy. This procedure is also often performed immediately following a breast biopsy. Under general anesthesia, an incision somewhat smaller than the one seen on the right in Fig. 16–8 is made through the skin, and the breast is removed, leaving the pectoral muscles intact. With a simple mastectomy, there is no surgery performed under the arm, which means healing is usually more rapid and there is no swelling of the arm. After the breast has been removed, the skin is closed; because there is less tension on the skin, complications are rare. Women are able to return to work much more rapidly. The scar is less horrifying and breast augmentation is possible. Some physicians work directly with plastic surgeons and initiate augmentation surgery in combination with simple mastectomy, starting to rebuild the breast at the same time the cancer is removed. Women who have had only simple mastectomy seem, according to studies published throughout the world, to have the same survival rate as those with radical mastectomy, and have less psychological trauma.

Simple or Radical?

Today's woman is much more aware of her own body and, particularly, to the threat to life inherent in breast cancer. It is increased awareness and knowledge that have women examining their breasts on a regular basis. Ninety percent of all breast tumors are discovered by women themselves, and as women examine themselves with increasing regularity, breast cancers are being discovered in earlier, more treatable phases. If breast cancers are discovered early, either by regular breast examination or by mammography in high-risk cases, the indications for radical mastectomy are minimal.

The controversy over simple and radical mastectomy in the treatment of breast cancer continues in the United States. Most physicians in the United States today feel that until proven otherwise, it is better to overtreat breast cancer with a radical mastectomy rather than undertreat it with a simple mastectomy. They fail to realize that after a radical mastectomy, the psychological scars can be as extensive as the physical scars.

The survival rate for early breast cancer is the same for radical as for simple mastectomy. There is an important number that does not show up in the statistical tables, and that is the number of women who find and fail to report a breast tumor because of the fear of radical mastectomy. Perhaps many women die because of this.

Simple mastectomy may be the preferred treatment for even more advanced cancers, due to the advances in radiation and chemotherapy.

The majority of women with breast cancer in Europe are treated by simple mastectomy. Doctors in the United States have reserved judgment until a strict comparison study of the two methods has been performed. This study is now in progress, under the direction of Dr. Bernard Fisher of the University of Pittsburgh. At present, it involves 1,700 patients at thirty-four medical centers throughout the country. The study was begun in 1971, and although it is still too early for a judgment, which is usually based on five-year survival rates, there are strong indications that radical mastectomy offers *no* advantage over simple mastectomy.

One interesting study was performed in Illinois, where radical mastectomy was generally carried out before the war. During the war, most trained surgeons were drafted. Many of the remaining surgeons did not know how to perform radical mastectomies, so instead performed simple mastectomies. Statistics have shown that patients treated with simple mastectomy had the *same* survival rate as those who were treated with radical mastectomy before and after the war. All these indications point toward simple mastectomy as the treatment of choice in breast cancer. Hopefully, this point will one day be fully proved.

KELOIDS

No chapter on operations would be complete without some discussion of keloids. Keloids are ugly scars produced by a healing abnormality after surgery. The development of keloids has nothing to do with the surgical technique of the physician; it is probably genetic.

Though there is no known cure for keloids, plastic surgery techniques are being developed to remove them. Many patients go to surgeons to have keloids removed only to have them return immediately. It is essential that this type of procedure be performed by a surgeon with special training and expertise in keloids, to ensure that the operation is not futile.

One technique for dealing with keloids involves steroid injection combined with excision of the scars. This has been found to decrease the re-formation of the keloids in many cases.

If keloids are removed surgically, a rim of keloid tissue should be left beneath the epidermis. Since no new tissue has been cut into, this prevents the formation of new keloids; they will not form from an incision in the scar tissue. This process, combined with steroid administration, is often very effective.

chapter 17

CIRCUMCISION

MALE CIRCUMCISION

Between the time a boy is born and the time of his first locker-room shower, he might never question the physical normalcy of his penis gland. It's there, it functions, it's even fun to play with, but it must be kept faithfully behind a zipper. Yet as soon as he walks into that shower uncircumcised and confronts a mass of ten or fifteen circumcised boys, he may be in for a shock. It is exactly this type of psychological trauma which constitutes the major arguments, pro and con, surrounding circumcision.

Throughout the history of circumcision (literally meaning "to cut around"), the operation has been performed more as a ritual or duty than for medical reasons. In the Old Testament, it was deemed as a "blood for life" sacrifice. It was feared, by mothers, especially, that the gods would take revenge on an uncircumcised baby. In certain Middle Eastern tribes, as stated in the Bible, the newborn boy was a threat to the father's prominence in the hierarchy of the family, and circumcision became a jealous act of revenge, a "taking away."

Even in the Hebrew religion, where circumcision as a practice still prevails, the ceremony derives from religious beliefs rather than from any untoward hygienic concern. The Jewish *briss* of today, a circumcision on the eighth day of life, dates back to the Mesopotamian practice thousands of years ago. Today circumcision is practiced by Europeans and Americans, independent of religion.

Procedure

Basically, the operation is simple. A Gomco clamp is secured around the tip of the infant's penis gland. The foreskin is cut after it is stretched and tightened over the gland to prevent blood from reaching the area. The incision is then covered with a Vaseline gauze, and the cut is completely healed seven to eight days later. It is rare for infection to invade the area, but when it does, it can be serious because the baby is sometimes too weak to fight back. There have even been cases when a child has died from just such an infection.

If a male has a circumcision later in life (usually stemming from insecurity at being different), the operation is more complex. An anesthetic is needed, and the healing may take weeks, not days. Still, the surgical procedure is basically the same.

Side Effects

In terms of the physiological side effects of circumcision, there are two major considerations: (1) the relationship to cancer in women; and (2) the effect on the man's sexual ability.

It was first believed that circumcision was a link to cancer in women, especially after several reports emerged claiming that Jewish women had fewer cases of cancer because their men were circumcised. It was felt that *smegma* (the secretion of the sebaceous glands) which developed beneath the foreskin would damage the woman's cervix during intercourse.

However, recent research has denied this association. Rather, it is generally agreed that cancer of the cervix is connected to women who are more sexually active and who began having intercourse at an early age. This is not to say that women should curtail their sexual activity, but that there is a greater likelihood of a virus being introduced through frequent intercourse, and that annual Pap smears are strongly advised. Also, the earlier a woman bears a child, the greater her susceptibility.

The low rate of cervical cancer among Jewish women with circumcised mates might merely reflect marriage later in life. According to Orthodox customs which demanded virgin brides, this would indicate coitus later in life. It also indicates a limited number of sexual partners for the woman—another factor in cervical cancer.

The second myth regarding the circumcised man is that he is sexually superior to the uncircumcised man. After circumcision, the glands become firmer and, therefore, are not so easily stimulated. The correlation, of course, is that it takes longer to ejaculate a circumcised organ, and this accounts for the prevalence of this myth. Not true! There are no medical indications that this is fact. Many circumcised men have problems with premature ejaculation. It is interesting to note that in Europe, where the majority of men are not circumcised, there are generally fewer sexual problems. Most sexual problems, though, originate in the mind, not the genitals.

Women, for the most part, don't seem to care if their men are circumcised. In fact, a recent survey showed that most women could not even tell if their men were circumcised. On an erect penis, the foreskin usually pulls over the gland, making circumcision difficult to determine.

Still, the sexual-superiority myth continues. It must be said time and again that there is no association between circumcision and sexual prowess. If there is an association, it is psychological, not physiological.

When to Circumcise

When confronting the decision of circumcision for the newborn boy, parents should consider the community in which he will be raised. If he is to be reared in a place where most of the men are circumcised, then the child should probably be circumcised. Con-

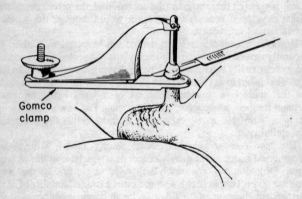

ABOVE
Fig. 17–1: The physician places the base of the Gomco clamp at exactly the level at which he wants to perform the circumcision. If the doctor wants to remove a small amount of foreskin, less tissue is pulled up through the clamp. When the Gomco clamp is properly placed, the foreskin is squeezed at the area where the cut will be carried out by tightening the screw on the Gomco clamp.

RIGHT
Fig. 17–2: Degrees of Circumcision. The drawing to the right shows a penis that could either be semi-circumcised or an uncircumcised penis with a natural shortening of the foreskin. An uncircumcised penis is shown in the upper left corner and a typical circumcised penis is shown below.

versely, if he is to grow up in a European culture, he should probably be left uncircumcised.

Semi-Circumcision

There are alternatives to full circumcision. Essentially, these are described by the amount of foreskin removed. In Europe before the war, Jews concerned with recognition often underwent this half-circumcision. In this procedure, only half of the foreskin is removed. The procedure is enough to satisfy the religion, but equally important, the skin can be pulled over the gland without risk of an infection underneath. This enabled many Jews to escape detection at a time when their religion brought them much persecution.

Today, Orthodox parents who don't want their sons to feel embarrassed, yet who want to complement community standards, may choose a semi-circumcision.

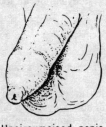

Uncircumcised penis

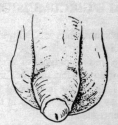

Semi-circumcised or uncircumcised penis with natural shortening of the foreskin

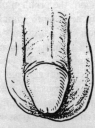

Circumcised penis

Prevalence of Circumcision

Years ago, only Jews and a few other groups performed circumcision with any regularity. Nowadays, circumcision is common not only to Jews but to all Americans—Catholics, Protestants, blacks, Chinese, and so on.

In Europe, most men are still uncircumcised, but the procedure is catching on. It is estimated that within twenty years, most European men will also be circumcised.

Circumcision, as you can see, is a matter of community standards and practice, and not a gravely important medical issue.

Tissue Research

Unfortunately, it has been the practice, up to now, to discard the foreskin removed during circumcision. This has been an enormous waste, since it is all fresh tissue. Only recently, researchers have found that this tissue can be used in laboratory analysis. Hopefully, new means of treatment will be aided by studying this all too often discarded yet plentiful tissue.

FEMALE CIRCUMCISION

Although most men are unaware of the fact, a woman can also be circumcised.

There are several types of women, unable to achieve orgasm during intercourse, who feel that the foreskins, or hoods, over their clitorises are too large. In the instance of a woman who rarely masturbates, the hood may cover the clitoris in the same way the foreskin covers the male penis gland.

Many women decide to have this hood surgically removed. This operation is also performed with the aid of the small Gomco clamp. Yet even after removal of the hood, the problem of difficult orgasm remains. These women probably need more stimulation in order to achieve orgasm, and circumcision will *not* usually help.

Sex researchers have found that many women do not directly stimulate the clitoris while masturbating. The women still achieve orgasm, though, because the surrounding tissue is high in nerve supply. These nerves usually lead to arousal of the clitoris. Because of this, female circumcision is not advocated by many doctors.

In Western cultures, most female circumcisions are performed exclusively for sexual reasons. This is not the case in parts of Africa, including Egypt, where circumcision of a woman is part of a religious custom. In many of these cultures, circumcision qualifies a woman to act as a temporary man while the men are away from the family, either foraging or at war. It is a circumcision based on a supposedly practical need rather than a sexual consideration.

Clitoridectomy

There is an operation performed, mostly in North Africa, that is called a *clitoridectomy*. This is, simply, removal of the clitoris.

When the North African man goes to a war, he performs a clitoridectomy on his mate, thinking it is then safe to leave her alone. The only problem with this is that nerve sensations remain even after the clitoris is removed. These nerves lead directly to the sex centers in the brain and do not stop the woman from having, or enjoying, intercourse.

Justice, it seems, sometimes triumphs in these backwardly chauvinistic societies.

chapter 18

BREAST EXAMINATION

Many observers feel that the most profound economic, religious, ethical, and personal symbolism revolves around the female breast. From the minute we are born until the second we die, we are confronted with the symbolism of the breast. Madison Avenue uses the breast to sell a wide variety of products—from toothpaste to motorcycles. Society implies that a "real" woman is one who has a perfectly proportioned body, one with relatively large breasts. Breasts signify femininity, motherhood, sexuality, the girl next door, beauty, wealth, power, and fame, among many other positive attributes.

Is it any wonder that most women are absolutely traumatized with the thought of one day losing one or both of their breasts? For years, women have been taught that their worth resides, in large part, with their breasts. One day, these women are told they have cancer and a breast must be removed. The women lose not only the breast; they often lose their sense of self-worth and of their place in the world.

Ironically, it often is just the fear of losing the breast that ultimately causes the trouble. Many women are so frightened by the thought of breast cancer that they hide from it in hopes that the threat will go away. In so doing, they completely fail to provide themselves with adequate protection, protection that has been proven time and again to thwart the invading cancer.

That protection is *self-examination,* and if you don't think it is important, consider this: Breast cancer, which, if detected early enough, can be completely cured, is the leading cause of cancer death in women and the leading cause of death in women between the ages of thirty-nine and forty-four. If it is discovered very early, the breast can even be saved, but this can only happen if a woman sees her doctor for a regular checkup, if she uses the available diagnostic techniques at suggested intervals, and if she employs *monthly* self-examination.

THE IMPORTANCE OF SELF-EXAMINATION

Obtaining a complete cure depends heavily on finding the cancer in time—while it is still treatable. Over the past twenty years, diagnostic techniques have improved greatly, making early diagnosis much more possible. But, even more important, in recent years women are becoming much more aware of self-examination, which makes early diagnosis much more probable. Still, there are too many women who rely solely on yearly or six-month checkups for breast cancer detection. That is a great mistake. A doctor may discover the disease at that time, but it might be too late. Instead of removing a very small tumor with almost assured success, the surgeon will have to operate more widely and the patient will have to wait . . . and hope. Interestingly, most breast lumps *are* discovered by women, themselves.

High-Risk Women

While self-examination for every woman cannot be overemphasized, it is especially important for women who fall into a high-risk category. Generally speaking, a woman has a higher than average risk of developing breast cancer if she has a strong family history of breast cancer, a chronic cystic breast condition, a history of premalignant breast lesions, a history of breast cancer, a late menopause, previous exposure to high doses of X-rays, or various conditions such as Stein-Leventhal disease, in which high estrogen levels are produced.

Women who are obese tend to produce high levels of estrogen; this, in turn, causes greater stimulation of the breast glands, thereby placing obese women in the high-risk category. And finally, women who take hormone replacement or estrogen hormones after the change of life might fit into the high-risk category. Of course, being in a high-risk group does not necessarily mean that a woman will develop cancer. It means only that her chance is greater than those not in the group.

Feeling the Cancer

Many women think that it isn't necessary to examine their breasts. They reason that if they had cancer, they'd feel it. Nothing could be further from the truth. When a woman has a tender lump in a breast, it is quite often not cancer, but a cyst or a breast gland that is developing and stretching the tissue. Since breast cancer grows slowly, it usually does not pull on the nerves; it therefore causes little pain. In other words, breast cancer does not hurt.

What to Look For

Of course, examining your breasts is not particularly helpful unless you know what you're looking for. Basically, you should notice any dimple on the skin, any nipple discharge, any nipple that was previously normal and has suddenly started to become inverted (or pulled in), any discoloration or abnormality of the breast tissue or the nipples, any type of ulceration of the skin, or any persistent lumps, either in the breast area or in the armpits. These symptoms warrant immediate attention and further examination by a physician. Remember, they do not mean that you definitely have cancer—they mean only that you might. The sooner a doctor can diagnose the abnormality, the sooner proper treatment can be carried out.

PROCEDURE FOR SELF-EXAMINATION

Every woman should understand how her breasts are affected by the natural functions of the female body. While she is in the fertile age and having menstrual periods, her breasts undergo natural hormonal changes throughout the month. The feel of her breasts, therefore, changes during the course of the cycle.

Immediately after the menstrual period, the hormone level is at its lowest. This is the ideal time for a self-examination, because there is usually less tension and swelling in the breasts. Later in the month, the estrogen level begins to increase. By the end of the month, both estrogen and progesterone reach their highest levels. This, in turn, causes tension in the breasts as they prepare for possible conception. All the milk glands enlarge, sometimes creating pain and tenderness. For some women, the breasts become more cystic as the body becomes more edematous (swollen with water). Since hormonal influence is high, this is the worst time for self-examination.

Consequently, women are advised to examine their breasts once a month, after each menstrual period.

Technique of Self-Examination of the Breast

The procedure for self-examination has two parts. Both are easy to follow and neither takes a great deal of time.

In the first part, you are looking for any changes in appearance that your breasts may have undergone since the last time you examined

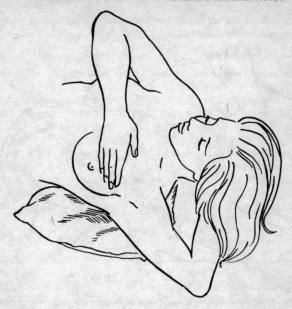

Fig. 18–1: Breast examination should be done both lying down and sitting up. When lying down, a pillow should be placed underneath the shoulder of the breast being examined. When the left breast is examined, the left arm should be placed behind the head. The right hand should examine the left breast and visa versa. The fingers of the examining hand should be kept flat and touch each area of the breast gently.

them. You should sit or stand in front of a mirror, with your hands at your sides, and take a few minutes to look at your breasts. Become familiar with their appearance. Is there any unusual dimpling or puckering of the skin? Have the superficial blood vessels gotten larger, or have they increased in number? Has the shape, size, or contour of your breasts changed?

Next, raise your hands over your head. Ask yourself the same questions. Then, observe your breasts with your hands on your hips.

A positive answer to any question is a warning sign, and you should see your doctor as soon as possible. The abnormality may not be serious, but only a physician can diagnose with certainty.

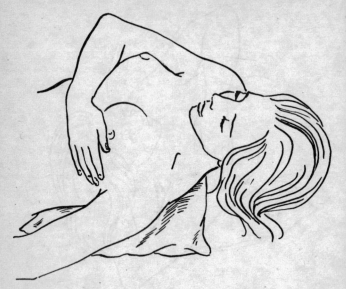

Fig. 18-2:   In order to examine the armpit properly, the arm should be lowered and placed along side the body.

The purpose of the second part of the exam is to find any new lumps or thickening in the breast. You should lie flat on the floor, or on a bed, placing a pillow or folded bath towel under your left shoulder. Place your left hand under your head and the palm of your right hand over your left breast. With the right palm, move the breast around. This is done to ensure that the whole breast can move freely around the chest wall.

Then, keeping the fingers of your right hand flat and together, gently place them at the twelve o'clock position on your left breast. Using small circular motions, rotate your hand gently over the area —this is to feel any abnormal lumps that may be present. Once you have determined that there is or is not a problem, move your fingers a few inches clockwise and repeat the circular motion. Be sure that each new position overlaps the old, so no area is missed.

When you have completed the circuit, returning to the twelve o'clock position, move your fingers slightly closer to the nipple and

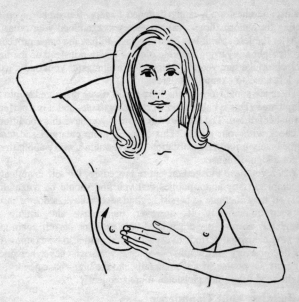

Fig. 18-3: In the sitting position, if the right breast is examined, the right arm should be placed behind the head. The arm should then be lowered down along side the body and the armpit thoroughly examined for any enlargement of the lymph glands.

begin again. In other words, you are now moving in a circle within the circle you just made. Continue this pattern until the entire breast, including the nipple, has been examined. When you finish with the left breast, follow the same procedure on the right breast, placing your right hand behind your head and using your left hand to examine the breast.

After each breast has been covered thoroughly, the armpit areas should be examined. The lymph glands are located here, and sometimes cancer spreads through the lymph channels into the glands. The procedure is similar to that for breast examination. Lie down and put your left arm alongside your body. Then place the fingers of your right hand on your left breast at the three o'clock position. With the same circular motion, rotate your hand as you move toward the left armpit. When you reach the armpit, be sure to press the entire area against the chest wall, using flattened fingers. Remember, you are feeling for abnormalities, just as when you examined your breasts.

After the left armpit has been checked, follow the same procedure for the right side, using the nine o'clock position instead of the three o'clock. Make sure you put your right arm alongside your body, using the left hand to examine the area.

There are some women who have breast tissue that spreads into the armpit area. This is called *accessory breast tissue*, and it is a perfectly normal condition. The best way to know if you have this condition is to check with your doctor. This tissue is more enlarged and tender immediately prior to menstruation. You shouldn't worry about this; it is not a sign of cancer.

When you have finished the entire procedure, the self-examination is complete. Any abnormalities that you find should be reexamined daily. If they continue to persist beyond several days, a doctor should be seen immediately. If, however, the breasts and armpits are completely normal, a woman need only examine herself again after the next menstrual period. Every woman should also be examined by her doctor every six months, or once a year, whichever her doctor suggests. Of course, if a woman falls into the high-risk category, she might need to see her physician more frequently.

Building Your Confidence

Too many women secretly believe they cannot give themselves adequate examinations. If you are one of these women, there are two steps you can take to build confidence in your ability.

First, the next time you see your doctor, ask him to observe you as you perform a self-examination. A physician is in the best position to see if you are doing it right and to correct any faults. A doctor who is truly concerned about the health of a patient should be happy to do this.

Secondly, give yourself an examination several times a month over the first two or three months. As you do this, try to develop a sense of how your breasts and your entire body change from the beginning of your menstrual cycle to the end. Although some of the changes are very subtle, many women become surprisingly sensitive to them. They soon know how the feel of their breasts fluctuates naturally during the course of their cycles. This kind of familiarity enables a woman to distinguish more easily between a normal and an abnormal change. Becoming an expert on the subject of your own breasts should build confidence in your ability to perform regular self-examinations.

BREAST EXAMINATION PLUS

The importance of self-examination should be emphasized over and over again. Most breast tumors are found by women themselves, yet if the cancer could be detected even sooner, chances of recovery would be greater.

It is now known that cancer of the breast starts as a so-called *in situ* cancer. It may take years before it develops into a tumor or spreads to the lymph glands. While in the *in situ* stage, the cancer is usually not large enough to be detected by a physical examination alone. Yet this is the ideal time to find it. Consequently, researchers have been developing and improving several diagnostic tools and techniques geared specifically toward the earliest possible detection of breast cancer. These techniques include *mammography, xeroradiography, sonography,* and *thermography.* Because a woman will probably be exposed to one or more of these new detection methods, she should understand and be familiar with each of them.

Mammography

Perhaps the best known of all the new techniques is mammography. A *mammogram* is a soft-tissue X-ray of the breast. Screening women this way has proven effective in finding breast cancer before they are large enough to be felt. Some physicians consider this method the closest thing to a Pap smear for breast cancer.

The mammogram gives a picture of the breasts. This picture shows the location and extent of any suspicious lesions. The physician can, if necessary, perform a biopsy to confirm any suspicion and base treatment on these findings. Early cancers found using this procedure are curable in 85 to 95 percent of the cases. If the cancer is found in a more developed stage, but while it is still confined to the breast, the five-year survival rate (the number of patients still alive five years after discovery of the cancer) is 84 percent. If, however, cancer is discovered after it has spread to the lymph nodes, the five-year survival rate is only 55 percent. Obviously, the benefit of mammography is that it enables the physician to detect cancer while it is still small. The smaller the growth the less radical the surgery, and the better the chance a woman has to recover fully.

Unfortunately, mammography has one major drawback. The procedure exposes breasts to radiation. While the amount of radiation received during one mammogram is low and not itself considered dangerous, the effect is cumulative—if a woman is exposed to a small dose of radiation every year for ten years, at the end of those ten years, her breast tissue reacts as if it has been exposed to the *sum* of all the small doses. Some people fear that the amount of exposure could cause cancer in yet another ten years or so. This does not mean that a woman will necessarily develop radiation-induced cancer if she is regularly screened by the mammogram. It only means that she increases her chance of developing such a cancer. Because of this, a woman and her doctor must weigh the possible benefit against the possible risk before deciding on mammography.

Is the choice haphazard?

No. A woman falling into the high-risk group is advised to get a mammogram on a routine basis, the frequency of which should be determined by her doctor. Since she runs a greater chance of developing cancer, the opportunity of finding it in time, if in fact it does develop, far outweighs the possible danger that could occur ten or twenty years later.

For the average woman not in the high-risk category, the use of the mammogram should be governed by her age. As a rule, it is rare for a woman to develop breast cancer before the age of thirty-five. At thirty-five, the risk increases. The older she gets, the greater the risk. Statistically, women between the ages of thirty-five and fifty account for approximately 25 percent of the cases of breast cancer that occur each year. The other 75 percent occurs in women over fifty. When you relate those statistics to the risk of getting radiation-induced cancer, a logical course of action emerges.

Generally speaking, the under-thirty-five woman not in the high-risk cancer group does not need to be routinely screened by a mammogram. It may be advisable for women over thirty-five but only if the benefits of the examination outweigh the risks of the radiation. Finally, some women over fifty should probably have mammography done every year. Remember, as a woman gets older, her chance of developing breast cancer increases. Because of this, the risk of having a cancer that needs to be detected is greater than the risk of getting cancer from mammogram radiation.

In other words, mammography is simply a matter of playing the odds that are in your favor.

Xeroradiography

Another technique beginning to gain as much popularity as mammography is called *xeroradiography*. Developed by Xerox, this diagnostic tool combines X-ray with the Xerox copying technique.

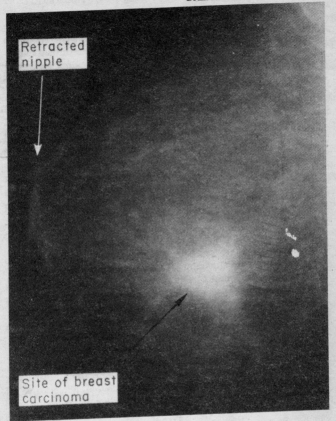

Retracted
nipple

Site of breast
carcinoma

Fig. 18–4: Mammography. It is easy to see how cancer shows a completely different configuration from the surrounding breast tissue. Cancer of the breast causes tissue changes which often pulls the skin of the breast to an extent that the skin becomes retracted. In this X-ray, the nipple is retracted.

Recent studies have shown that diagnoses made from xeroradiography closely correspond to follow-up biopsy diagnosis in determining the difference between malignant and benign lesions of the breast. In other words, xeroradiography is an extremely effective diagnostic tool.

The pictures produced by the *xeroradiogram* are clearer than those produced by the mammogram, and the edges of lesions are much more distinct. For this reason, many researchers believe that xeroradiography is superior to mammography. However, other specialists contend that there is no difference between the readings each method provides, claiming that while xeroradiography may provide a clearer picture, anyone properly trained to read mammography will find that it records the same information.

It is still unclear whether one method is superior to the other, but development of the xeroradiogram has created a much-needed atmosphere of competition. As a result, manufacturers of each method are doing more research to improve their respective techniques, each trying to get better readings while utilizing less radiation. This research should provide superior X-ray type diagnostic devices within the next few years.

Sonogram

Other researchers are trying to develop diagnostic devices which do not involve the use of radiation. One such device is the *sonogram*. This method uses sound as the determinant agent. Several studies done in Great Britain, Japan, and the U.S. suggest that sonography might be a very effective way to detect breast cancer in the future. (Sonography is described in greater detail in the fibroid tumor section in Chapter 13, Uterine Abnormalities.)

Thermography

Another relatively new method of diagnosing breast cancer is *thermography*, which operates on the theory that all objects give off infrared energy. A *thermogram* takes a picture of these infrared emissions, which vary depending on the temperature of the body from which they come. Since cancer is comprised of rapidly dividing cells requiring a greater blood supply than normal, a cancerous area generates more energy and heat than surrounding tissue. Therefore, when thermography is used to screen the breasts, any cancerous area appears hotter than normal.

Thermography gives physicians a greater indication of where to look for abnormalities, but it cannot pick up very early *in situ* cancer, as can mammography and xeroradiography. For that reason, it should not be used alone, but rather as a supplementary diagnostic tool.

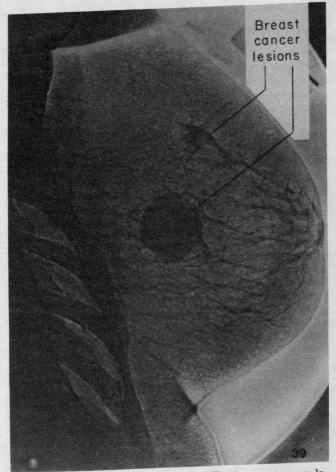

Fig. 18-5: Xeroradiography. The picture illustrates two cancer lesions, clearly separated from the other breast tissues. One can see tissue bands between the breast cancer lesions and the nipple, which is slightly retracted. (Reproduced by permission of Daniel S. Cukier, M.D.; Sharlin Radiological Associates, P.S., Hackensack, N.J.; and Xerox Corporation, Xeroradiography, Pasadena, California.)

Blood Sample Diagnosis

Besides trying to improve already existing diagnostic techniques, researchers are always looking for new and better methods. Several studies are presently being done to see if cancer can be diagnosed from blood samples. These studies are still in a preliminary stage and are not yet of any clinical value.

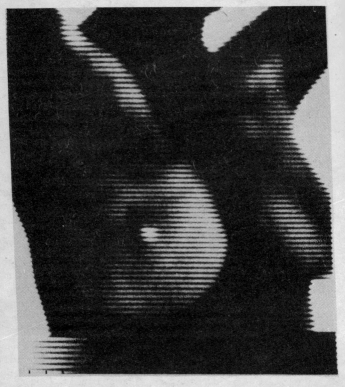

Fig. 18–6: Thermography. The picture illustrates a normal thermography; the darker area shows higher temperatures.

Government Projects

In 1972, the National Cancer Institute and the American Cancer Society, in conjunction with the United States government, set up twenty-seven screening centers throughout the country. These screening centers are participating in the National Breast Cancer Detection Demonstration Project. Mammography, xeroradiography, and thermography are among the many diagnostic tools that are being tested for effectiveness. From 1972 to 1978, 270,000 women in the over-thirty-five age range took part in the program to determine a more definitive choice between the methods.

Biopsies

Many women want to know what happens if an unusual mass is discovered during examination. There are several different, though related, procedures that can be followed. If the abnormality is slight and the physician doubts malignancy, the patient is usually sent for an X-ray, or maybe an X-ray in combination with thermography, for further analysis. However, if the mass is distinctly abnormal, a physician may feel that a biopsy is in order. In such a case, mammography may or may not be used to help define the area on which the biopsy will be performed.

A biopsy is a medical technique used to examine body tissue. In cases of possible breast cancer, an extremely small piece of the suspicious tissue is removed and sent to a pathological laboratory. The tissue is then cut into extremely thin layers, and various dyes are applied to stain the cells of each section. These dyes show whether cysts or cancerous growths are present. By examining the various dyed sections under a microscope, the nature of the growths can be diagnosed. Biopsy is at present considered the only definite way to determine whether a growth is cancerous.

If the mass appears highly suspicious and possibly malignant during an examination or X-ray, a biopsy is performed in a hospital. In this country, it is normal for the surgeon to send a sample of the suspicious tissue to the hospital's pathological laboratory during the course of the operation. The tissue will be examined in the lab, and the physician will know if the mass is malignant within a few minutes. If it is, the patient usually has an immediate mastectomy —the breast with the malignant tissue is removed.

Although it has been the standard for years, this procedure has recently come under attack. Some people believe a less extensive operation with postoperative chemotherapy would be just as effective as mastectomy. However, if the mass is so large that it can be felt and it is suspected of having spread to the lymph glands, a mastectomy is in order. If the operation is very extensive, radiation and chemotherapy may still be needed afterward to obtain a complete cure.

FIBROCYSTIC BREAST DISEASE

There are several disorders besides cancer which affect the breasts. Cystic disease is one of the most common of these, occurring in approximately 15 to 20 percent of women between the ages of twenty and fifty. There are several varieties of fibrocystic breast disease, each with a different name and somewhat different symptoms. Among the various types are *cystic mastitis, chronic cystic mastitis,* and *fibrocystic disease.*

The exact cause of cystic disorders is unknown, but they usually occur during a woman's reproductive or estrogen-producing years. Fibrocystic breast disease is a condition created by a hormone imbalance, and increases sharply in women over the age of thirty-five and in their forties. Some women develop a chronic cystic condition, while others experience cystic conditions only just prior to menstruation. While some women suffer slight discomfort, others experience extreme pain. The pain can be so severe that a woman can hardly wear a bra or other clothing on the breasts, particularly just prior to menstruation, when the hormone level is highest. Sometimes a cystic condition makes a breast feel very granular. At other times, as in the case of fibrocystic disease, the masses tend to be more solid (a woman with this type of cystic disease runs a higher risk of developing breast cancer. Therefore she should examine herself more often and more carefully. After the age of thirty-five, she should have a biyearly X-ray of the breast in combination with thermography).

Aspiration

If a patient has a tendency toward cystic breasts, she may occasionally feel the development of a cystic mass that causes extreme pain. In these cases, the mass can be *aspirated* (drawn out) by a needle. This is usually done in a doctor's office.

The procedure is quite simple. A needle is inserted into the cyst, and the fluid is drawn out or aspirated. If it is suspect, the fluid drawn from the cyst is sent to a cytology laboratory to be analyzed for cancer cells. If cancer lines the cyst, the cancer cells expel into the cyst fluid. Therefore, they are present in the aspirated matter. Aspiration is, in fact, a sort of needle biopsy.

Many physicians prefer not to perform needle biopsies and will only aspirate an area if they are certain the patient forms cystic masses. In these cases, aspiration takes pressure off the breast and alleviates pain. Although aspiration can provide a rough screening for cancer, most doctors continue to perform surgical biopsies for cancer diagnosis.

Treatment of Fibrocystic Breast Disease

Traditionally, physicians have felt that because water retention causes tenderness in the breasts, women with cystic tendencies should take diuretics. Diuretics cause the body to lose water, thereby reducing tenderness. Other physicians believe a woman with cystic tendencies should be placed on a low-dose hormone pill. This keeps the hormone balance at a steady level throughout the month, rather than allowing it to fluctuate naturally. For a woman with cystic disease, this can alleviate some problems. (This has been confirmed by the recent studies of oral contraceptives.) Yet, while low-dose hormone pills are prescribed for some women, others are treated with Enovid, a birth-control pill containing a rather high amount of estrogen. Women on Enovid also experience improvement of their conditions. Most doctors will not recommend this treatment because of the dangers of the high estrogen content in these pills. Because of problems with these pills, Danocrine (danazol), the first and only drug to be approved by the FDA for fibrocystic breast disease, is the treatment of choice.

Caffeine and Vitamin E

Caffeine has been shown to stimulate the development of fibrocystic breast diseases. Women suffering from any of these conditions should eliminate caffeine from their diets entirely by avoiding coffee, tea, cola drinks, and chocolate. It takes several weeks after all caffeine has been eliminated from the diet for the beneficial effects to become evident.

Vitamin E, on the other hand, has proved effective in alleviating the symptoms of fibrocystic breast disease. The required dosage is 1,000 units daily. If these conservative measures fail, treatment with danazol (Danocrine) may be indicated.

Danazol: the Treatment of Choice for Fibrocystic Breast Disease

Recently a new antigonadotrophic hormone called danazol (Danocrine) has been developed. An antigonadotrophic hormone stops stimulation of the ovaries and is usually used to treat endometriosis. Aside from its intended use, though, danazol, in doses of 200 or 400 milligrams daily, has been proved effective in relieving cystic mastitis. The reason is simple: Danazol decreases FSH and LH in the pituitary gland. FSH sends the signals which cause an egg to be produced in the ovaries. Once the egg has been produced, LH signals the release of that egg. When a woman takes danazol, her ovaries receive less stimulation as a result of the decreased levels of FSH and LH. As a consequence, there is less estrogen production and no cyclic variation in the hormone level. This causes a decrease of the breast's cystic glands. Moreover, Danocrine blocks the estrogen receptor in breast tissue, producing a direct beneficial effect. Danazol has cured cystic mastitis in 87.5 percent of women tested, and it has been approved by the Food and Drug Administration for use in treating cystic diseases. This recent approval will allow many women with cystic tendencies to enjoy the benefits of danazol.

OTHER BREAST ABNORMALITIES

Of course, not every irregularity in breast appearance means that something is wrong. Breasts come in different shapes and sizes and, for peace of mind, women should know some of the more interesting variations.

Some women have unevenly sized breasts, a condition similar to men who have one testicle larger than the other. This characteristic is usually hereditary. Such women are completely normal and function every bit as well as women with evenly matched breasts. As a matter of fact, their breasts are just like other women's; they're just not evenly matched. This difference hardly needs to be corrected surgically.

It is also considered normal for some women to have inverted nipples. Generally if a woman is born with an inverted nipple, it is a genetic factor, and should not cause concern. It does not change sex characteristics or affect pleasure.

However, if a woman has had a converted nipple that *becomes* inverted, she should see her doctor. It could be a sign of some abnormality developing inside the breast. Such a condition should be examined and treated accordingly.

Other women are born with several nipples. In such cases, the nipples start where the breasts are usually located, and two or three additional nipples are located on each side of the abdomen, going down toward the pubic hair. The condition seems to be a throwback to our evolutionary predecessors, but it is not rare or dangerous. However, if one or more of the extra nipples is large and causes psychological trauma, it can be removed by a plastic surgeon. Still, such an operation is not considered necessary for good health.

MAINTENANCE OF HEALTHY BREASTS

Good health care should be constant practice for everyone. Ultimately we are all responsible for ourselves; we can't rely on doctors to provide miracle cures when we notify them too late about specific abnormalities or diseases.

Concern for health is the most important weapon in the fight against disease. Monthly self-examination of the breasts and regular check-ups with your physician should be routine parts of your life. It is important not to allow fear to get in the way of common sense. Remember, what you don't know can hurt you, especially if you neglect it. Cancer of the breast is cured every day of the year, and it is beaten by those women who discover and recognize the disease while it is still in its early stages.

chapter 19

CORRECTIVE BREAST SURGERY

Many women are unhappy about the appearance of their breasts. Some who feel their breasts are too small undergo all forms of exercise and/or hormone treatments to enlarge the breasts and often finally decide that such efforts yield no results. Some of these women decide to have silicone injections or implantations, only to find that the silicone injections are frequently harmful. In some instances, the breasts become very hard and lumpy, resulting in fear of having them touched or caressed.

Other women, who consider their breasts to be great beauty assets, find that after childbearing, their breasts often become softer and start to sag. This often causes unhappiness. Some women feel they are not as attractive as before, and so decide to have corrective breast surgery.

Quite a few women have been happy with the results of corrective breast surgery. It should be emphasized, however, that if you decide to have breast augmentation surgery, you should be sure you choose a very competent surgeon, one familiar with the latest developments in this field.

In the last few years, surgical corrective procedures of the breast have developed into a fine art. Pendulous breasts can be made smaller; sagging breasts can be elevated; ugly scars can be excised, and small breasts can be enlarged. Most of these operations must be considered major procedures, but not in the risk-to life category. Nevertheless, because these major procedures require general anesthesia, which in itself entails a certain risk to life, breast surgery should not be performed on every woman wishing a correction for minor abnormalities or a reduction of slightly large breasts. Nor should it be performed to enlarge breasts that can be considered normal. However, a great number of women can and have benefited from the techniques of corrective breast surgery.

Today the desire to beautify the breasts is not limited to any particular age group. Young and old alike display great interest in the possibility of help through plastic surgery, and such help should not be denied any woman on the basis of age. On the other hand, the general state of a woman's health should be considered before any final decision is made. The most important consideration is the type and extent of the breast deformity. Remember, one should never undergo breast surgery for a minor defect.

Another equally important consideration is the emotional stability of the woman. It has been found that insecure, maladjusted, and unstable women are usually poor candidates for corrective breast surgery. Such women tend to expect the operation to cure emotional ills unrelated to the shape or size of their breasts. It should be pointed out that no plastic surgeon, no matter how good he is, can change your life. Only you can do that. Many plastic surgeons, especially if they are honest and competent, soon become familiar with the psychological problems of their patients and know beforehand who should or should not be subjected to breast reduction or augmentation surgery. When in doubt, many plastic surgeons refer patients for psychiatric evaluation prior to any surgery.

Finally, this type of surgery should only be performed by very skilled plastic surgeons—surgeons who are highly specialized in these procedures. Women should seek a physician who wants to do a good job, who carefully evaluates his patients, and who tries not only to increase the beauty of the breast, but who also takes into account the psychological stability of the woman. Obviously, plastic surgeons who are just looking to make money should be avoided.

It is, of course, difficult to find the right and most competent plastic surgeon. Referrals from friends who have had plastic surgery performed and were satisfied with the results could be good leads. It is probably a good idea to try to find a plastic surgeon who is associated with a teaching institution, since they are generally familiar with the most up-to-date procedures and also are not likely to recommend unnecessary surgery. For more concrete guidance, a woman considering corrective breast surgery can write to the American Society of Plastic and Reconstructive Surgeons (29 East Madison, Suite 807, Chicago, Illinois 60602) and request a list of qualified plastic surgeons in her area.

UNDERDEVELOPED BREASTS

Usually a woman's breasts are fully developed by the time she is sixteen or seventeen years old. Of course, some women's breasts develop later in life, and this is usually determined genetically. In

428   IT'S YOUR BODY: A WOMAN'S GUIDE TO GYNECOLOGY

other words, if your mother developed late, you might also develop late. Sometimes, however, the estrogen hormone, which gives the secondary sex characteristics in women and is the stimulus to breast growth, is not released normally, and therefore does not trigger the development of the breast or the growth of pubic hair. If this is the case, a physician can administer hormone treatments, which sometimes help trigger the growth and development of the breast and other secondary sex characteristics. Birth-control pills containing a high level of estrogen usually increase the size of the breasts. When this type of birth control is discontinued, the breasts generally return to their original size. Pregnancy also stimulates hormone production, causing the breasts to increase in size. Again, the breast size usually decreases after pregnancy, or after a woman has finished breast-feeding.

Breast Exercises

Advertisements for various types of breast-development techniques and exercise programs erroneously lead many women to believe that it is relatively easy to increase breast size through these methods. As a result of these advertisements, many women spend a great deal of money only to discover that the promised results are never achieved. There is no exercise that will increase the actual amount of breast tissue. All exercise and breast-development techniques can do is strengthen and firm the pectoral muscles, which support the breasts. Good posture, with the back straight and the shoulders back and down, also greatly improves the breast contours by giving them better lift.

Many women wonder what breast developers actually are. They are merely exercise props. Many consist of a strong rubber band with two handles; others consist of an exercise bar which is held with both hands to emulate the movements of isometric exercises for strengthening the pectoral muscles. Some breast-development courses include additional devices, such as plastic cups containing tiny jets through which water is emitted in order to massage the breasts, and various kinds of moisturizing and massage creams for the breasts. Needless to say, these extras are completely useless as far as increasing the size of the breasts is concerned. Most breast-development programs include a booklet illustrating various exercise movements which should be performed with the aid of the rubber band or the exercise bar. Many also contain a nutritional guide, since proper nutrition may affect the fatty deposits in the breast tissue. Once again, it should be pointed out that no breast-development technique or exercise program can actually increase the amount of fatty tissue in a woman's breasts. This is a genetically determined characteristic.

Instead of spending money on these so-called breast-development programs, it would be much more reasonable for a woman to do some isometric exercises especially geared to developing the pectoral muscles and strengthening the back muscles for good posture. These exercises are often featured in various fashion and other women's magazines. Isometric exercises work on the principle of opposing muscles which are so contracted that there is little shortening but great increase in the tone of the muscle fibers involved. Pushups are another way of strengthening muscles in the back, chest wall, and upper arms. Swimming is also an excellent all-purpose exercise which improves the tone of the muscles that support the breasts. Remember, though, there is only so much that exercise can do to change the size of the breasts, since it can only firm the muscles which support the breasts.

Who Should Have Breast Augmentation?

As the saying goes, it is not how much you have, but how you use it that counts. It is time for women to start looking at themselves in a more positive light and not allow their self-esteem to be unduly influenced by the male fetish of large breasts, an attitude prevalent in the United States. It is perfectly understandable that a woman wants to be attractive and feel good about her appearance. This can, however, often be achieved through dieting and proper exercise. Also, the right clothes can do a great deal to enhance a woman's figure. Unfortunately, many women go to great lengths to appear younger and more attractive to men. For this reason, many women resort to all kinds of breast-development courses, exercise programs, and even plastic surgery to achieve this goal. It should be pointed out, however, that a majority of men do not look at a woman's breast size when they first meet and are attracted to her. They are usually more interested in the qualities that make up the total person. A woman should try to be pleased with herself as she is, and not necessarily look to a plastic surgeon as soon as she notices minor wrinkles or sagging.

If you are extremely unhappy with the size of your breasts, try to delay any surgical procedures until you have finished childbearing, since too many women who have breast augmentation before they become pregnant find that they need additional surgery after childbearing. Breast size has nothing to do with erotic sensitivity or pleasure. Only those women who feel their breast size has become a burden to them should consider breast augmentation, and then these women should realize that the results of breast augmentation are not always what they expect them to be.

Silicone

One of the first methods of breast augmentation was the injection of liquid silicone into the breast. This created a cystic mass inside the breast, which enlarged the breast and kept its contour up. Some of the first women to have this procedure performed were go-go dancers, belly dancers, stripteasers, and others whose livelihood depended on their physical assets. However, by looking closely at these women, one could see that the breasts did not move naturally, and furthermore, they were as hard as rocks when touched. Many of these women did not want anyone to touch their breasts for fear of being ridiculed.

Worse still, when examined under research conditions, the injected silicone was found to be very dangerous. It formed a hard mass encapsuled inside the breast tissue, making it impossible for a physician to examine the breast or to determine if cancer was present.

Even though they were widely used for mammary augmentation, liquid silicone injections involved several other serious hazards. Since liquid silicone is really a foreign substance injected into the tissue, all types of foreign-tissue reactions could occur. There was a fear that it could even cause cancer, and if cancer did occur, that it could not be detected. Often a solid tumor developed around the injected silicone and created a nodule so painful that surgery for removal of the mass was necessary. The silicone often migrated into the lymphatic tissue and bloodstream, and from there to other parts of the body, where it could also form tumors. Liquid silicone has, by mistake, been injected into blood vessels, and in some instances, it has even traveled to the heart. There was a recent report of a nightclub dancer who died a few hours after a silicone injection. For a variety of reasons, silicone was found to be dangerous in an injected form and was finally taken off the market by the Food and Drug Administration. Silicone injections are now illegal.

However, silicone itself is a substance which is extremely body friendly—if it is put into the body, there is usually no body reaction against it. Silicone does not react completely like another foreign body, and it has many advantages over other substances, such as plastic, since it can be implanted into the body for longer periods of time. Silicone is now used as a prosthesis in the replacement of hardened arteries, as well as for other types of corrective surgery.

Eventually breast implants of a hard, silastic material (also called silicone) were developed in the shape of a cup. A surgeon could perform an incision underneath the breast and implant these cups in such a way that they would not move around in the body. These cups would then stretch out the breasts, thereby uplifting them and giving them better contour. This operation was performed on many thousands of women throughout the United States and Europe, particularly on well-to-do women or those in the public eye. These women found that such silastic implants improved their appearance and also uplifted their self-image.

A major problem, however, was that these implanted masses were very hard. Although thousands of women who had these hard silastic implants found pleasure and happiness after the surgical procedure, many were afraid that as soon as a man would touch them, even while dancing, he would feel the hard cup. Subsequently, there was a great deal of psychological trauma for some of these women. Although many women felt improvement in their appearance, they were often afraid to tell a man, particularly a new boyfriend, that they had silicone implants in their breast—justifiably so, it seems, since many men were repelled by the new breasts and felt as if they were making love to a rubber doll, not to a woman. This caused uneasiness for both the men and the women involved.

Soft Silicone Implants: A Real Improvement

A new type of silicone has recently been developed by the Dow Corning Corporation. This silastic is made of low-viscous silicone gel which is so soft that it approximates normal breast tissue. This gel is poured into a very strong, thin cover, which prevents it from leaking out. It is then implanted into the breast, where it will stay *in situ* (i.e., it will not leak into other areas or be absorbed by the bloodstream and then transported to other parts of the body).

This new type of soft silicone is available in different shapes (including round) and sizes, all approximating various breast shapes. This soft silastic has been used by certain specialists for several years and has been very successful. Since it is implanted underneath the breast next to the chest wall and is completely surrounded by breast tissue, it is impossible for a layman to feel any difference between the implanted soft silastic and normal breast tissue.

Still, many institutions and clinics do not use the soft silicone extensively, and many physicians are still inserting the hard silicone. Women should be alerted to the fact that soft silicone is now available, and many specialists, particularly plastic surgeons special-

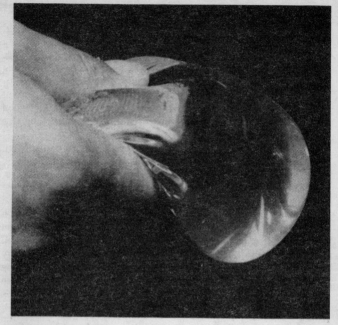

ABOVE

Fig. 19–1: A soft silicone breast implant. The silicone is smooth and easily conforms to the pressure of the hands. This implant comes in many various sizes and shapes.

BELOW

Fig. 19–2: The position of a soft silicone implant inserted through an incision in the inframammary fold underneath the breast. (Courtesy of Dow Corning Corporation.)

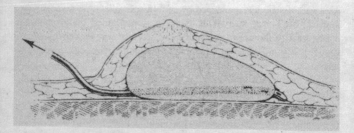

izing in soft-silicone breast implantations, have gained great knowledge and skill in the implantation of the soft material. Further, these specialists have become very knowledgeable in using the right size and shape implants so as to create the most natural look for each woman.

If you are planning to have a silastic implantation, you should ask for the soft silicone. It is ideal for breast augmentation if the breast sags too much or if it is too small, or after breast surgery, biopsy, or maybe even after mastectomies. The hard implant should only be used in very special cases. It can cause great unhappiness, and you should refuse to have the hard silicone implanted unless it is absolutely necessary.

Implanting the Soft Silastic

The implantation of the soft silastic is essentially performed in one of two ways. The silastic can be inserted through an incision underneath the breast, in the so-called inframammary fold (the fold between the chest wall and the breast). This incision is usually not seen, because the breasts tend to fold in that area. The operation is performed under either general or local anesthesia. Under a local anesthetic, you normally receive premedication, such as morphine or Demerol, and thereafter, local injections of Novocaine. The physician then makes an incision in the inframammary fold, inserts the silicone prosthesis underneath the breast tissue at the chest wall, and closes the incision with a few sutures. He then places a tight bandage around the breast to prevent bleeding and to ensure that the implants remain in the right position. A small tube is often placed through the incision in order to drain off any blood which otherwise could form a hematoma. The new, soft silastics do not tend to slide once they are placed in the proper position.

The majority of physicians prefer to perform this procedure in a hospital under general anesthesia. By doing this, a physician can better determine correct size and can more easily mold the breast, placing the silastic implant in exactly the right position, without causing unnecessary harm or pain to the patient. Usually the patient is released from the hospital one to two days later. The patient is asked not to move around too much during the first week, giving the implantation time to rest and heal inside the breast without causing any harm, unnecessary bleeding, or damage to the tissue.

If a woman has a large enough areola (the pigmented area around the nipple), plastic surgeons often make a circular incision on the edge of the pigmented area and insert the silicone through this incision. A small pocket is made from the incision into the chest wall so the silicone implant is placed right at the chest wall, underneath the milk glands. The incision usually heals well and is hardly visible after the operation.

Many women have been pleased with the results of the soft silastic implants; however, it must be noted that the results are not always satisfactory. Many other women have had to undergo repeated operations because they were dissatisfied with the appearance and size of their silastic implants, or because of complications, such as hardening of the silicone or scar tissue which subsequently developed around the implant. In order to ensure the best possible results, a woman should try to find the most competent and experienced plastic surgeon she can. The final result of a soft silastic implantation will depend upon the original size of your breasts, areola, and nipple, and upon the extent of enlargement that you desire.

Replacing Hard Silicone Implants with Soft Ones

Any type of silastic that has been inserted into the breast can usually be fairly easily removed and replaced by another type. Many women have already had the hard silicone replaced by the soft gel. The results have often been excellent. Furthermore, if a woman has already had implantation of either the hard or soft silastic and feels that the size is not right, the implants can usually be removed and replaced.

One such patient recently came to my office. Before the examination she told me she had had the hard silicone removed and the soft inserted, and was very pleased with the results since her breasts now felt completely normal. I asked two nurses to examine her, pretending that I thought the patient had a breast tumor. Both nurses examined the patient's breasts thoroughly, and could not feel a tumor. Later on, when I told them the woman had had soft silicone implanted, they could not believe it, because to them, the breasts felt perfectly normal. Several other patients have also said that after they had soft silicone implanted by specialists, even their own gynecologists could not detect that they had implants.

Is the Silastic Implantation Dangerous?

The soft silastic has not been found to be dangerous. It is a product which does not give a foreign-body reaction, and it can be easily implanted into the breast. If the soft silicone is implanted in a lower

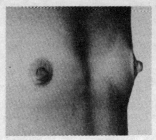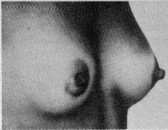

ABOVE
Fig. 19-3: A woman before and after soft silicone implantation. This woman had almost no breast tissue prior to surgery, but by implantation of a small cup, the breast is given sufficient enlargement to create a natural look. (Courtesy of Robert G. Schwager, M.D., attending plastic surgeon at New York Hospital, New York City.)

BELOW
Fig. 19-4: A woman before and after a breast augmentation with implantation of soft silicone. The silicone was inserted underneath the breast, in the inframammary fold, and a smooth, natural curve has been achieved. (Courtesy of Robert G. Schwager, M.D., attending plastic surgeon at New York Hospital, New York City.)

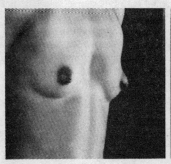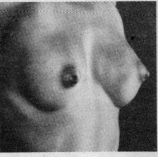

incision, in the inframammary fold, it is put underneath the breast tissue so that the tissue completely surrounds it. A physician examining the breast can still detect cancer, either manually or by mammography. Soft silastic implants have never been shown to cause cancer in any laboratory studies. If the implantation is done by a qualified and experienced physician, there should be no major complications. For these reasons, it can be safely stated that the new silastic should not be dangerous to women.

Breast-Feeding after a Silastic Implant

A woman who has a silastic implantation performed through an incision in the inframammary fold underneath the breast will still have normal breast tissue and can, therefore, breast-feed, since such an incision leaves the milk gland intact. Normal breast examinations and mammography are also the rule. On the other hand, a woman who has an implantation through an incision in the nipple might have difficulty breast-feeding, since some of the ducts leading the milk to the nipple might have been cut during this procedure.

BREAST REDUCTION

For every woman who is unhappy because she feels that her breasts are underdeveloped, there is another woman who is burdened by overdeveloped breasts. There are numerous reasons why women with very large breasts are unhappy, and each individual case is different. Many problems which women with overdeveloped breasts face can be attributed to the trauma which our breast-oriented society imposes upon women in general.

Many women become so concerned with breast size that they diet extensively, hoping that a drastic weight loss will also reduce the size of their breasts. Unfortunately, this doesn't happen consistently. Girls in their teens are often alarmed at the rate at which their breasts develop, because the breasts undergo continuous growth during this period. This growth is accompanied by increased vascularity, which, in turn, can make the breasts feel very heavy. Naturally, this feeling is quite different from what a young girl experiences in her early teens. A woman's breasts do not reach their maturation until she is about twenty years old.

Because of the breast-oriented society in which we live, many women become so concerned and emotionally upset about the size of their breasts that they decide to have reduction surgery at an early age. These women often feel very uncomfortable, since they think people are always staring at them. Instead of being known for their personality, intelligence, and other qualities, such women feel that

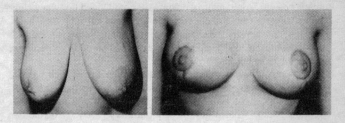

Fig. 19-5: Breast reduction. The picture to the left is before and to the right is after breast reduction, *mammaplasty*. This woman complained of heavy, large breasts which became increasingly troublesome after childbirth. She also developed large stretch marks in the breasts. She underwent breast reduction surgery by a modification of the *dermal mastopexy* operation. This is a procedure developed by Dr. Dicran Goulian, Jr., professor and chairman of the department of plastic surgery at the New York Hospital–Cornell University Medical Center, New York City.

Dermal mastopexy is a procedure in which the areola and the nipple are moved upward on the breast and excessive skin tissue is excised. This procedure stretches the skin on the breasts and makes the breasts look healthier and younger without damaging the milk glands. This procedure has been referred to in lay terms as a "breast lift." The patient in the illustration had a modest breast reduction in association with the mastopexy. The breast tissue removed is usually a small part of the mass. Most of the resected tissue is excessive fat. The scars had not completely healed when this picture was taken a few weeks after the procedure. The scars subsequently become lighter and more difficult to notice. The milk glands have not been damaged during this procedure and the patient will be able to breast-feed if she has a child. The stretch marks which were seen before the procedure have become less conspicuous because of the tightening process. (Courtesy of Dicran Goulian, Jr., M.D., chairman of the department of plastic surgery, New York Hospital, New York City.)

they are only known as "the girl with the big breasts." Most girls are aware that breast size is genetically determined, so if their mothers and grandmothers have very large breasts, this is often an additional incentive to seek breast-reduction surgery at an early age.

Aside from the emotional discomfort which hypertrophic breasts may inflict upon a woman, there can also be considerable physical discomfort. Pendulous breasts can be so heavy as to cause strain on the back muscles by pulling the shoulders forward, thus contributing to poor posture. Also, many women have complained that the weight of their breasts causes their brassiere straps to cut into their flesh. This, too, can be very disagreeable. Furthermore, some women with pendulous breasts tend to adopt poor posture in an effort to minimize the size of their breasts.

Most women have some slight variation in the size of their breasts, with the left breast tending to be somewhat larger than the right. Although this slight variation is perfectly normal and usually goes unnoticed, some women have a very marked asymmetry of the two breasts. Again, if a woman is emotionally mature and has a healthy amount of self-confidence, this asymmetry should not be a source of concern, although it does cause psychological trauma in some women. Women should not be too concerned about a slight variation in the size of their breasts, since this is much more common than most people realize. However, if the asymmetry becomes too great a problem, plastic surgery to even out the two breasts through reduction of the larger breast might be warranted.

Before making a definite decision regarding breast reduction, women should remember that this type of surgery does not always produce satisfactory results. Since the breast is composed of fatty tissue, any reduction in its size often entails the removal and replacement of the nipple. This means that several incisions must be made in the breast. Although the breast might have a better overall appearance, upon close examination, there will often be scars, because fatty tissues tend not to heal well. These scars can be very ugly and can cause unhappiness, despite the fact that a woman can be pleased with her improved overall appearance.

Sadly, breast-reduction surgery is often performed very early in a woman's life, sometimes while she is still in her teens. This is a time when most people have not yet found themselves emotionally. Physiologically, although a girl may be fully grown by the time she reaches her teens, she might still have baby fat. Frequently when a woman reaches her twenties, she loses this baby fat and her body assumes its normal size and proportions. If breast-reduction surgery has been performed while a girl is still in her teens, she might find later that, as she loses weight, her once overly large breasts become too small. There are even cases in which women who have had breast-reduction surgery in their teens have subsequently undergone silastic implantation to increase the size of their breasts. For this reason, breast-reduction surgery should not usually be performed until after a woman has borne children. Following childbearing, the tissues are more relaxed, especially when the breasts are large, and the breasts might then start to sag. If the breasts sag after bearing children, corrective surgery might be in order.

Is Breast-Reduction Surgery Necessary?

The possibility of breast-reduction surgery should be very carefully evaluated. If a woman feels that her breasts are too large or asymmetrical, she should try to focus on the other beauty in her life instead of letting this bother her unduly. Furthermore, large breasts should not usually cause a woman to suffer from poor posture if she has the discipline and determination to exercise in order to strengthen her back and to correct her posture.

Some women have been conditioned by religious upbringing to feel ashamed of their large breasts. This is strictly a matter of cultural conditioning. In some countries—for example, in France—women have not been negatively conditioned in this manner, and every Frenchwoman is generally happy to show how well endowed she is by maintaining erect and good posture.

Before deciding to undergo breast-reduction surgery, a woman should first carefully evaluate the reasons she feels such an operation is necessary. She should also be well aware of the fact that she will most likely be left with many scars in the breast after such an operation. Also, a woman should first try to camouflage her breasts with the right kind of clothes.

A woman should not have any kind of corrective surgery performed on her breasts unless they really are damagingly large. If she does decide to have such an operation performed, she should go only to the very best plastic surgeon she can find—to a physician very experienced in this specific procedure.

It is only after a woman has had at least one child that she should consider breast-reduction surgery, and then only if the breasts begin to sag to such an extent that they cause the woman psychological trauma. At this time, a woman might have a breast-reduction operation, or perhaps a breast lifting. In any event, a woman should not have either of these operations performed while she is in her teens unless her breasts are unusually hypertrophic or asymmetrical.

Does Breast Sensitivity Decrease after Breast-Reduction Surgery?

Breast-reduction surgery is a procedure in which most of the fatty tissue and all of the nerve endings in the breast are removed. The

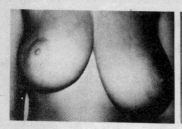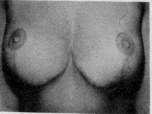

Fig. 19–6: Breast reduction in a patient with marked breast asymmetry. The picture illustrates the breasts of an eighteen-year-old woman who complained of breast hypertrophy and marked asymmetry, the left breast being much larger than the right. Her breasts were very heavy and the veins very visible; the veins can just be seen on the picture before surgery. The picture to the right shows the results after breast reduction surgery. Both breasts were reduced in size; they are now equal in size and have a natural look. The fresh scars are still visible beneath the left breast. The patient has subsequently undergone further correction of these scars — and is very pleased with the operation, claiming both physical and emotional satisfaction. (Courtesy of Dicran Goulian, Jr., M.D., chairman of the department of plastic surgery, New York Hospital, New York City.)

nipple is also generally removed and replaced. Consequently, some women do not have any feeling or sensation of sexual arousal in their breasts following surgery. This deprives these women of so much sexual pleasure that they find it more difficult to achieve orgasm, or orgasm must be reached without breast stimulation and satisfaction.

Also, some women become so emotionally upset following breast-reduction surgery that they feel they can no longer show their scarred breasts to a man, and therefore have turned to lesbian relationships. It must be made clear, however, that this usually happens only to women who have always attached too much importance to the appearance and/or sexual appeal of their breasts.

If a woman feels the need for any correction of her breasts, especially if she is still in her teens, it might be wise to try to accomplish this through exercise rather than with an operation which could leave her with unattractive scars, and which could also cause a possible loss of much sexual pleasure by desensitization.

CAN STRETCH MARKS BE REMOVED?

Many women find that as the milk glands grow during pregnancy, the breasts enlarge so much that stretch marks appear. This is more likely to happen to girls who become pregnant in their teens. When a woman has reached her twenties and her body is fully grown, there seems to be a lessened risk of stretch marks. Nevertheless, many women who become pregnant in their teens and early adult lives find that their breasts have been disfigured by stretch marks. This may cause problems with their sexual partners.

There is presently no medication to prevent or remove stretch marks. Many women apply vitamin E cream, other creams, baby lotions, and a wide variety of other products to their breasts during pregnancy to prevent stretch marks, but this has never been scientifically proven to be effective. The best way to avoid stretch marks is to wait until you are in your twenties to have children. If you already have stretch marks, there is no way, surgically or otherwise, that they can be removed. If the stretch marks bother you, you might try getting a light suntan on your breasts. When the skin is lightly pigmented, these marks are less visible.

REMOVING SCARS OR BURN MARKS

Some women, particularly those who have undergone breast-reduction surgery, find the surgical scars so unattractive that they cause great unhappiness. Such women return time and time again to plastic surgeons for removal of the scars. If a surgical scar is really wide and disfiguring, a competent plastic surgeon can usually minimize it. Still, as the doctor is again making an incision and suturing the skin, there will be one remaining scar. By closure with finer sutures resulting from modern plastic-surgery techniques, though, the final scar should have a much better appearance. If a woman has problems with scars, she should make sure that she goes only to the best plastic surgeon. It is generally better to go to plastic surgeons associated with large medical institutions, since they know about the latest developments in this area. In this way, a woman can usually be assured of excellent results. Remember, though, there will always be one remaining scar.

RECONSTRUCTION AFTER A MASTECTOMY

Much research has been done to develop implants for women who have undergone mastectomy. Some women who have undergone radical mastectomies, entailing the removal of all of the muscle under the chest wall and in the armpit, have so little tissue left underneath the breast that it is very difficult to insert any kind of silicone. Women who have undergone such major surgery have usually had a very extensive type of cancer, and in such cases, the woman's health is undoubtedly more important than aesthetic considerations.

Nonetheless, as newer developments and understanding of cancer progress, there is hope of finding new ways to cure breast cancer. Perhaps by removing a lesser amount of breast tissue and at the same time giving chemical or radiation therapy, breast implants could be cosmetically utilized. In fact, research centers are now developing varying types of breast-augmentation techniques in combination with mastectomy to rebuild the removed breast.

Reconstructing the Nipple Following Mastectomy

One of the major difficulties in breast augmentation after or in combination with mastectomy is the nipple. The nipple is usually removed along with the excised breast, and to rebuild a new nipple is virtually impossible. However, a nipple can be reconstructed using tissue from the vulva, and occasionally a new breast can be built using tissue from a woman's own body or through augmentation with soft silastic. A breast can occasionally be built up after mastectomy so it has approximately the same size as the other breast when a bra is worn. It is, however, impossible to rebuild a breast that is exactly like a woman's own breast and that will look the same in the nude. Most breast reconstructions involve several surgical procedures. If there is some tissue left underneath the mastectomy scar, a small silastic implant can possibly be inserted, and this can subsequently be replaced with larger implants until the right size is achieved. A nipple can then be constructed from genital tissue. Since it is often difficult to achieve the same size breast, though, plastic surgeons often perform a reduction on the woman's other breast to equalize more or less the size of the two breasts.

Several European surgeons who have been performing less extensive mastectomies are saving sufficient skin tissue to enable them to reconstruct a new breast. They are creating a nipple by placing sutures underneath the skin in a circular mode to form a nipplelike protrusion. They then simulate the areola by tattooing this area in the same color as the other side.

Future Developments for Breast Reconstruction Following Mastectomy

More than a thousand women in the United States, and many more worldwide, have already undergone breast augmentation after mastectomy, and almost 90 percent of these women have been satisfied with the results. However, in order to achieve the most satisfactory results with breast-reconstruction surgery, it is crucial to save the woman's own nipple during mastectomy, if it is at all possible. Since cancer involves the nipple in only about 10 percent of all breast cancer cases, it is often possible to save the woman's nipple.

In order to obtain optimum results from both cancer treatment and breast reconstruction, during mastectomy it is important for the cancer surgeon and the plastic surgeon to work as a team. Usually when a woman discovers she has breast cancer, she becomes so frightened that her first reaction is to go to a surgeon and have a mastectomy performed as quickly as possible, so as to safeguard her health. This is a perfectly normal reaction.

However, after such women have fully recovered from cancer surgery and look every day at the resultant scars, they become concerned with the appearance of their bodies and wonder whether it would be possible to have reconstructive plastic surgery to minimize the mastectomy scars. They also wonder if the excised breast can be reconstructed.

Unfortunately, it is very difficult to achieve satisfactory results in breast reconstruction following mastectomy if the woman and her doctors have not planned on this possibility before performing the mastectomy. Because of this, it is strongly suggested that whenever a woman is confronted with the dilemma of breast cancer, she should concern herself not only with the mastectomy procedure, but should also investigate the possibility of having reconstructive breast surgery performed concurrently. Several medical centers are presently investigating various types of combination mastectomy/reconstructive surgery procedures, but such centers are few and far between, since this possibility is still in the very early stages of development. At the present time, most doctors are not likely even to consider the possibility of breast reconstruction in combination with mastectomy. Still, these new developments hold great promise for the future.

Some experimental techniques of reconstructive plastic surgery following mastectomy involve the removal of the nipple and the areola (the pigmented area surrounding the nipple) during the actual mastectomy. A piece of this tissue is then checked for cancer. If it is free of cancer, the nipple can be temporarily grafted onto other parts of the patient's body, such as the abdomen or the buttock, where it would remain to draw nourishment until such time as it can be transferred back onto the newly reconstructed breast. When the mastectomy scar is completely healed and there is no more sign of cancer, the breast reconstruction could be initiated.

This type of breast-reconstruction plastic surgery involves several stages of surgical intervention. First a roll of skin and fatty tissue must be obtained by making a transverse incision in the lower part of the abdomen, where it remains until the scar has healed. The next step involves freeing a part of this roll of skin and fatty tissue from the lower part of the abdomen and swinging it into the position of the mastectomy scar, where it remains as a tube of tissue connecting the abdomen, from which it draws nourishment, to the mastectomy scar, where hopefully it will "take." When good vascularity between the mastectomy area and the skin and fatty tissue roll has occurred, the skin and fatty tissue can be detached from the abdomen and then, in the next operation, rolled up and formed like a breast. The final stage in this type of breast-reconstruction plastic surgery is to move the nipple back from the area where it has been receiving nourishment to the newly reconstructed breast. This particular technique looks promising, but several other ideas for breast reconstruction are also presently being developed.

Several European centers, in order to reconstruct more natural-appearing breasts, perform less radical surgery than in the United States. They rarely remove the pectoral muscles, which United States surgeons often do. Therefore, they have much greater success then their United States counterparts in breast augmentation.

There is much hope that in the future, women will be able to achieve satisfactory cosmetic results following mastectomy.

chapter 20

CANCER

Cancer is a frightening, costly, and painful disease which strikes indiscriminately. Medical researchers are now stating that we are in the midst of a cancer epidemic. The cancer rate in America has almost tripled since the turn of the century, and what had been a one-percent yearly increase since 1933 jumped to a five-percent increase in 1975. Approximately 650,000 new cases of cancer are discovered each year, and about 365,000 (over half) of them are fatal. Cancer strikes one out of every four people today, touching two out of every three families. More than 1,000 people die every day from cancer—more than one every minute and a half. As you can see, the chances are that *you* will not get cancer, but the odds are extremely slim.

On the other hand, some 222,000 Americans are cured of cancer every year because of early detection and improved treatment techniques. Cancer is no longer the certain death it was only a few years back, but it still sends a deserved chill through us when we encounter it. Probably because of the quickened pace and complexity of modern life, which affect our environment, eating habits, and life-styles—all of which may contribute to cancer—cancer is definitely on the rise. The only method to guard against it is *constant vigilance* and *early detection*.

WHAT IS CANCER?

Cancer is a disease in which normal cells start to grow uncontrollably. There are more than one hundred different forms of cancer; it is found in all the organs, as well as in the bones and in the blood. The disease is older than man. Evidence of this disease has been found in dinosaur fossils. The Egyptians wrote about it in their papyrus scrolls, and Hippocratic surgeons studied it in Greece.

The causes of cancer have baffled scientists through the ages and even today are only scarcely understood. For instance, we know that

445

cigarette smoking contributes to lung cancer, but we still don't know exactly why. The first documented indirect cause of cancer was discovered by Sir Percival Pott in 1775. He noted a high incidence of cancer of the scrotum in chimney sweeps who had undergone prolonged exposure to soot. Soot is closely related to tar, and the sweeps were suffering from the same type of cancer that afflicts the lungs of smokers today.

Any cell in the body has the capacity to become cancerous, but once it does, its descendants exhibit some of the normal functions of the cell from which they originated. Thus if cancer begins in the liver and spreads to the kidneys, the tumors in the kidney will have liver characteristics, and doctors will be able to determine where the disease originated.

WHAT CAUSES CANCER?

It is possible to be exposed to a carcinogenic, or cancer-causing agent, and not develop the cancer for twenty or thirty years. Obviously this makes it extremely difficult to isolate the causes of cancer. Researchers are often criticized for introducing absurdly large amounts of questionable substances into laboratory animals to see if cancer develops. The resultant data are thought by some to be irrelevant because of these distorted quantities. But researchers have no choice. A well-controlled experiment over a period of twenty years is not feasible. In the face of the rush to add more and more preservatives and additives to our food and to stretch the limits to which we can pollute our air and water, criticism of these experiments is not completely valid. There is growing concern nationwide, however, that these critics (who themselves can offer no conclusive data to refute opposing research) are quick to criticize on the side of danger rather than safety—and when you're dealing with the environment, mistakes are irreversible.

So the debate rages. Some researchers are trying to find psychosomatic causes for cancer. Others look into cyclamates and other artificial sweeteners. Still others suspect the key will be found in the genetic code. A few causes have been positively identified, like the chimney sweeps' soot, radiation following the bombings of Hiroshima and Nagasaki, prolonged exposure to the sun, and, most conclusively, cigarette smoking.

The effects of these agents on tissue are not fully understood, but the mechanism is usually described as *irritation*. Cigarette tar clings

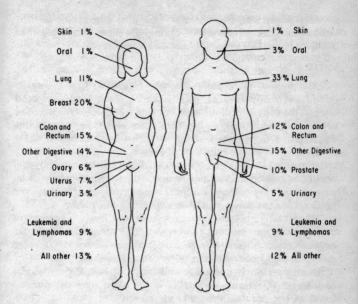

Fig. 20-1: Cause of Cancer Deaths in 1976.

to the lungs and irritates the cells. A chronic inflammation may occur and persist for as many years as you smoke, until one day the cells begin to transform into abnormal cells—the start of cancer. The ultraviolet rays of the sun irritate the skin, and the same process may occur. Certain industrial pollutants carcinogenically irritate the liver, while others cause cancer of the kidneys.

Of course, with over a hundred varieties of cancer, all of them may not stem from the same cause. Some scientists believe cancer is a virus that can be cured as soon as an effective vaccine is developed. Others believe it is a physical reaction to emotional stress. These theories are not mutually exclusive.

Still, even though the *how* of cancer is unknown, the *what* is becoming clearer every day. Because of this, cancer prevention is probably far ahead of cancer treatment, or could be if people would heed the warnings. Unfortunately, they generally do not, endangering not only themselves, but whomever else they may expose to their carcinogens. One of the major causes of cancer today is human indifference and irresponsibility, as well as ignorance.

Tobacco

Sixty million Americans still smoke cigarettes. Considering its proven and well-publicized links to cancer, emphysema, and heart disease, the popularity of cigarette smoking is baffling. True, nicotine is physically addicting, but that didn't stop almost half the doctors who smoked from quitting when they first learned that smoking caused cancer. As the militancy of nonsmokers increases and they realize that smokers are giving them cancer and causing them physical discomfort, which is a violation of their natural right to breathe clean air, smoking may undergo a cultural transformation and become less fashionable, less accepted, and less appealing to children.

Unfortunately, this process has not yet begun. Today, 33 percent of all cancers in men are lung cancers, while 11 percent in women are lung cancers. It is feared that since more women are smoking tobacco today, the incidence of cancer in women will increase.

It seems peculiarly ironic that while science has finally made steps to solve this centuries-old puzzle, at the same time the problem increases because the facts are being ignored.

Cigarettes are especially toxic in an urban environment, where the air is already filled with potential carcinogens. In conjunction with alcohol, the chance of getting cancer is up to 1,500 percent greater for someone who drinks and smokes as for someone who neither drinks nor smokes. Too much liquor alone is related to cancer of the mouth, throat, esophagus, larynx, and liver. When liquor is linked with tobacco, the danger expands to many other types of malignancies. The agents goad each other on to progressively more destructive acts.

Pipe and cigar smoking are less harmful if the smoke is not inhaled, though the danger to nearby nonsmokers is as great. However, pipes lead to higher incidences of cancer of the mouth and lower lip, while cigars have been linked to cancer of the bladder.

Stress

Though there is no conclusive evidence to prove it, stress is thought by many physicians to be a key factor in the development of cancer. Stress is known to stimulate the body's production of steroids, particularly cortisone. These chemicals inhibit the functioning of the body's immunity system. If cancer is a virus or some other entity that can be fought by the body's immune system, stress clearly can open the door for the development of tumors by stripping the body of its protective antibodies. The solution to this threat is simply to relax. Sleep more, cut down your work regime, and act decisively to clear up personal problems. However, if you find this difficult, *learn* to relax through such techniques as yoga or transcendental meditation. Try to organize your life so that it will become more enjoyable.

The Cancer-Prone Personality

Although there is no conclusive proof, many studies have found that certain personality types are more prone to cancer than others. Women who cannot cope with stress and who suppress extreme feelings of anger and other deep emotions were found in one study to have a high susceptibility to cancer of the breast, while women who expressed their emotions freely, were more assertive and spontaneous and generally more relaxed were less likely to develop the different types of gynecologic cancers. It is interesting to note here that many women develop cancer during periods of severe life stress such as divorce, separation, or the death of a loved one. It is the cancer patient's inability to deal with her personal problems successfully that, many times, triggers a malignancy. Therefore, if there is such a thing as a cancer-prone personality, and evidence is pointing in this direction, women should make every effort *not* to bottle up any strong feelings. There are books and training courses now available that teach people how to be more assertive. There are different techniques for achieving deep relaxation.

Good nutrition is an important factor that is very often forgotten in fighting stress. Perhaps in the future, doctors will give immediate attention to a patient's psychosocial problems, thus creating another means of early detection and a more favorable prognosis.

Genetic Factors

Cancer can run in families. This does not mean that if someone in your family has it you are going to get it, but your chances are greater. It is estimated that there is a 15 to 20 percent genetic factor in breast cancer, which means if a relative has it, 15 to 20 percent of your chances of getting it are genetic. Of course, this factor is not fully understood. The cancer could actually be in your genes, or there could simply be a genetic weakness in your immune system. The problem could even be in the traditional eating habits of your family.

Some cases, however, have definitely been related to genetic, rather than cultural (eating habits, sleeping patterns, etc.) factors. Patients suffering from Down's syndrome or mongolism (a condition of mental retardation caused by chromosome abnormalities) have been found to exhibit at least eleven times the normal risk of developing leukemia, a cancer of the blood.

Two or more first-degree relatives with the same or related kinds of cancer (cancer of the breast, for example, is related to cancer of the colon or the uterus), can be considered evidence of inherited cancer or susceptibility to cancer.

Diet

In the past decade or so, there has arisen in our culture a stereotype known as the health-food nut. She is generally considered to be a fanatic with a make-believe cause. Ironically, as so many people ignore science's warning about tobacco, so do they ignore the warnings about diet. In fact, animal fats, additives, preservatives, and overprocessed foods like white bread may contribute, directly and indirectly, to half the cancers in women and almost a third of those in men.

Dietary causes of cancer are especially acute in countries like the United States, where the diet is rich in soft foods such as meat, white bread, and all white-flour products, refined sugar, and related overprocessed foods without roughage. These factors are related to cancer of the colon, stomach, esophagus, breast, liver, and uterus.

The Western world is especially afflicted by cancer of the colon, due to a lack of fiber in its diet. Until recently, fiber was largely ignored as a nutritional requirement because it provides no nourishment—it does not contain protein, sugar, starch, fat, vitamins, or minerals, it is simply roughage, the plant food we do not digest. A person living in the West consumes four to six grams of fiber daily, while his or her African counterpart consumes five times that much. In fact, Africans very rarely developed any type of cancer until they started to eat the Western diet; then cancer began to appear where it had been virtually unknown. Experiments have shown that this Western diet results in more than twice as long a transit time for stool —about seventy hours as compared to thirty—which means bacteria have more time to multiply and harmful substances are held against the intestinal wall for a longer period. This leads not only to cancer, but possibly also to benign tumors, polyps, and appendicitis. The easiest way to get more fiber in your diet is to eat fresh fruits, vegetables, and raw salads and substitute whole-grain flour, cereals, and bread for refined flour, processed cereals, and white bread. Whole bran is especially high in fiber content if it has not been ground and reconstituted, as it is in many of the popular bran breakfast cereals. Your local health-food store is the best source for obtaining raw, unrefined bran.

Fatty diets have been linked to cancer of the breast and of the bowel. This is evident when you compare the high rate of bowel cancer in the United States, with its meat-oriented diet, with the low rate in Japan, with its staple diet of fish. The Scots, who consume 20 percent more beef than the neighboring English, have one of the highest bowel-cancer rates in the world. The current suspicion is that fats overstimulate hormone production, causing unrestrained growth of some cells, especially of the breast, prostate, and uterus. Throughout the world, there is a five to ten times difference in the death rate from breast cancer between countries with low-fat diets and those with high-fat diets. The solution here is to eat less meat and saturated fats and more fish, fowl, and polyunsaturated fats. At the same time as we cut down our use of saturated fats, we should also curb our intake of protein. We are too obsessed with eating large amounts of protein, thinking it will improve our health, when just the opposite may be happening. It has been found that overeating of protein causes deficiencies of vitamins B_6 and B_3 and magnesium, as well as pancreatic enzymes—deficiencies which are considered among the reasons for cancer development. It is this overindulgence in protein and the body's inability to digest and utilize it that may cause cancer.

Overeating has also been related to the increase in the occurrence of cancer, as well as heart disease and diabetes. Statistics from the Metropolitan Life Insurance Company have shown that the prevalence of these conditions is much higher among the overweight than among those of normal weight. This fact was clearly demonstrated in the hunger years during and after the world wars, when there was a sharp decrease in cancer. However, when food rationing ended and people again started to overeat, the incidence of cancer started to increase sharply, going back to the prewar levels. Smaller, more frequent meals would be a healthier way to live rather than our standard three-meals-a-day routine. In Europe, the main meal or course is served in the afternoon, in a leisurely fashion, allowing plenty of time for rest, relaxation, and good digestion. Americans might learn something from this—with our fast-food restaurants, we often eat not only in fifteen minutes, but many times, standing up! To make matters worse, we eat our main meal in the evening and then most likely retire for the night. This is the typical pattern of eating for the American people. The results can only be tragic, as we are surely starting to learn.

Preservatives and Dyes

To add insult to injury, the meats of which we are so fond—and which probably are giving us cancer—are impregnated with dyes, growth hormones, additives, and preservatives which are also probably giving us cancer. A controversy surrounding the chemical preservatives and dyes known as sodium nitrite and sodium nitrate, has developed. You will find these two in most processed meats —salami, bologna, bacon, ham, smoked meats, corned beef, pastrami, hot dogs—to enhance their color and inhibit the growth of the deadly bacteria that cause botulism. Although not carcinogens by themselves, sodium nitrite and sodium nitrate combine with *amines* which are found in the body to form *nitrosamines,* which have proven to be highly potent carcinogens in animals. Food processors complain that the threat of cancer is minimal compared to insurance against botulism, but consumer advocates insist that no one knows just how serious the cancer threat is, since the incubation period is so long, and that we are better off safe than sorry.

Interestingly, we swallow as many natural nitrites daily in our saliva as are found in a pound of bacon, but they are combatted by vitamin C, an important intake. Both vitamins C and A are known to reduce various cancer risks.

There is a continuing controversy over the Food and Drug Administration's ban on cyclamates and red dye #2, once one of the most prominent dyes in our diet. Though there have been conflicting studies over cyclamates, red dye #2 was shown to be carcinogenic after having been in our food for decades. Other dyes have yet to be properly tested. In the case of some preservatives, processors argue that the choice is between the lesser of two evils; in the case of mere colorings, this argument is hardly relevant. In essence, we are exposed daily to various possible carcinogens for the sake of marketing techniques.

It is interesting to note that diethylstilbestrol (DES) is one of the hormones injected into cattle to fatten them up. Traces of this hormone are found in all beef products that reach the market. This hormone is banned in twenty-one countries, and eleven European countries refuse to import our meat as long as DES is used. Young girls reach puberty at a much earlier age than they used to, and many young men are becoming increasingly more feminine. Several scientists now wonder if this could be due to the DES found in meat, considering that Americans are big meat-eaters. This is presently under further scientific investigation. In Europe, the grave consequences of DES have already been considered. Why have we closed our eyes to the danger to the American public?

Health-food stores are still too expensive and offer too limited a selection for many people, but by carefully reading labels in your supermarket, it is often possible to choose between two products that are almost identical except for their chemical additives. This is especially true of bread, cereal, canned goods, cheese, frozen goods, condiments, snacks, pastries, and salad dressing.

In addition to these chemicals, some foods contain known carcinogens in the forms of pesticide residues, trace elements picked up from the soil, and a poison called *afflatoxin* produced by mold. Washing all fruits and vegetables carefully, while not completely purging them of these chemicals, at least gets rid of those that are not ingrown.

Excessive alcoholic intake is associated with an increased risk of cancer of the esophagus. This is especially acute if the drinking is mixed with smoking. In general, moderation is wise not only in drinking but in all food consumption. The body reacts differently to all vitamins and minerals, fats, starches, and sugars. If our hormonal balance is to be maintained, these nutritional elements should remain relatively well balanced. A moderate diet and plenty of exercise will keep the body working properly and strengthen the immune system which helps prevent cancer.

Drugs

Many experts consider carcinogenic drugs far more dangerous than the carcinogenic chemicals we find in our food, mainly because the drugs are ingested in larger doses. But the drugs, despite the risk of cancer, are often necessary to treat some other disorder. Your doctor must carefully balance the various dangers in such cases and should warn you about any risks you may be taking.

More frightening is the case where the drug is not essential, and is found, in retrospect, to cause cancer. This happened in 1971, when it was discovered that the daughters of women who had taken synthetic estrogen diethylstilbestrol (DES) during early pregnancy were more susceptible to an often-fatal vaginal cancer. A few decades ago obstetricians felt that DES was a cure for women who repeatedly miscarried. The treatment is no longer prescribed, but women who were given DES during pregnancy should be aware that their daughters should be checked frequently for carcinoma of the vagina.

Recent studies have suggested that the use of estrogen by middle-age women to alleviate the symptoms of menopause increases the risk of uterine cancer. It might also be linked to breast cancer. Women who have undergone hysterectomies need not worry about uterine cancer, but other women should be aware of the danger because this treatment is still widely prescribed. Estrogen helps maintain the hormonal balance, which some researchers feel helps prevent cancer of the ovary, a far more serious disease than cancer of the uterus. The estrogen treatment keeps a woman's skin, vagina, bones, and organs healthier, slowing the deterioration of the aging process somewhat. The first symptom of uterine cancer is bleeding, so if a woman is aware of this and watches for it, early treatment is almost always successful. Again, careful weighing of risks and benefits must be made, and the patient should be able to make a well-informed choice. Many doctors suggest that women who take hormone replacements should have biopsies taken from their uteri to detect any abnormalities about once a year when they have their Pap smears.

There have also been reports linking certain birth-control pills to uterine cancer. However, only ten to twenty such reports have been confirmed out of fifty million women who use the pill. Still, these reports generally stem from high-estrogen-containing pills. Most of these brands have been taken off the market. Women on the minipill, which contains low hormone levels, have never been shown to develop increased risk of cancer.

Drugs used to prevent rejection of organ transplants have also been found to cause cancer. Among more than six thousand kidney-transplant recipients, the risk of lymphatic cancer was found to be thirty-five times greater than normal. These drugs are designed to counteract the body's immune system, a system thought to be a key element in cancer prevention. In these cases, there is usually no choice but to use these drugs, but your physician should watch carefully for any signs of tumor development.

Before any drug goes on the market, it is first tested on animals, then on a controlled group of human beings. The U.S. Food and Drug Administration is responsible for evaluating and licensing drugs for general or prescription use on the basis of these tests. Unfortunately, the agency cannot possibly keep up with the hundreds of drugs introduced every year, and must often rely at least in part on data supplied by the manufacturer. Because it can take so long for cancer to develop, the carcinogenic implications of any new drug are never completely understood until the drug has been in use for several decades. Thus no drug should be considered entirely cancer-safe, and no drug should be taken unless its use is specifically indicated by symptoms.

X-Rays

Are X-rays miracle viewers or zap guns? This question has plagued the scientific community since Roentgen first discovered X-rays in 1895, but only recently have the negative charges been substantiated. There is no longer any doubt that X-rays and similar forms of radiation can cause leukemia and other cancers if received in high enough doses. Survivors of Hiroshima and Nagasaki have shown significantly high incidence of leukemia and cancer of the breast, bowel, and brain. The radiation from an atomic explosion and that from an X-ray machine are fundamentally the same.

Recently researchers have found that children in the 1940s and 1950s who were treated with radiation for tonsillitis, enlarged thymus glands, and skin conditions such as acne have increased risks of thyroid and skin cancer. The threat is real, but no one knows yet how dangerous it is. There is no doubt that X-rays are one of the physician's most valuable tools for diagnosing and treating a vast range of diseases, disorders, and traumatic injuries. Are they worth the risk?

Some researchers feel that a single dose of X-rays will age the cells it hits by a year. Others feel that routine X-rays are perfectly harmless as long as they are spaced sufficiently to give the body a chance to recover. Many physicians frown on X-rays of men and women during the reproductive years because of the increased chance of leukemia in the offspring. For this same reason, and because of the danger of damage to your own reproductive system, you should have a shield over your abdomen whenever you have X-rays taken, even by a dentist.

Surely, no matter how slight the danger may turn out to be, caution is indicated. Your physician should not order any routine X-rays, including chest X-rays, unless you have symptoms that require X-rays for diagnosis. If he does prescribe X-rays, you should question him about their necessity.

The Environment

In the air we breathe, the water we drink, the food we eat, the products we use, and the materials with which we work, there are about 1,400 chemicals that are now suspected of causing cancer. Many experts link these substances to the five-fold increase in the cancer rate in 1975. Previous years had registered increases of only about one percent.

The dangers of pollution are impossible to escape, although they can be controlled to an extent. Country air is safer than city air, for example. Choosing not to smoke cigarettes, not to live near a fume-infested freeway, or not to use aerosol sprays all help.

Perhaps the most susceptible to environmental dangers are certain industrial workers who must work in atmospheres thick with carcinogenic dust and gas. The list of these occupations grows every day. Painters are exposed to chromates that are linked to lung cancer. Rubber workers have a risk of leukemia from exposure to benzene. Lung cancer and lymphoma occur in high rates among workers exposed to inorganic arsenic, a major chemical in over forty processes from tinting windshields to spraying roses. Like vinyl chloride, found in many plastics, arsenic has been linked to liver cancer. For eighty years, benzidine, which is used in dye making, has been known to cause bladder cancer. Benzidine has been withdrawn from the market in Great Britain, the Soviet Union, and several other countries because of its carcinogenic properties, but it is still widely used in the United States.

Many occupational carcinogens work in concert with other agents —asbestos workers radically increase their chances of getting lung cancer if they smoke.

These industrial pollutants make their way into surrounding communities all too easily. Epidemiologists in South Africa and England have found *mesothelioma* (cancer of certain abdominal linings) in a number of men and women who had never been inside an asbestos plant, although asbestos was indicated as the cause. In the United States, people living in communities with smelting facilities have higher-than-average lung-cancer rates. In three Ohio towns where vinyl chloride was used in industries, researchers found a mysterious series of deaths from cancer of the central nervous system in adults and numerous birth defects in children.

Employers should be aware of these dangers and should be legally bound to minimize them as much as possible. Unfortunately, enforcement of such safety regulations is almost impossible, so employers must police themselves. This is not a question of expense, it is a question of human life. Employees should also be aware of the chemicals with which they work and should see a doctor regularly to check for signs of any cancer that those chemicals may be suspected of causing.

The Sun

One of those things we all know but which we all hate to think about is that the sun causes skin cancer. A committee of the National Academies of Science recently estimated that among white people living along the fortieth parallel, 40 percent of all melanomas and 80 percent of all other types of skin cancer could be attributed to ultraviolet rays. Most skin cancer is slow-growing and has a low mortality, but not all. *Melanoma,* one of the deadliest, kills 75 percent more people in the span of states running from Louisiana to South Carolina than it does in the northern latitudes from Washington to Minnesota.

It is possible that ultraviolet light interferes with the body's defense system against cancer, a system still unknown to immunologists. This theory would explain why the worst form of human skin cancer, malignant melanoma, shows up as often on unexposed skin as on exposed, yet the source is probably the sun. On the other hand, other forms of skin cancer affect only the areas exposed to the sun. Perhaps the rays initiate cancer by various means.

The danger of skin cancer from the sun is real, but you don't have to stay indoors for the rest of your days. Unless you work in the sun (in which case you should shade your face with a hat), normal outdoor activities should not expose you to a dangerous extent. Excessive sunbathing, however, may do more to your skin than add color.

TYPES OF GYNECOLOGICAL CANCER

Breast Cancer

Breast cancer accounts for 20 percent of cancer deaths in women. This is the most common form of cancer among women, especially those over forty-five years of age. It has been linked to various causes, from obesity to not breast-feeding, but very little progress has been made in the understanding of the causes of breast cancer. It is generally considered a disease of various origins. Breast cancer will kill approximately thirty-three thousand Americans this year. One of every fifteen women will develop breast cancer during her lifetime, but usually not before age thirty-five. In 1975, about ninety thousand new cases were diagnosed in the United States.

Causes
Though the causes of breast cancer are elusive, it is known that a history of the disease in the family not only increases a woman's

possibility of getting cancer, but also of developing it earlier and in both breasts instead of one.

Other women in the high-risk group include those with polycystic ovaries (Stein-Leventhal disease). In this condition, the ovaries become enlarged, producing a higher amount of estrogen than normal. It is possible that because the hormone levels with this condition are high throughout these women's lives, this overstimulation of the breasts can subsequently lead to the development of cancer. By the same token, estrogen-replacement therapy for menopausal women might increase their risks of developing breast cancer. Obesity and heavy fat intake can also increase the risk of developing breast cancer. The explanation is that fats overstimulate estrogen production and that the prolonged effects of hormones cause an irritation of the breast tissue which subsequently can lead to cancer. In animals used in experiments, fats have been found to be directly related to development of breast cancer.

There have been studies that maintain that breast-feeding lowers the incidence of breast cancer, though other studies have contradicted these findings. The theory here is that the milk glands, if not used as nature intended, can cause an irritation leading to cancer. Recent studies have shown that the incidence of breast cancer is more common in the United States and the United Kingdom than in developing countries. These studies concluded that these differences were not related to the number of children or the length of breast-feeding, but rather to the age of a woman at her first childbirth. Women who have their first child at age thirty-five or later have a risk of developing breast cancer three times higher than that of women who have a first child before their eighteenth birthdays. This is why some researchers believe that oral contraceptives, which simulate pregnancy to a certain degree, might protect a woman from developing breast cancer. The birth-control pills result in a steady hormone level and prevent the natural hormone fluctuation with the cyclic breast stimulation.

Stress can also increase the chances of breast cancer by overproducing steroids which depress the body's immune system. This overproduction has led some researchers to recommend treatment with vitamin A or bacillus Calmette-Guerin (BCG) injections, both of which can increase immune responses.

Symptoms and Diagnosis

The best way to detect breast cancer in its early stages is by conducting regular self-examinations. If a woman is in a high-risk category, she should see a gynecologist twice a year. A breast tumor most frequently begins as a *painless* lump in the upper outside quadrant of the breast (see chart in Chapter 18, Breast Examination). As the lump grows, the overlying skin tends to be pulled inward and eventually dimples. Skin discoloration can occur when the cancer is more advanced, and the nipple sometimes retracts. Any of these signs should prompt an immediate examination by an expert. The fact that the lump is usually painless leads many women to ignore the problem until it is too late. Breast cancer grows slowly, so it does not pull unduly on the nerves. Small, painful lumps are usually harmless cystic milk glands, common in many women in their fertile years and especially before menstruation.

Women with cancer in the family and who are overweight or over forty years old should have yearly or biyearly mammography or thermography exams in combination with breast palpation. Early discovery almost always leads to successful treatment. More than 90 percent of all breast cancers are discovered by women themselves. If a suspicious breast lump is found, a breast biopsy is indicated to confirm the diagnosis (see section on Breast Biopsy).

Treatment

There are three basic treatments for breast cancer—surgery, radiation, and chemotherapy. The correct treatment, or combination of treatments, depends on the spread of the cancer. If the disease is caught in the early stages, the tumor can usually be removed surgically. If during surgery cancer is found in the lymph glands, it may have spread even farther, and surgical removal is not enough. Then radiation or cobalt therapy is needed to kill the cancer throughout the lymphatic system around the breast. Occasionally chemotherapy is also added to the treatment schedule.

There is considerable controversy about the various cancer treatments, none more heated than that about radical or simple mastectomy (surgical removal of the breast). If cancer is suspected, a biopsy should be performed. This is often done in conjunction with preparations for mastectomy. If the tumor is benign, the operation is over. If it is malignant, the surgeon may perform an immediate mastectomy. At this point, the surgeon must decide whether to remove the bulk of the breast in a simple mastectomy, or the entire breast with its underlying muscles and the lymph nodes in the armpit by a radical mastectomy (see Chapter 19, Corrective Breast Surgery).

The radical mastectomy allows a pathological examination of the entire breast area to determine the extent to which the cancer has spread. This gives the physician data to use in prescribing further treatment. Many doctors believe, however, that once the main tumor is removed by a simple mastectomy, the body's natural antibodies can effectively fight the remaining cancer. The debate continues, and worldwide research is being conducted in an attempt to settle the question. A woman can be sure of getting the best treatment by choosing a physician or medical center that is thoroughly up to date on the latest research. There are only three centers in the United States with facilities and staff capable of treating every form of cancer as proficiently as possible: the Anderson Hospital and Tumor Institute in Houston, Texas; the Roswell Park Memorial Institute in Buffalo, New York; and the Memorial Sloan-Kettering Cancer Center in New York City. If it is impractical to visit one of these centers, they can probably direct you to the best facilities in your area.

If the breast cancer is localized without any sign of spread when it is removed, the five-year survival rate is between 75 and 80 percent. If it has spread to the lymph nodes, the cure rate is somewhat lower. Some physicians have suggested removing the ovaries in women under fifty to decrease estrogen stimulation which could promote cancer in the remaining breast, but most breast-cancer specialists do not recommend this anymore.

Some researchers recommend radiation therapy *instead* of mastectomy in treating localized breast cancer. In one study, more than one hundred patients with localized tumors who either were too old or who refused surgery were followed for more than two years. Every patient was given an average dose (5000 rad) of radiation over a period of five weeks. The results showed that the cure rate for radiation alone was as high as the best rate obtained by radical surgery. A group of French physicians has also reported the same successful cure rate with radiation therapy alone in a large group of patients which has been followed for many years. Of course, the danger here is that the physician may underestimate the extent of the tumor. If the tumor has spread and a radical mastectomy is performed, followed by radiation therapy, a New York study found the cure rate to exceed 90 percent. Some experts support radiation therapy as a means of preventing recurrence of the cancer, but chemotherapy is generally considered more effective.

According to Italian researchers, a new three-drug treatment —*cyclophosphamide, methotrexate,* and *5-fluorouracil*—after surgery has produced a great reduction in breast cancer recurrence. However, doctors in the United States who have been using this treatment caution that the Italian tests were limited to 207 cases, and that the results are not yet conclusive. Without chemotherapy, the recurrence rate when there are no cancerous lymph nodes found is 24 percent within ten years; with cancerous nodes, the rate jumps to 86 percent. The Italian study noted a recurrence rate of only 5.3 percent with the treatment, compared to 24 percent recurrence in a similar group who did not receive the three-drug chemotherapy, but these statistics were collected after only twenty-seven months. Further testing is being conducted in the United States now, and a four-drug program is also being studied.

The drug BCG (bacillus Calmette-Guerin) has shown spectacular results when used in combination with a three-drug chemotherapy program for recurrent breast cancer. In a study group of twenty-one patients in the United States who received three-drug therapy alone, three died and six relapsed. But of fourteen patients who received the three-drug therapy plus BCG injections, there were no deaths and only one relapse. BCG is thought to build up the body's immune system.

Chemotherapy may be an unpleasant experience. The treatment often causes vomiting, gastrointestinal pain, and loss of hair. But it is certainly preferable to the alternative of recurring tumor.

Cancer of the Cervix

In the past decade, deaths from cancer of the cervix have decreased from approximately eighteen thousand to nine thousand per year. Epidemiologists have ascribed this reduction to two causes—a greater awareness among women, and the Pap smear, which detects the cancer very early. This is the only cancer with a decreasing death rate.

There are great disparities in the cervical cancer rates of various ethnic groups. For example, 3.6 Jewish women per 100,000 suffer this disease, whereas for Puerto Rican women the rate is 98 per 100,000. Black women have a rate of 48 per 100,000, as opposed to 14 per 100,000 white women. No one knows why these differences exist. Some experts contend that the factor is cultural—some races traditionally have children earlier, for example, which increases their chances for cancer of the cervix. Others believe that the problem is a genetic weakness in the immune system. The mean age for development of cervical cancer is between the ages of forty and fifty. This type of cancer, however, is not uncommon in women under the age of thirty-five.

Causes
Though not much is known about the causes of cervical cancer, there are numerous indications linking it to sexual intercourse.

Prostitutes have an extremely high incidence of cervical cancer, while nuns have an extremely low incidence. It has been shown that cervical cancer is more prevalent in women who experience early sexual activity, childbirth at an early age, and/or numerous sex partners. It is possible that the penis secretes an inflammatory substance. The longer that sex has been engaged in, the more this irritant has been working on the cervix. Just as the irritation of the sun causes skin cancer and the irritation of tobacco causes lung cancer, so might the irritation of this still-unidentified penile factor cause cancer of the cervix. In the past, this irritant was thought to be *smegma,* a whitish, cheesy secretion from the penis which collects under the foreskin. Circumcision prevents this accumulation of smegma. Since Jewish men are circumcised, this seemed to be the logical explanation for the lower incidence of cervical cancer among Jewish women. However, even though a large number of men in the United States are circumcised today, there has not been the expected decline in cervical cancer. In fact, studies have been performed comparing the incidence of cervical cancer among women with circumcised mates to the incidence among women with uncircumcised partners, and when the groups were matched for age, initiation of sexual activity, childbirths, and number of sexual partners, there were no significant differences between the two groups. Circumcision in the male does not appear to protect his sexual partner from cervical cancer. In retrospect, it was felt that the low incidence of cervical cancer among Jewish women was due to infrequent premarital sex, later marriage, and having a single sexual partner.

The irritant might be directly related to the sperm itself or to sexually transmitted diseases such as herpes simplex Type II (see Chapter 7, Venereal Disease). During pregnancy, there is an increase in the vascularity of the cervix, often leading to the development of cervicitis, which can reoccur with each pregnancy. Chronic cervicitis may predispose a woman to cervical cancer, and this could be the reason for the higher incidence of cervical cancer among women with many children.

If a woman leads an active sex life or began having sex at an early age, she needn't change her life-style, but she should have regular Pap smears at least once a year.

Symptoms and Diagnosis

Early cervical cancer is asymptomatic and can only be detected by a Pap smear. Cancer of the cervix usually starts as an inflammatory reaction which, over the years, develops into a slight abnormality of the cells in the cervix. This abnormality, called *dysplasia,* can either heal spontaneously or develop into cancer. The development of the cancer usually takes several years and the Pap smear, analyzed in a competent laboratory, can detect dysplasia before it develops into cancer. This very early detection in the precancerous state should lead to colposcopy or biopsy of the cervix to verify the diagnosis, so that appropriate treatment can be instituted even before the cancer develops. If cervical cancer is detected in the precancerous state or in the cancerous state, but before it has had a chance to spread, a well-trained specialist will be able to remove the cancer surgically with an almost 100 percent cure rate.

In 1975, forty-six thousand new cases of cervical cancer were diagnosed. There were nine thousand deaths reported to have stemmed from the disease. Many researchers agree that no one should die from cancer of the cervix, especially since modern techniques are effective in diagnosing and treating this type of cancer. Deaths from cervical cancer are almost always the results of diagnoses made too late. Your only insurance is to see a specialist who keeps up with the latest research in the field, and to see him regularly. A woman must have Pap smears at least yearly as soon as she becomes sexually active. Women in high-risk groups should consider having Pap smears every six months.

Treatment

If cervical cancer is detected in its *in situ* state, it is usually removed with a *cone biopsy,* in which a wide, cone-shaped piece of the cervix is excised. If the patient has had children and intends to have no more, some physicians advise removing the uterus to ensure that the cancer will not spread.

If the cancer is more advanced, it can be treated by an extensive hysterectomy, either alone or with the addition of radiation or cobalt therapy. Cobalt treatment must be performed by a specialist. If it is not properly administered, cobalt can cause extensive tissue damage of the bowels, the vagina, or the bladder. The American Cancer Society can recommend a suitable treatment center or specialist.

Cancer of the Uterus

Uterine cancer is on the rise. In 1975, there were 3,300 deaths from this disease, predominantly in the white population (as opposed to cervical cancer, which appears more often in black and Puerto Rican populations). The average age of development is fifty-seven, with 75 percent of all cases occurring after fifty and only 4 percent occurring before forty.

Causes

The incidence of cancer of the uterus is higher in women who have not borne children and in obese women (especially those with hypertension and diabetes). No one knows the link between the absence of children and uterine cancer (nuns have a high rate of occurrence of this disease), but obesity is linked to high estrogen production, which is thought to overstimulate the uterus, becoming a carcinogenic irritant.

A woman who is twenty to fifty pounds overweight increases her chances of developing a uterine tumor by 300 percent, while a woman who is more than fifty pounds overweight increases her chances by 900 percent.

The racial differences in the uterine cancer rate (or endometrial cancer, cancer of the uterine lining) are now thought to be largely a matter of diet. Asian women, who have a relatively low incidence of endometrial cancer and a high incidence of stomach cancer while living in their native countries, tend to have a higher incidence of endometrial cancer, consistent with the American norm, after one or two generations in the United States. This could be due to the high caloric and cholesterol intake in the American diet, which, again, affects estrogen production.

Women with Stein-Leventhal disease (polycystic ovaries), who have higher estrogen levels, also run an unusually high risk of having endometrial cancer. Women with polycystic ovaries should be aware of this threat and respond to any abnormal bleeding by seeing a doctor for an endometrial biopsy.

Millions of American women have been taking estrogen for years to prevent such menopausal symptoms as drying of the skin, backaches, or fatigue. Naturally, since various cancers (including that of the uterus) have been linked to estrogen, this treatment increases the risk of tumor growth. This is a calculated risk that you and your doctor must ponder carefully. Again, if you are undergoing estrogen treatment, you should have any abnormal bleeding checked out immediately. When endometrial cancer is diagnosed early, the cure rate is almost 100 percent.

Symptoms and Diagnosis

If abnormal bleeding occurs in any of the instances already discussed, or anytime after menopause, a biopsy of the endometrium or a D&C should be conducted to investigate the cause. Pap smears are adequate for cervical cancer but detect uterine cancer in less than half the cases. Endometrial biopsies can occasionally be performed in the doctor's office, but many physicians prefer to conduct a D&C in a hospital with the patient under general anesthesia. This gives the doctor an opportunity to check the uterus for any abnormality or enlargement. If there is a cancer development but the uterine cavity is less than eight centimeters deep, the cancer is usually in the early stages and can be fairly easily treated by hysterectomy.

Treatment

In general, to treat endometrial cancer, surgery is combined with radiation therapy. This varies from case to case and from institution to institution. The aim of the radiation is to shrink the uterus and block the lymphatic system to prevent the tumor from spreading. An abdominal hysterectomy and bilateral oophorectomy, in which the uterus and both ovaries are removed, is then performed. This is usually accompanied by radiation treatment of the vagina to prevent the cancer from spreading there.

If the tumor has already spread deep into the uterine wall or to the lymphatic system, it is very difficult to cure, since it may have spread into surrounding organs as well. This situation would call for chemotherapy in the hope of eliminating the cancer wherever it has spread. The treatment of endometrial cancer should be guided by a cancer specialist.

Adenomatous Hyperplasia

Adenomatous hyperplasia is a condition characterized by an overgrowth of endometrial tissue; it occurs most frequently in women in their forties and in postmenopausal women. The symptoms are intramenstrual or postmenopausal bleeding. It is probably caused by a hormone imbalance that results in the endometrium growing but not being sloughed regularly. The condition is diagnosed by microscopic examination of endometrial tissue obtained during curettage. At times, this curettage proves to be not only diagnostic, but also curative, and the symptoms do not recur after the surgery. At other times overgrowth returns and leads to endometrial cancer in 10 to 12 percent of all women affected. Prolonged progesterone treatment, however, has been effective in the control of adenomatous hyperplasia in some women. In cases of recurrent adenomatous hyperplasia, when less conservative approaches have failed, hysterectomy may be justified in the woman who either has completed her family or is postmenopausal.

Cancer of the Ovaries

Although the incidence of carcinoma of the ovaries is lower than the incidence of cervical and endometrial cancer, there are almost as many deaths from ovarian cancer as from uterine malignancies. The reason for its unusually high mortality rate is simple. There are no early symptoms, so early detection is rare. By the time cancer of the ovaries is discovered, it has often spread too far to be contained.

Causes

Unlike most other gynecological cancers, ovarian cancer is probably not influenced by estrogen. There are no known high-risk groups for this type of cancer, either, and it seems unaffected by diet. Some researchers suspect that the gonadotrophins LH and FSH irritate the ovaries, causing them to become cancerous. If this is true, estrogen might very well inhibit ovarian cancer, but there is no conclusive evidence to back this up yet. Tests are presently being conducted.

Symptoms and Diagnosis

Cancer of the ovaries is estimated to be responsible for 6 percent of all cancer deaths in women. Ovarian cancer seems to be more prevalent after menopause, although it can occur during the childbearing years. The disease is varied, with different types of tumors causing different types of symptoms, but usually it starts with gas pain and abdominal distention. The ovaries are aligned very closely with the intestines, so that, when cancer inflames the ovaries, the intestines are disturbed. Any continuing, unusual gas pains should be checked by a *gynecologist;* an internist might evaluate the symptoms without a diagnosis for months. Following gas pains, weight loss and fatigue occur, all relatively vague symptoms. Unless the physician is specifically looking for ovarian cancer, it will often go undiagnosed.

After menopause, many experts believe the ovaries shrink because they are no longer needed. They should be difficult to palpate (hard to feel during a pelvic exam). If a postmenopausal woman comes to her gynecologist with gas pains and her ovaries are easy to palpate, an *exploratory laparotomy* should be conducted to examine the ovaries for possible cancer. Many deaths from ovarian cancer could have been avoided if the patient had visited her gynecologist more often. After menopause, a pelvic exam should be conducted at least once a year, perhaps even twice a year if gas pains are felt, since ovarian cancer develops quite rapidly.

Scientists are presently working on blood tests (similar to the CEA [carcino embryonic antigen] test for cancer of the colon) and urine analyses to detect ovarian cancer. Development of these tests is especially critical for this disease, since early detection is so difficult. At the moment, an ovarian biopsy is the major diagnostic tool, and that is performed only if ovarian cancer is suspected.

Treatment

Carcinoma of the ovaries is generally treated by a *total hysterectomy* and *bilateral salpingo-oophorectomy* (removal of the ovaries and fallopian tubes). Removal of the omentum (a fatty fold of abdominal lining attached to the stomach) is also recommended, since it is often a site for cancer spread. Total abdominal radiation should follow surgery, often accompanied by chemotherapy.

Cancer of the Vulva

Cancer of the vulva accounts for about 5 percent of all gynecological cancers. The prognosis is relatively good once the diagnosis has been made.

Causes

As with most cancers, the cause of cancer of the vulva is unknown. It strikes most often in postmenopausal women, who are susceptible to basal cell carcinoma, or skin cancer, which is what cancer of the vulva actually is. The average age of contraction is fifty-nine.

Symptoms and Diagnosis

Cancer of the vulva frequently starts with white lesions or other abnormalities and itching of the vulva. If a woman experiences these symptoms, she should consult a gynecologist. The diagnosis can only be verified by pathological examination of a biopsy from the vulva.

Treatment

Surgery is generally required to treat cancer of the vulva, but in the early stages, a wide excision is almost always successful. When the cancer is more developed, there is some controversy about whether the lymph nodes in the groin should be removed during a *radical vulvectomy* (removal of the entire vulva), but this question must be evaluated in every individual case. Chemotherapy has also successfully effected cure in some cases.

Cancer of the Vagina

Vaginal cancer is rare; it accounts for less than 2 percent of all genital cancer in women. This type of cancer is most common after menopause. It is often an epidermoid cancer, developing in the outer skin layer of the vagina, though it can also spread from the uterus and other areas. Of particular concern is the incidence of this cancer in children. In 1974, an estimated 3,600 deaths were reported in the United States from cancer in children under fifteen. Though most of these deaths were caused by leukemia or neoplasm of the brain and central nervous system, up to 5 percent were due to cancers of the female genitalia.

Causes

The cause of vaginal cancer in adults is unknown. The cause of vaginal cancer in children might be linked to genetic abnormalities, though no one knows exactly how or why. These cancers may develop while the child is still in the uterus (when the child's immune system is not yet fully developed) or might be related to complications during pregnancy or drugs taken by the mother.

Diethylstilbestrol (DES) is an estrogen-type hormone that was used years ago to treat repeated miscarriages. It was later found to cause *cancer* of the vagina in the daughters of women who took DES during pregnancy. If a woman was given DES during pregnancy, her daughters should be considered to have a high risk of vaginal cancer and should have regular gynecological checkups twice a year with Pap smears and possible colposcopy.

Symptoms and Diagnosis

Early cancer of the vagina is asymptomatic but can be detected by a Pap smear. Thus, Pap smears should be performed even in women who have had hysterectomies. If a young girl experiences any abnormal vaginal bleeding, she should be taken to a pediatrician immediately for further investigation. This is especially crucial if the child's mother was given DES during pregnancy. Clear-cell carcinoma can be detected either in a Pap smear or a colposcopy, followed by a biopsy if any abnormalities are found.

Treatment

If vaginal cancer is discovered early, it can be removed by local excision. More extensive cancer requires more extensive surgery, though some vaginal carcinomas also respond to radiation therapy. Clear-cell carcinoma of the vagina usually requires extensive surgery and should only be treated by a cancer specialist.

CANCER PREVENTION

The National Cancer Institute estimates that 25 to 30 percent of all cancer deaths in the United States could be prevented through more conscientious use of early detection techniques and changes in the American life-style. Many of the 80,000 lung cancer deaths every year could be prevented by putting an end to cigarette smoking. This would also tremendously reduce the 13,500 deaths annually from cancer of the mouth and the esophagus. Of these 13,500 deaths, 5,000 could be prevented by a reduction of alcoholism. Almost a third of the 30,000 colon and rectum cancer deaths could be prevented by switching to a diet lower in animal fats. And 5,000 of the 18,000 bladder and liver cancer deaths could be prevented by better controls over industrial pollution. Obviously, we are not going out of our way to protect ourselves against this group of diseases. Cancer is still on the increase, despite constantly improving detection techniques and treatments. Cancer claims over 1,000 lives daily.

How to Prevent Cancer

The future is promising for progressively more effective cancer treatment, and there are certain steps you can take today to lessen your chances of developing the disease. There are numerous substances in our world that are known to be cancer producing. You are probably familiar with at least a few—industrial pollutants, many food additives and preservatives, animal fats, talc, and so on. By limiting your voluntary exposure to these carcinogens, you improve the odds against getting cancer. The key here is the use of the word *limiting*, not *avoiding*. Animal fat probably does not cause cancer, but *excess* animal fat does.

Tobacco is another story. There is *no* safe amount of tobacco. Every cigarette is carcinogenic, not only to you, but to your children, to your friends, or to strangers near you. If you must smoke, don't mix tobacco and alcohol.

If you live near an industrial area, there's not much you can do about the air, but you can drink bottled water to protect yourself against potential polluted municipal water supplies.

Excessive radiation is known to predispose a person to the development of cancer; therefore, overexposure to the sun and to unnecessary X-rays should be avoided.

It is fairly well known that if a close member of your family has developed a particular type of cancer, your chances of developing this cancer are increased, and you should take particular precautions. For example, if your mother or aunt had breast cancer, you should be especially faithful in performing breast self-examinations every month, keeping your weight within reasonable limits, taking oral contraceptives with low levels of estrogen, and being cautious about postmenopausal estrogen-replacement therapy.

Anticancer Diet

The anticancer diet is simply a well-balanced diet—balanced not only among the four food groups (meat, dairy foods, fruits and vegetables, and grain), but balanced within each group. As a general rule, don't eat red meat any more than you eat chicken or fish. Enjoy a vegetarian meal once in a while. Most people use approximately half of their food calories on fats, both animal and vegetable. Beneficial effects could be expected if the fat calories were reduced to one third. In general, polyunsaturated oils and margarines should be substituted for saturated fats whenever it is possible to do so. A link has recently been established between nitrosamines, which are present in all processed meats, and the development of cancer. Therefore, nitrosamines should be avoided. Avoid cholesterol-rich foods such as organ meats, liver, and egg yolks, particularly if you have a high level of cholesterol in your blood. Increase the amount of fibrous food in your diet by eating more raw fruit and vegetables, as well as more dry cereals and unadulterated whole grains. A bran supplement can be added to the diet, but if bran is added, be sure to increase water consumption to prevent bowel problems. Substitute brown rice for processed rice and whole-grain breads and flour for white bread and processed flour. If it is possible, reduce sugar intake. Yogurt, but only yogurt with live cultures, may be an important source of protein in the diet. A study of mice showed that yogurt had some effect in the prevention of the growth of cancer tumors in mice. The intake of all vitamins should be watched, but particular attention should be paid to vitamins A and C, which appear to have some anticancer properties. Try to buy food with the fewest additives and preservatives. Whenever possible, buy fresh food without any artificial ingredients. And remember, drink plenty of water. Watch not only what you eat but how much you eat. Obesity results in excessive estrogen production, which predisposes a person to the development of breast and uterine cancer.

Early Diagnosis of Cancer

You may have noticed a common phrase in the treatment of every form of cancer mentioned in this chapter (and in every form of cancer not mentioned): early diagnosis. This is the determinant between life and death in many cases. Early diagnosis can mean the difference between a simple procedure and major surgery. It means shorter recovery time, less expensive treatment, less psychological trauma. It is the strongest weapon in the war against cancer.

The seven warning signs of cancer listed by the American Cancer Society are:

1. a change in bowel or bladder habits
2. a sore that does not heal
3. unusual bleeding or discharge
4. a thickening or lump in the breast or elsewhere
5. indigestion or difficulty in swallowing
6. obvious change in a wart or mole
7. nagging cough or hoarseness

These should be memorized, and at the appearance of any of these signs, a physician should be consulted.

Women must become aware of their bodies and heed the warning signs. Any abnormalities should be questioned, and most should be looked into by a gynecologist. Routine checkups should be scheduled at least once a year, and self-examination should become a frequent habit. If you've but one life to live, you should live it in health.

The Future—Cancer-Preventing Agents?

Researchers at the National Cancer Institute and elsewhere are looking into the possibility of vaccinations against cancer and of pills that can be taken daily to prevent cancer. The main thrust of the research is aimed at three chemical agents: vitamin A, Laetrile (vitamin B_{17}), and a compound called 13-CIS-retinoic acid.

Vitamin A

Vitamin A has been proven to stimulate greatly the immune response in doses of more than ten times the daily requirement. These extremely high doses of vitamin A have been successfully used as an anticancer agent in about 1,100 German patients. Not only did the vitamin A seem to prevent tumors, but those patients who had developed cancer before being treated showed a much higher survival rate. Unfortunately, high doses of vitamin A cause hypervitaminosis, which can result in headaches, dizziness, diarrhea, change in skin coloring, edema behind the eyes, and liver damage. Because of this, the dosage must be carefully controlled by a physician. Large amounts of cod liver oil containing vitamin A might diminish the problem of toxicity.

13-CIS-Retinoic Acid

This chemical compound is a member of the chemical family of *retinoids*. Retinoids, although they show no effect on cancer that has already developed, appear to regulate cell growth in the epithelial (lining) tissue of organs such as the lungs, the breasts, the bladder, and the prostate gland. These organs are the site for development of 70 percent of all human cancer. The specific retinoid—13-CIS-retinoic acid—is the only one of these compounds considered safe for human use. By regulating this tissue growth, retinoids have reduced cancer development in laboratory animals. The prophylactic effects of this drug are presently being investigated in humans.

Laetrile–Vitamin B_{17}

Laetrile, the controversial anticancer substance, has received a great deal of recent publicity. There have been tests with this drug for more than twenty-five years and no valid scientific evidence yet exists to prove its value in the treatment of cancer. However, there have been reports in the media and publications on cancer cures and remissions following treatment with Laetrile. There are a number of organizations attempting to have Laetrile made generally available in the United States. The Food and Drug Administration has not legalized Laetrile since it feels that there is no dependable scientific evidence of the efficacy of this drug and its release might prevent some people suffering from cancer from receiving the necessary, early, effective treatment.

Laetrile is available in Mexico (and a growing number of states) and people have gone there to receive the drug. At the present time the proponents of Laetrile have shifted the emphasis from Laetrile as a cancer cure to Laetrile as a cancer preventative and/or a means for slowing the growth of the cancer.

The Food and Drug Administration will probably not release Laetrile without documented proof of its effectiveness.

BCG (Bacillus Calmette-Guerin)

One of the most promising anticancer treatments is the injection of BCG, an antituberculosis agent. BCG strengthens the immune response. When it is used in conjunction with chemotherapy, BCG has drastically reduced the death rate in cancer patients. Research is presently being conducted to determine the possible prophylactic properties of BCG. If cancer is caused by a virus—herpes II has been linked to cancer of the cervix—BCG could turn out to be an essential component of a cancer vaccine.

Vaccination

When you receive a vaccination against a disease like polio or smallpox, you are actually being given a small dose of that disease. Your body reacts by producing antibodies to fight whatever you've been infected with. These antibodies, once in the bloodstream, protect you against the disease, sometimes temporarily and sometimes for life. The chances of developing such a vaccine for cancer are encouraging. The field of immunology is progressing by leaps and bounds, and some experts believe certain types of cancer will eventually be as rare as polio. Anticancer vaccines would be especially valuable for the elderly, who are highly susceptible to cancer, since the immune system deteriorates with age.

Whether the answer is BCG, vaccination, pills, or vitamins, cancer prevention is certainly in its infancy. The prognosis for the future, based on the successes of medicine in the past, is good. The answer may be a long time in coming. Still, it will come.

chapter 21

SEX

WHAT IS NORMAL SEX?

People have sex for one or more of three simple reasons: to have children, to express their love, and to have fun and relax. The variety of ways in which sex can fulfill these needs is astonishing.

No one can define *normality* with exact precision, especially when dealing with a sociopsychological phenomenon such as sex. Still, the lesson of history is clear: Sex has always existed, and so has almost every imaginable sexual act. For example, group sex was a normal feature of life in the days of Imperial Rome, incest has been a traditional practice of royalty since the Egyptian pharaohs (Cleopatra was a descendant of six generations of brother-sister marriages), sadism and masochism were common in early religions and familiar fairy tales (such as Cinderella, who willingly suffered torment and humiliation from her stepmother and stepsisters). Homosexuality has been common in tribal societies around the world. Homosexuality was also common in Greek mythology; even Zeus was so inclined. Indeed, in ancient Greece, a homosexual relationship was a standard, respected part of the total education of any well-bred young man.

The lesson of nature is equally clear: There is nothing "unnatural" about any of this. Whales and porpoises enjoy group sex. Homosexuality is everywhere in the animal kingdom; monkeys are the gayest. Zebras and wild horses kick and bite each other bloody as a prelude to sex. And in the Vienna zoo, a white peacock and a Galapagos turtle were observed trying to mate.

So what is "normal"?

The answer is that normal sex is any kind of sex that is felt to be normal by the participants. Oral sex and masturbation are criminal acts (sometimes even for married couples) in more than forty states, yet the Kinsey Report found that 95 percent of American men and 85 percent of American women qualify for a prison sentence under these laws. It could be normal for a couple to enjoy group sex, as long as neither partner is *forced* to participate. Homosexuality is normal sex for homosexuals but not for heterosexuals.

Anything can be normal sex if there is love and understanding between the partners. When it is abnormal to one of the partners, it becomes abnormal sex. Unfortunately the Judeo-Christian morality of Western society—and particularly our own American Puritan heritage —has rigidly opposed the enjoyment of human bodily functions and sensations. This narrow attitude has influenced every area of our modern lives. Our schools, churches, laws, manners, and dress all inhibit us. It is no surprise that our beliefs are in confusion between what we are told and how we feel.

PSYCHO-SEXUAL PROBLEMS

Masters and Johnson, the leading sex therapists in America today, have stated that approximately half of the marriages in this country have or will have sexual problems.

And the fact is, *most sexual problems start above the waist*. That is, most sexual problems are not physical, but psychological. Our upbringing has taught us to feel guilty about sex. Now, in our sex-oriented world, we feel anxious about meeting our own and our partner's sexual expectations. Evidence shows that sexual problems are not usually manifestations of profound emotional disturbance. To the contrary, they occur regularly in people who function normally in all other psychological aspects.

The cause of many sexual problems is simply lack of information. With sex as highly visible in our society as it is today in books, magazines, movies, plays, songs, on TV, and right there on the street, it's hard to believe anyone could still be handicapped by an ignorance of basic anatomical facts. Yet doctors and sex therapists see couples who have been married several years and have never had intercourse because they don't know how. More commonly, a man might not know that it takes a woman much longer to become sexually aroused than it does himself; a woman might not know that a man's sexual abilities change throughout his life. Lack of information—lack of sex education—works differently in different people, and can cause problems in a number of different areas.

Guilt

Sex therapists treat many patients who are inhibited by guilt and who never suspect it as the root of their problem. Moreover, they are surprised when the therapist points it out. One of the most frequently observed sexual dysfunctions in men, for example, is premature ejaculation, which often originates in guilt feelings. Guilt is both a cause and an effect of lack of information; a misunderstanding that produces a sexual problem which is itself misunderstood.

Frustration

A lack of information can obviously frustrate a couple who want a full and fulfilling sex life. Gaining knowledge can bring a second frustration—the sense of having missed something—which may lead the woman or man or both to blame their relationship and look elsewhere for a second youth.

Overexpectation

Many women are looking for the perfect, sublime orgasm that everyone is talking about. These women often feel cheated when they don't achieve it. Many women react to their first sexual experiences by thinking, "Is that all?" They wonder if they have an average amount of sex. Yet studies consistently show that how often people have intercourse has nothing to do with how much they enjoy it. Like sexual problems, sexual pleasure also starts above the waist—with an open, understanding attitude between the partners. This is a statistical fact. People often expect too much of sex because they don't know what to expect.

Insecurity

Many couples are so anxious to please each other sexually that each member will ignore her or his own enjoyment to concentrate on the other's. Men worry about achieving an instant erection. Women worry about faking orgasm. It's unfortunate when sex becomes a theatrical performance striving to attain a glossy ideal, with an audience of two critics who don't know any better.

Hidden Problems

Many people are unaware that certain diseases (like diabetes), medications (such as those used for hypertension), and alcohol abuse can seriously impair sexual pleasure. The first step in treating any sexual problem is a complete physical examination, to determine if the problem stems from physiological causes.

Embarrassment

Many sexual problems could be avoided if the couple openly discussed their attitudes and preferences, learned about each other's bodies, considered new ideas—in short, exchanged information about themselves. Too often, embarrassment prevents this. People are ashamed to reveal their ignorance. Or they are confused about what they do know. This embarrassment complicates old problems, creating new ones.

The First Step to Solving a Problem

A lot of sexual problems can be cured simply by education. This education should start at an early age and continue until death. Parents should be open and honest with their children, explaining to them what happens in sex and what doesn't, what to expect and what not to expect. Schools should supplement and reinforce parental teachings, supplying, perhaps, facts which are not within parental grasp. As an adult, it is vital to continue seeking information—from lovers, friends, books, or anything else. There is nothing you shouldn't know about sex, and no information you should greet with a less-than-open attitude. After all, how can anyone enjoy sex before knowing what is possible and what isn't? In the limited space of this chapter, we will offer a closer look at the exotic cornucopia of sex and the basics, too —what happens and what doesn't, what's possible and what isn't.

One thing that isn't possible is for a peacock and a turtle to mate. What's important, and perfectly normal, is that they tried. All the information in the world will be useless if your mind isn't open to receive it. Relax, feel good, and expand. Learn to enjoy sex for the beautiful experience it is.

YOUR BODY

It's sexy, all right . . . but what, exactly, *is* sexy about it? And why?

People are different and fashions change, in sex as in any other preference. Ancient religious cults featured vaginas and penises as powerful symbols and images. In eighteenth-century Europe, women's ball gowns were tailored to extreme décolletage in order to display their powdered nipples. In the Roaring Twenties, women bound their breasts and men ogled their "gams" instead. Modern American men seem to admire most a woman's breasts. The girl from Ipanema, or anywhere else in South America, wears a *tonga*—a string bikini—when she walks down the beach because Latin men are more stimulated by a woman's buttocks than by any other part of her body. Turnabout is fair play, and a majority of young American women who were questioned in a recent survey agreed that they liked *men* with trim buttocks.

Fads and fancies come and go; the truth is, as the old saying goes: What you have isn't as important as how you use it.

The Vagina

People come in all sizes, and so do their sexual organs. In general, the larger a woman is, the deeper her vagina will be; the important fact, however, is that most women, large or small, can usually accommodate any size penis.

After all, the vagina is an amazing organ. Its ability to stretch and then return to its normal size is astonishing. One month it can accommodate a baby's passage. The next month it is large enough to accommodate only a penis.

The vagina's ability to stretch is always present. Because of this, if a woman complains that she has difficulty accepting a very large penis, it may be simply that she needs a greater amount of stimulation, since the vagina actually increases in size the more excited a woman becomes. More frequent intercourse will also cause a woman's vagina to enlarge.

When a woman first starts having intercourse, she might face a different problem—the size and type of her hymen. Since, like everything else, the hymen ring inside the opening of the vagina varies from woman to woman—from a tight, thick membrane to an open, thin one—some women will be more stretched than others, will experience greater pain, and will be harder to penetrate. If a woman is young and just beginning to have sex, then some sort of external lubrication (with, for example, K-Y lubricant or baby oil) should help the immediate problem, and intercourse will probably become easier with the passage of time. In more serious cases, where penetration may be impossible, the surgical procedure called hymenectomy is advisable. This is merely a matter of surgically opening the hymen ring, requiring a short hospital stay.

Often the complaint is just the opposite. A woman, especially after bearing several children, will feel stretched to such a degree that she is unable to squeeze tightly around a man's penis and has less pleasure during intercourse. Sometimes this is the result of a traumatic or prolonged childbirth, and the solution lies only in a surgical procedure (a posterior repair) which tightens the vaginal muscles, returning the vagina to normal size. If, though, a delivery has been uncomplicated, with good obstetrical care, the vagina usually returns to its normal size by itself. A simple exercise can help most women keep their vaginas in tone.

The Kegel Exercise

Today many people are concerned with physical fitness. They jog, visit health clubs, or do exercises at home to keep healthy. A woman's vagina is an opening covered with muscles that respond to exercise like other muscles and should be kept in as good condition. The Kegel exercise was developed by the late Arnold Kegel, a California gynecologist. Dr. Kegel initially used his technique for older patients who couldn't retain their urine. The purpose of the exercise was to strengthen the muscles around the vagina. Dr. Kegel found that after doing the exercise for a while, women experienced a greater capacity for orgasm, even when they were previously unable to achieve one.

The Kegel exercise is easy. Squeeze your buttocks together and draw in your pelvis: the contraction you feel is the *pubococcygeus* muscle. Try to keep this muscle contracted for three seconds, then relax for three seconds, then squeeze again. Women sometimes have trouble contracting the muscle for three full seconds in the beginning. The Kegel exercise starts with three three-second contractions at three different times during the day and increases up to twenty three-second contractions at a time. The Kegel exercise can be done while you're walking, riding the subway, or sitting in a car, and the improved vaginal control it brings means better sex for you and your partner. To check the progress of this exercise, you should occasionally insert a finger into your vagina and squeeze, determining if you are exercising the right muscles and monitoring the increased pressure on your finger. The same exercise can be used to great benefit during intercourse. All you do is replace your finger with a penis. Some stripteasers have gained such control that they can pick up dollar bills with their vaginal lips.

Vaginal Malformations

All kinds of malformations can exist in the vagina, as in any organ. In rare cases, a woman may even be born *without* a vagina or uterus, and yet possess other normal sex characteristics such as breast development and pubic hair. In these cases, doctors can create an artificial vagina with skin taken from the inside thigh. If the uterus is absent, the woman is not able to have children, but the artificial vagina will respond sexually like a normal vagina, with normal secretion, orgasmic contractions, and pleasure during intercourse. This is the same type of vagina that is created in men who undergo sex-change operations.

The Clitoris

From various specific research, including the implantation of electrodes in the vagina, modern sexologists have determined that the crucial factor in producing female orgasm is stimulation of the clitoris. The clitoris is a tiny vestigial penis, a bundle of nerves with a head and shaft which gathers and transmits impulses to the sex centers of the brain, where orgasmic responses are controlled. The clitoris has six to ten times more nerve endings than the tissue which surrounds it. It is so sensitive that some women find direct touch painful, preferring to masturbate or be stroked around or near the clitoris instead.

The in and out movements of a man's penis during intercourse pull the vaginal lips and tissue around the clitoris, and a woman may therefore conclude that her arousal is linked to the penetration of her vagina rather than, as is the case, to the stimulation of her clitoris. Also, a woman will feel a pleasurable sensation deep in her vagina as it secretes and enlarges with her excitement, and may identify this as the source of her orgasm, although the transmitter and pacemaker of her sexual response is really the nerve center of the clitoris.

The Penis

There is no connection between a man's race or body size and the size of his penis. It's like his nose—it all depends on genetics. Large and small penises seem to run in families. A large unerected penis may give a man a psychological boost, but what counts is, of course, the size of the erected penis, and this does only vary slightly from man to man. Studies have shown that a large flaccid penis may only increase slightly to its erected state, while a small flaccid penis often can more than double its size to an approximately equal erection. The average size of an erect penis is between six and seven inches, regardless of its size when it is flaccid.

The more sexual stimulation and intercourse a man has, the larger his penis will become. Mood and health also affect a man's sexual response; a man's erection can increase or decrease by an inch from day to day. Finally, a whole group of devices guaranteed to increase penis size is available in sex shops and through magazine advertisements. While these devices may be pleasurable to use, they are only a gadgety excuse to stimulate the penis, and this stimulation can be achieved more simply and economically by masturbation and intercourse.

Men worry about these things, but women seem to agree that the size of a man's penis has little to do with his ability to be sexually satisfying. A man can best satisfy a woman by understanding a woman sexually and preparing her for intercourse.

Silicone Implantation in the Penis

As is the case with the vagina, there are surgical procedures available to correct or rebuild the penis. Silicone implantations have been performed, mostly in urology departments for patients whose penises were partly excised due to cancer. In order to allow the patients sexual satisfaction, doctors will implant silicone rods in the penis to produce a permanent stiffness (although true erection, a raising of the penis, will not usually occur). Men with small penises sometimes inquire about this operation, but urologists are reluctant to perform it except where severe corrective surgery has been necessary.

The Breasts

A woman's breasts are a very sensitive erogenous area for the woman and an important sexual attraction for many men. Some women feel such excitement having their breasts stimulated that they can reach orgasm; some women actively dislike it. In either case, a woman's breasts will swell and become fuller, and the nipples will become erect during arousal.

The size of a woman's breasts has as little importance as the size of a man's penis. A woman may worry that her breasts are too small, or too large, or different sizes, instead of simply enjoying them for the pleasure they can give. In fact, the erogenous focus of the breast is the nipple and surrounding area, which is equally sensitive no matter what the size of the breast.

A common complaint of women is inverted nipples, which they fear may be a deformity or a block to sexual pleasure. Not true. Inverted nipples are considered to be well within the limits of normal breast variation, and in no way affect the quality of sensation a woman feels in her breasts.

The breasts are among the most blatantly obvious sex characteristics, which certainly accounts for much of their attractiveness to men. Furthermore, the mother's breast means warmth, nourishment, and safety to the infant. This sensual bond can easily carry into adulthood on a subconscious level. For whatever reason, many men substitute the part for the whole, and respond to the woman in terms of her breasts. Some men prefer women with big breasts, on the theory that quantity means quality, while others always want small-breasted women, expecting them to be more sexually diverse. Both attitudes miss the point completely.

As women and their sexual partners mature, and sex becomes a regular feature of their lives, the emphasis on breasts, big or small, seems to fade. The entire range of sexual experience becomes available, and a woman's breasts are only one of many means of enjoyment.

The Buttocks

One recent theory has proposed that as human beings evolved into using a face-to-face position in intercourse, women's breasts grew larger and rounder to replace the twin globes of her buttocks as a sexual lure. This may be only anthropological speculation, but the sexual function of the buttocks (the rump of animals) is undeniable. Almost all male animals approach and mount the female from the rear. The persistence of the hourglass shape as an ideal woman's figure suggests the strong sexual power not only of the breasts but of the buttocks as well among human beings since antiquity. Clothing from bustles to bikinis has served to accentuate the appeal of the buttocks.

The buttocks are a sexual feature of both women and men, which seems to clarify and confuse their function. Much of the enjoyment of anal sex, which is practiced by heterosexuals and homosexuals alike, is undoubtedly provided by the visual and tactile stimulation of the buttocks. The confusion of gender may add to the excitement for some people, but the simpler truth is that the anus and buttocks are an extremely sensitive area for everyone.

THE ORGASM

Our present knowledge of human sexual orgasm comes largely from the excellent and extensive research carried out by Masters and Johnson during the past two decades. These two pioneers investigated the physiological functions of orgasm in more than six hundred women and men from eighteen to ninety years of age.

Masters and Johnson divided the orgasm response into four phases: the excitement, the plateau, the orgasm, and the resolution.

The Excitement Phase

This is the initial phase of sexual response, characterized in the woman by vaginal and clitoral response. Lubrication or wetness and enlargement of the vaginal lips occur within thirty seconds after the initiation of any form of effective physical and/or psychological stimulation. This stimulation can be caused by anything from erotic

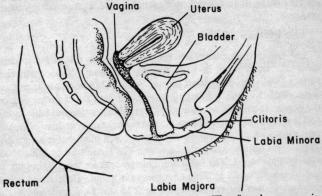

Fig. 21–1: Female Pelvis: Normal Phase. The female organs in cross-section, in a normal resting phase before sexual stimulation. The uterus is in the anteverted position. The vagina is relaxed.

fantasies to direct sexual contact. In some, but not all, women, there is an increase in the size and hardness of the clitoris. These changes are partly caused by vasoconstriction (a narrowing of the blood vessels), which holds blood in the vulvar area.

Blood continues to be pumped into the vulvar area and causes a swelling of the vulva and the lower part of the vagina. There is also an enlargement and lengthening of the upper part of the vagina. Uterine contractions increase. All these changes enable easier penetration, since the vagina is now opened, softer, wetter, and lengthened to accommodate a fully erect penis. These changes take place even in women who have had hysterectomies, in women after menopause, and in women with artificial vaginas. There is also often a noticeable increase in the size of the nipples as the breasts become aroused in this first phase.

The initial physiological response to sexual stimulation in a man is the erection. Younger men can achieve an erection from fantasy or other indirect causes, while older men need more direct stimulation, such as masturbation or oral sex. Blood is pumped into the penis and held there by vasoconstriction, and the penis erects as it fills with blood. At this time, the man's scrotum contracts and elevates. There is an increase in his heart rate and breathing, which also occurs in women. Although direct manipulation can make a man's nipples harden, there is no consistent breast response in men during intercourse.

The Plateau Phase

The bodily changes already begun continue in this phase to their most advanced state in both women and men. Vasoconstriction further swells the outer third of the vagina. This results in increased wetness of the labia, allowing easier penetration and a firmer grip on the penis. The upper two thirds of the vagina continue to balloon out and lengthen. The uterus elevates, and contractions occur with greater frequency, which the woman experiences as a pleasurable sensation. The clitoris retracts and rotates upward. The significance of this is not clearly understood. The labia will change in color from light pink to red to deep purple as they engorge with blood. Heightened blood pressure causes the vessels on the neck to stand out noticeably. The breasts continue to swell, becoming largest immediately prior to orgasm. The areolas around the nipples also swell so that the nipples appear to retract. Breathing pattern and blood pressure increases in both women and men.

During the plateau phase in men, the erection is complete and the penis extended to its maximum size. The testes are elevated and engorged with blood and about 50 percent larger than in their resting state. A few drops of clear fluid, probably expelled as a lubricant by the Cowper's gland, may appear on the head of the penis. There may be some darkening in color of the penis corresponding to the darkening of the vaginal labia. The pupils dilate and the nostrils flare in both sexes. Lightheadedness frequently occurs in both partners during this phase.

The Orgasm Phase

The characteristics of orgasm are identical in all women and are always triggered by direct or indirect stimulation of the clitoris. The variety of ways this may be achieved probably explains the different abilities to reach orgasm in various women. The uterus rises and regular contractions occur every 0.8 second, which is the same rhythmic frequency as the ejaculations of the man's orgasm. These contractions may create a suction in the vagina, and a woman may feel air being drawn into her during this phase. The woman's anal sphincter tightens. Her toes curl, as do the man's. In women just prior to or after childbirth, there may be a small secretion of milk from the

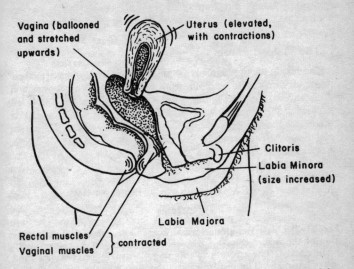

Fig. 21-2: Female Pelvis: Orgasmic Phase. The upper portion of the vagina balloons out during orgasm, and the uterus has risen from its resting position to an upright position. The vaginal muscles which surround the lower portion of the vagina contract, and both the uterus and the vagina have rhythmic contractions occurring every .8 seconds. The labia minora swell and increase in size; the labia majora spread slightly apart. The clitoris rotates and retracts upward and the rectal sphincter muscles contract. During sexual intercourse, a man can usually recognize the orgasmic phase, since the upper part of the vagina usually becomes larger, and he should be able to recognize the squeezing of the lower vagina.

breasts due to their enlarged state at orgasm. Pulse rate and breathing are elevated. The clitoris retracts further under the foreskin. Maximum sensation and intensive pleasure occur at orgasm, which rarely lasts longer than ten or fifteen seconds.

During orgasm, the man ejaculates semen in regular spurts every 0.8 second. These contractions are so strong that semen can be ejaculated a distance of several feet from the penis. The scrotum contracts and the testes elevate. His anal sphincter tightens. Pulse rate and breathing are elevated and blood pressure increases to its highest

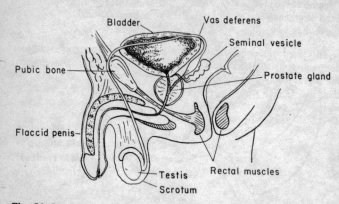

Fig. 21–3: Male Genitals: Normal Phase. The anatomical relationship of the male genitalia is shown, in cross-section, in the normal resting stage. The scrotum in this stage is usually relaxed and the testes hang low. The picture clearly demonstrates the vas deferens, which leads the sperm from the testes to the prostate gland, where both urine and sperm pass through the penis via the urethra.

Fig. 21–4: Male Genitals: Orgasmic Phase. The penis is erect and the muscles of the scrotum are contracting, which lifts the testes during the preorgasmic and orgasmic phase. The rectal muscle is contracted and the urethral bulb dilated.

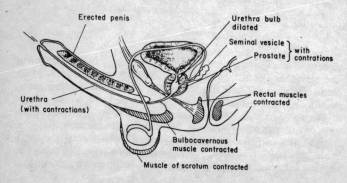

level. There is a necessary interval between orgasms for all men, which is brief in the prime of adolescence and becomes greater as the man ages.

The Resolution Phase

This final phase begins with the fading of the woman's uterine contractions and release of the vasoconstriction, draining blood from the pelvic area. This phase continues until the pelvic organs return to their resting state, and heart rate, breathing, blood pressure, and skin vascularity are again at normal levels. This takes up to a half an hour. The drop in blood pressure initiates a sense of easeful fatigue and relaxation.

Corresponding changes occur in the man. The erection fades, the testes relax, and the bodily rhythms slow until functions return to normal and the man grows drowsy.

COMMON VARIATIONS IN SEXUAL RESPONSE

A significant number of women do not reach orgasm during intercourse. They can reach the plateau phase and are not able to relieve the tension created in their bodies. In many such cases, a woman needs longer or greater or more direct clitoral stimulation. It is not possible for all women to achieve an orgasm by intercourse alone, and masturbation, the use of a vibrator, or other means of additional manipulation of the clitoris might be necessary.

A woman must be frank with her partner if she needs extra or special attention. All too often a woman fakes orgasm rather than suggesting her particular needs, thus depriving herself of the profound delight of a successful orgasm, and depriving her partner as well of the opportunity to enjoy further sex play with her.

Pelvic Congestion

A woman who remains too long in the plateau phase, or who cannot go beyond it to orgasm, often experiences restlessness, the inability to sleep, and severe backaches from pelvic congestion. In the plateau phase, blood is pumped into the vagina and uterus. This causes a swelling (or *edema*) of the pelvic organs—a pelvic congestion. The rhythmic contractions during orgasm, as well as the cessation of the vasoconstriction, relieve tension by pumping the blood out of the pelvic tissues and allowing fresh oxygenated blood to reach the area. When this buildup of fluid, or *edema*, is unrelieved, it creates a physical tension in the body which quickly becomes a psychological tension, too. In many cases of pelvic congestion, researchers have found a woman's uterus can be enlarged to twice its normal size by fluid. Clearly, the woman's body is in a state of stress. A woman may complain of pains, discomfort, or exhaustion and blame it on family, friends, or work, and not realize her tension has this sexual basis. Pelvic congestion is both unpleasant and unhealthy—and it's unnecessary, too, considering the simple remedy, which is orgasm, either through intercourse or masturbation.

Frequent intercourse without orgasm results in a greater incidence and more severe symptoms of pelvic congestion. Because of this, prostitutes are especially vulnerable to this malady.

Multiple Orgasm

Once a woman has achieved one orgasm she has a good chance to enjoy multiple orgasms—a whole series of successive orgasms during a single act of intercourse. For men, as mentioned, the interval in the resolution phase between one arousal and another becomes longer as they age, and many older men are only able to reach one orgasm during a session of sex. A woman, though, does not descend from her orgasm directly into the resolution phase the way a man does. A woman goes to the plateau phase first. So, by continuing stimulation, she can be brought rapidly back to the orgasm phase. This can be repeated many times. Five or six orgasms are common and ten to fifteen are possible. There have been occasional reports regarding women who have reached up to a hundred orgasms. Needless to say, the validity of such reports is difficult to confirm. The ability to achieve multiple orgasms continues in women throughout their lives.

Status Orgasmus

Sadly, there can be too much of a good thing. *Status orgasmus,* or persistent orgasm, is a physiological state caused by rapidly reoccurring orgasms between which there is no relaxation or plateau phase. This results in a sharply increased heart rate (often over 180 beats per minute) and a sharp, cramplike pain in the vagina caused by a lack of relaxation and a lessened supply of oxygen. A woman may feel this painful sensation during prolonged intercourse and think she is being hurt by the size of the man's penis, when in fact her vagina is cramping from status orgasmus.

Can Orgasm Initiate Labor?

Since orgasm involves multiple contractions of the vagina and uterus, it is similar to, and can in fact initiate, labor. Also, the semen ejaculated by the man during intercourse contains hormones called *prostaglandins*, which are known to cause uterine contractions, reinforcing the woman's natural response. Therefore, doctors often tell patients who have a tendency toward premature labor to avoid masturbation and intercourse in the last weeks of pregnancy. On the other hand, midwives in certain countries traditionally urge pregnant women to have sex if their babies are past term, as a way to induce labor.

Does a Hysterectomy Affect Sexual Response?

Many women who undergo hysterectomy at first feel "desexed" by the operation. Many men wrongly think that the penis enters the uterus in intercourse, and that a hysterectomy removes the "pleasure zone" from a woman's body. As has been shown, orgasm depends on the clitoris, not the uterus. Once a woman realizes that her sexual satisfaction is unimpaired by a hysterectomy, she may even discover that her sex life has improved. This is particularly true of women who have experienced uterine problems and are now free of them.

The Grafenberg Spot

Dr. Ernest Grafenberg, a German immigrant gynecologist who in the 1920s developed one of the world's first intrauterine devices called the Grafenberg Ring, made a new discovery in 1950 in which he described an especially sensitive *spot* inside the woman's vagina that, when stroked, evoked an intense orgasmic response in the woman. Grafenberg described the spot being located in the upper front portion of the vagina, right above the pubis bone and the bladder. The Grafenberg spot, often referred to as the "G" spot, has been the cause of debate among sexologists for more than three decades. The reason for this dilemma is that if the "G" spot is a trigger point for orgasm, that means that vaginal orgasm can occur! Several sex researchers have, since Dr. Grafenberg's description of the "G" spot, examined hundreds of women and many of these sexologists agree that when this spot is touched, a strong orgasmic sensation is felt by the woman. The muscle contractions and sensations are so strong that some women have described an intense wetness, almost as if they were ejaculating, when the "G" spot is stimulated. The sexual response is so intense that women initially have an urge to urinate, but after a few seconds of continuous stroking, the sensation changes to a distinct sexual pleasure. The sensitivity of the Grafenberg spot, according to researchers who believe in its existence, is so great that many women will sense strong rhythmic muscle contractions during an insertion of a vaginal speculum. Other women will state that if the penis strokes this area during intercourse, their sexual orgasm is much stronger.

Dr. Alfred Kinsey claims that vaginal orgasms are biologically impossible. Masters and Johnson, however, concluded that clitoral and vaginal orgasm were not separate biological entities. However, several trained sexologists claim that they can easily locate the Grafenberg spot in most women and thus trigger a specific vaginal orgasm.

Many sex therapists are now realizing that by teaching women to locate and stimulate the Grafenberg spot, either by using a vibrator or by teaching her lover to manually stimulate the "G" spot, many women who usually never reach orgasm can now achieve great sexual satisfaction.

Whether or not the Grafenberg spot exists will hopefully be clarified in the next few years by our leading sexologists. Whatever their conclusion, each couple can conduct their own studies and determine if there is an area in the front upper part of the vagina that when stroked causes a deeper, more satisfying "inner orgasm," or if the woman still achieves the greatest satisfaction by clitoral stimulation.

SEX AND APHRODISIACS

Hormones and drugs are agents that act on the chemical balance of the body in many ways, one of which is to influence sexual ability and pleasure.

The so-called sex hormones are secreted by the sexual organs and by the adrenal cortex. Under normal circumstances, men and women will have some amount of hormones of the opposite sex in their bodies. Transsexuals (people who have undergone sex-change operations) are administered a large dose of the hormones of their adopted sex over a period of time in order to complete their conversions, and hormones are regularly used by doctors to treat lesser sexual deficiencies.

Female Hormones—Are They Aphrodisiacs?

The female hormones, *estrogen* and *progesterone,* control the regular menstrual cycle and stimulate the secondary sex characteristics in women. The influence of these hormones on behavior varies from woman to woman.

The first female hormone, estrogen, has some aphrodisiac effect, but not to the extent of the male hormones. Immediately prior to menstruation, when hormone levels are at their highest, most women experience heightened sexual desire and can achieve orgasm more easily. The same effects are reported in women taking birth-control pills containing high amounts of estrogen. After menopause, when the estrogen level decreases, so does sexual desire. At this time, if estrogen replacement is administered, it usually increases desire.

The second female hormone, progesterone, has a lesser aphrodisiac effect and, in some cases, can even inhibit sexual arousal. This has been found true in some women who take the minipill, which contains progesterone alone.

Male Hormones—An Effective Sexual Stimulant

Male hormones, known generically as *androgens*, are the most potent hormonal aphrodisiac for women as well as men. Androgens control the development of the secondary sex characteristics in men and maintain sperm production. They affect appetite and metabolism, as well as behavioral patterns like dominance and vigor. Every woman produces a small amount of male hormones in her ovaries. Women with large or polycystic ovaries produce more, which increases energy and sexual desire, but can cause side effects such as heavy facial-hair growth, low voice register, or more developed muscles. This last characteristic explains the furious controversy in athletics concerning the permissible level of hormone injections given a woman contestant.

It is known that women who, after menopause or after removal of their ovaries, subsequently lose all production of *testosterone* (the most common androgen) will lose some of their sexual drive as well. When women receive hormone replacement treatment after menopause, they're usually better able to reach sexual fulfillment, particularly if they also receive testosterone. Aside from being the strongest aphrodisiac in women, testosterone also strengthens bones and muscles and aids in the ever-constant battle against fatigue.

In men, the androgens again act as aphrodisiacs, and testosterone is employed in the treatment of male impotence.

Drugs and Sex

People use a variety of drugs to enhance their sexual performance or pleasure, from aphrodisiacs considered to have specifically sexual purposes to substances such as marijuana and alcohol, which seem to have a generally more pleasurable effect on all activities. The inclusion of the use of drugs in this chapter is intended to be informative only. It is not the authors' intention to recommend the use of such drugs.

Lovers in every society throughout history have sought the perfect aphrodisiac, a guaranteed stimulus to the sex drive. From *abelmosk*, *burra gokeroo*, and *cubeb peppers* right on through the alphabet to *rhinoceros horn, serpolet*, and *yohimbe*, everything has been tried by someone somewhere, including *strychnine*. Many of these substances do have some sexual effect (including strychnine). They also may have other, unpleasant effects (ditto). Most aphrodisiacs, however, are inert at best. The only boost they generally give the user is a psychological one—but that can be enough, since so many sexual problems are psychological in origin. Other aphrodisiacs produce a state of sexual stimulation by means that are distinctly harmful to the body, such as the most famous aphrodisiac of all, *Spanish fly*.

Spanish fly is not a medicine; it is used solely as an aphrodisiac. It is a toxic substance which causes sexual stimulation by creating an irritation and inflammation of the genitals and bladder. Unfortunately, this irritation and inflammation is as dangerous as it is stimulating, since it can result in permanent damage to the genitalia and kidneys. This damage can even cause death. Today there are many drugs which are being advertised and sold as Spanish fly. Most of them are not Spanish fly but substances such as cayenne pepper, which cause minor urethral irritation and mild sexual irritation. In most instances, these imitations are not dangerous.

As you can see, though, the quest for an ideal love potion should be pursued very carefully. Drugs which are used for an overall "high" will affect people sexually in different ways: What turns you on can turn someone else right off. A person can respond differently at different times to the same drug. A discussion of a number of popular drug substances in terms of their possible sexual effects follows. These drugs are *not* aphrodisiacs, because they are not used for strictly erotic stimulation, but in certain circumstances they may have sex-enhancing properties.

Alcohol

Alcohol is not a stimulant, but a depressant. However, it does not depress all parts of the brain equally and simultaneously. Rather, it produces a specific sequence of effects. First, it depresses the brain center which controls fear, and thus releases anxiety and inhibition. It is at this point that alcohol seems to cause sexual desire. While alcohol in small amounts can have a stimulating effect on both women and men, the borderline between freedom and intoxication is very fine. Higher doses of alcohol depress the brain completely and bring sedation and sleep instead of arousal. Chronic intake of alcohol decreases the hormone level and reduces sexual ability considerably; in men, it often leads to impotence.

Amphetamines

Amphetamines ("speed") are agents which stimulate the central brain. The claims as to the sexual effect of amphetamines vary from person to person. Some people report that amphetamines heighten their sexual desire and performance, and that they have trouble functioning without these agents. Other sources suggest that amphetamine users experience a diminishing of their sexual ability as their dependency grows, until finally they become too ill to have any interest in sex. The danger of amphetamines should be emphasized, since they have a debilitating, addictive effect.

Amyl Nitrite

Amyl nitrite is a *vasodilator* (an agent which opens the blood vessels) sold by prescription to relieve the pain of angina, or heart spasms. It comes in small glass capsules which are broken (or popped open, hence the popular nickname, poppers) and inhaled through the nose. Popped just before orgasm, amyl nitrite causes dilation of the blood vessels in the brain and intensifies all sensations, particularly sexual ones. The increased blood supply causes a hot feeling, which directly heightens erotic sensation for the few minutes the drug is effective. It also relaxes the vaginal and anal openings and permits easier penetration. There are usually no negative side effects from the use of this agent, although it is extremely dangerous for persons with low blood pressure and certain heart conditions. In high or frequent doses, it has caused several deaths.

Barbiturates

The so-called downers (sedatives, sleeping pills, and insomnia tablets) have an effect on sex somewhat similar to that of alcohol. At first and when taken in small amounts, these agents relax inhibitions for about an hour. During this time, sexual interest increases while a generally mellow feeling occurs. After a while, the entire body is relaxed—sexual desire diminishes, and sleep, or at least fatigue, comes. Another type of downer, chemically unrelated to barbiturates, is *methaqualone,* commonly available by prescription as Quaalude. Although many people have found that this drug can stimulate sexual desire and prolong intercourse, its long-term effects are similar to those of barbiturates. Addiction to downers of any form is not unusual, and chronic abuse is harmful to sexual functioning. Cases of death from downers mostly involve a combination of excessive drug use and alcohol intake.

Cocaine

Cocaine, a derivative of the coca shrub of South America and once the effective ingredient in Coca-Cola, is today the prestige item of the drug elite, no doubt in part because of its extremely high price. (Its use is, however, illegal in the United States.) Cocaine comes in the form of a white powder which is "snorted," or sniffed, up the nose; the more fashionable coke users snort the ingredient from miniature spoons—gold or silver—which have become a symbol of the user's membership in the drug community.

Cocaine has a vasoconstricting effect and is said to get rid of a cold in no time. The drug is not always effective as an aphrodisiac, but when it is, it stimulates the higher brain centers, the nervous system, and the musculature, giving a feeling of enormous energy (a "rush") which the user may wish to express sexually. A couple using cocaine can enjoy much prolonged intercourse. Cocaine may also be used as a surface anesthetic, applied to the head of the penis or clitoris, to decrease sensation (sometimes preventing premature ejaculation) and permit longer and more varied sexual activity. Chronic use of cocaine is not addicting, but can lead to psychological dependence, and will certainly damage the mucous membranes and olfactory nerves in the nose. There is also increasing evidence of other damaging side effects from cocaine and its use is not recommended.

Heroin and Methadone

Heroin users report that in the beginning, they experience exquisite sensation during intercourse. As they become hooked on the drug, however, they develop other needs, mainly the need to find enough money to support their habits. At first, heroin produces a "high." Later, an addict must continue and increase the dosage just to feel normal. If this is impossible, the addict will be subjected to debilitating physical anguish. Methadone, which is administered to heroin addicts as a replacement drug on the way to complete withdrawal, usually decreases sexual appetite in men. For this reason, many heroin addicts are reluctant to enter methadone programs. Women who take methadone do not report this sexual decline.

LSD

The effects of LSD vary tremendously from person to person and from experience to experience. LSD is a hallucinogen which has a centrally stimulating effect, and in erotic circumstances sexual activity can be, literally, fantastically enhanced; the user's experience becomes not simply more intense but of a different quality—a cataclysmic, cosmic, spiritual coupling. In less successful situations, this chemical substance can produce an equally cataclysmic feeling of terror, paranoia, and hysteria—the typical "bad trip." The after effects can be so horrendous, that the use of LSD should be condemned.

Marijuana

Marijuana is the dried flowers and leaves of the cannabis plant, from which is also derived the similar, but more potent, drug —hashish. Marijuana is a mild psychedelic with some history as a sex stimulant (aphrodisiac sweetmeats are made in India from cannabis seeds, musk, and honey). The drug combines the freedom from inhibition that alcohol offers with the exciting properties of amphetamines. While some users feel more sensuous, erotic, and aroused after smoking or eating marijuana, others feel no sexual enhancement or sometimes even a depression of sexual interest. Many studies of this substance have been prejudiced by official disapproval of marijuana, so scientific findings about its true effects are contradictory at best, and often useless. It seems to increase sexual enjoyment in most users, but this may well depend on prevailing psychological factors at the time it is used.

Tobacco

It is well known that smoking cigarettes will increase the risk of lung cancer, heart trouble, stomach ulcers, and other diseases. There have recently been further findings that smoking tobacco reduces sexual desire, probably because tobacco is a vasoconstricting agent and decreases the amount of blood reaching the sex center in the brain. Some smokers claim that after they stopped smoking they have noticed, among other benefits, a greater sexual arousal.

WHAT ARE THE BEST APHRODISIACS?

Nothing can replace, or be more effective, than the natural aphrodisiacs: health, happiness, love, and caring.

Love and Caring

One of the nicest ways to express love and caring is to approach them honestly. Unfortunately, this approach is often lost in modern society, where many feelings are measured only by the frequency and quality of intercourse. Intercourse (a longer discussion of which follows) is great—it is healthy and fun. But it is not the total expression of love.

Touching, for instance, is always a beautiful and effective means of expressing feelings. It can surpass intercourse in its emotional, if not physical, intimacy. An affectionate hug or a kiss on the cheek can be just as pleasing as intercourse—often more so. Too often, couples feel they must jump directly into bed and perform sexually dizzying feats to express their affection. This should not be so.

People should understand each other, should be open to each other, and should care for each other in all aspects of life—not just intercourse. By doing this, each partner can discover the most satisfying way of expressing his or her love at any given moment —whether it is a soft caress, a gentle word, or imaginative intercourse. Orgasm is not the best response; loving is, however it is attained.

Imagination

The more love and caring there is in a relationship, the freer each partner becomes. Each can discuss her or his individual responses to different stimulants, fantasies, or sexual techniques. This openness frees the imagination and better sex and a closer relationship result.

THE POSITIONS

For many couples, sex has become all too routine, with intercourse occurring at the same time of day or night and always in the same position. Here, freedom and imagination can certainly enhance the couple's sex life by breaking the monotony.

There are literally hundreds of positions for sexual intercourse. One new publication described a different position for each of the 365 days of the year. This might be a little too much variety for the average couple, but it is useful information because it provokes the imagination. It is easy for a couple to fall into a particular pattern of sexual behavior which might once have been exciting, but which over a period of time becomes dull. Their sexual pleasure fades, perhaps so slowly that they are unaware of it. They think this eventually happens to every couple, or perhaps they are too embarrassed to talk about it. What is important is not how many positions you regularly use in intercourse, but how willing you are to experiment.

However many positions there are, most couples will usually find a few that they most enjoy at any one time. They may have sex simply in a single position, or sample several positions before orgasm. There are plenty of illustrated sex manuals around that you can use to get ideas for new positions. First and most important, though, use your imagination.

The Missionary Position

There's nothing wrong with the good old missionary position (face to face, male superior); in fact, it has a lot to recommend it. Lying together this way, a couple has intimate visual contact. They can kiss and touch each other easily. They can speak directly to each other. This position offers many variations—the woman can squeeze her legs together or put them on his shoulders or around his waist. Despite its advantages, though, it need not be the only mode of lovemaking.

The Female Superior Position

As a woman's pleasure mounts, she may prefer to change places with the man and take the superior position. The woman, kneeling on top, positions herself and moves her body as she wishes to bring herself the most fulfilling sensation. By bending forward slightly, she can increase the direct stimulation of her clitoris for more intense pleasure; by sitting back she can moderate the stimulation and prolong the act of intercourse. The woman can control how much she is penetrated by the man's penis. She has the freedom to move up and down or circularly on the penis, at her own rate, at the angle she wants. For the same reasons, sex therapists often recommend this position to women whose partners are impotent or ejaculate prematurely.

The Sitting Position

Sex in a sitting position has many variables. A woman can either sit on top of the man, facing him in the riding position, or she can place her feet or knees on either side of the man, and her arms around his shoulders, giving her great freedom of movement in the squatting or kneeling position. The couple face each other, so all visual and psychological stimulations are in play. In either of these positions, the woman's back can be toward the man. This allows greater freedom of movement, but less visual contact. She can use the arms of a chair to push herself up and down.

A woman can also be penetrated by the man while she is in a sitting position—either in a chair or on the edge of a bed. The man can penetrate by kneeling on the floor when her knees are bent, sometimes even extending her legs over his shoulders. This last position favors deeper and harder thrusts since the man can balance his power by grasping the back of the chair.

Of course, what you sit on is important, too. A sofa is good, so is a small chair without arms—anything that allows a natural position for the woman and supports the man upright. Armchairs are generally unsuccessful for women unless the arms are low and padded, to reduce the pressure on the woman's legs, or so wide that the woman can keep her knees inside the arms. If a chair is placed in front of a mirror the woman may wish to sit facing away from the man so that both partners can see each other in the mirror.

The Kneeling Position

A kneeling position, with the man entering the woman's vagina from the rear, brings the woman's buttocks into view as a sexual stimulant to the man. This position allows the man to drive into the woman with some force, which may be an exciting mode of indirect stimulation to her clitoris. If still greater stimulation is desired by the woman, she can kneel against one or two pillows and her clitoris will be rubbed against them by the man's thrusts. In this position, the woman can reach between her legs and touch the man's scrotum to excite him.

The Standing Position

Some difficulty may occur with standing intercourse, since the man is often taller than the woman and must crouch slightly to enter her. The woman can assist by raising one leg and placing it around the man, thus changing the angle of her vagina and making it more accessible. Or the man may lift her off the floor by her thighs and move her on his penis as she holds him around the neck. This variation is fairly strenuous for both partners and is usually of short duration. If this becomes too strenuous, he can rest the woman on an edge of a table, continuing his standing position. When a woman is wearing shoes or boots—which excites many men—she will minimize the difference of height. This is especially true if she turns and bends over to be entered from the rear, a standing position which is most comfortable for both partners. In order to keep her balance, it may be necessary for the woman to rest her arms or upper part of her body on a table, counter, or chair. As with the similar kneeling position of rear entry, the woman can easily reach the man's scrotum and arouse him by gently fondling it.

Is There an Ideal Position?

The main problem with most positions in sexual intercourse is that the woman's clitoris is located high up in front of her vagina and therefore usually receives only indirect stimulation. This affects the amount of time it takes her to achieve orgasm. A more rapid, explosive orgasm can be achieved if the woman receives direct clitoral stimulation. Some sex researchers have suggested that the "ideal position" might be with the woman sitting on top of the man, but facing away from him. This allows her all the pleasureful freedom of the female superior position, combined with the ability to rub her clitoris on the back of the shaft of the man's penis, stimulating sensitive areas on both herself and the man. Furthermore, this position brings together the woman's vagina and the man's penis at the most natural and comfortable angle for both. The drawback in this and all positions in which the woman faces away from the man is the loss of visual contact and exchange of expressions.

There can be many variations on these basic positions, of course. It is not possible in this brief space to mention them all, nor to suggest that they are all necessary to a happy sexual relationship. A couple ought to feel open and adventurous enough with each other to try anything. But at the same time, they ought to feel equally free to be simple in their tastes and enjoy sex in as unsophisticated a way as they want. Variety is the spice of sex life, but simple, honest enjoyment is the meat and potatoes.

ORAL SEX

Cunnilingus, the oral stimulation of the vulva and vagina, and *fellatio,* the oral stimulation of the penis, are the main features of oral sex. It has been illustrated on pottery and described in poetry from the earliest known human societies, and appears in every culture on earth, from the most advanced to the most primitive. Only in Western, Judeo-Christian societies has oral sex been viewed with hostility and taboo. This has resulted in many people remaining ignorant of and superstitious about it. Oral sex occurs commonly in animals, birds, and reptiles, yet human beings often suffer guilty insecurity if they practice it and certainly lose a source of tremendous pleasure if they avoid it. Emotional conflicts about oral sex can create pain and stress in individuals of any age, seriously undermining a sexual relationship and bringing problems to a marriage.

The Kinsey Report sex researchers have confirmed that the higher a person's level of education, the more likely she or he is to perform and enjoy oral sex. This itself is a perfect example of the gain in pleasure from good sex education. Americans are becoming a highly educated people, and there is a new sexual frankness in today's society. No doubt oral sex occurs in well over 70 percent of the college-educated population—and this in spite of the prevalent legal penalties against it. More and more people are learning that oral sex is neither dirty nor unnatural, but rather a delightfully different and completely normal means of sexual enjoyment.

Technique of Oral Sex

The mouth is delicate, soft, flexible, and extremely sensitive—a perfect sexual organ. A very precise, subtle type of stimulation which is unavailable any other way can be achieved in oral sex. Most women enjoy having their vaginas licked and penetrated by their lovers' lips and tongues. Often, the lover separates or pulls the labia apart in order to gain greater access to the clitoris and, thereby, increases stimulation. Most women will be highly excited by having their clitorises caressed, although this degree of direct stimulation can prove too intense for some women. Sometimes during cunnilingus, a partner will feel like blowing into the woman's vagina to stimulate it: *This is extremely dangerous!* The pressure caused in the vagina can drive air bubbles into the blood stream, and there have been cases of women dying of embolism as a result.

Since the anus is an extremely sensitive area, many couples enjoy stimulating it by oral means *(analingus)*. As long as each partner is clean, this is not harmful. Lovers should be careful, though, to wash thoroughly before engaging in this practice.

Most men enjoy having their penises kissed, licked, and sucked, and many enjoy having their scrotums orally stimulated as well.

During this form of sex play, a man enjoys the wetness of his lover's mouth. For this reason, many women take extra care to lubricate the penis with a large amount of saliva. If a woman's mouth gets too dry, she can fill her mouth with lukewarm water and release it around the penis while it is in her mouth. Although a complete *Deep Throat* technique is unnecessary, most men enjoy a fairly deep penetration in the mouth. At the same time, most men do not like to feel a woman's teeth, however lightly, during fellatio. In extreme cases, this can develop into a psychological condition of fear known as *vagina dentata*, or "teeth in the vagina," which is common in the folklore of many countries. Some men are unable to ejaculate in a woman's mouth. This may be due to a psychological factor; at other times, it is caused by insufficient friction. This problem can be aided by either partner manually stroking the base of the penis during fellatio.

Gourmet Sex

The pleasure of oral sex has recently been aided by the availability of such accessories as flavored douches, sex creams and oils, edible body powders, and the like. Many people enjoy covering their genitals with these products and having their partner "eat" them. Any imaginative couple can easily discover other suitable substances for themselves.

Variations of Oral Sex

Oral sex may be a part of foreplay, as a prelude to intercourse. A woman and man may engage in it mutually, each partner both giving and receiving simultaneously, or by turns. A woman may perform fellatio on a man and bring him to orgasm so that he can then enter into the prolonged act of intercourse which she requires. In a similar way, a man may perform cunnilingus on a woman and bring her to one or more orgasms before finally entering her so that they can enjoy an ultimate orgasm together.

When oral sex is continued to orgasm, it is usually performed by one member of the couple on the other, because the extreme excitement of the orgasm makes mutual stimulation difficult. Unlike intercourse, oral sex allows the two distinct sexual pleasures of giving and receiving to be individually savored to the fullest.

Is Oral Sex Unhealthy?

A great deal of the difficulty that people have in accepting and practicing oral sex comes from the vague notion that it is in some way dirty. This attitude is based on the common confusion of the reproductive and excretory functions of the genitals—functions which are totally independent of each other. Assuming that both partners maintain basic bodily hygiene, there is no reason why the genitals should be unpleasant either to the taste or the smell.

The internal situation of the vagina makes it more susceptible to odor, but if the vagina is in a clean and healthy condition, this odor will be minimal, and not distasteful or harmful. By now, most women are probably aware that the various vaginal deodorant sprays on the market, which capitalize on the hostility of Western societies to any natural smells, can be unsafe to use. Vaginal deodorant sprays commonly cause irritation, which develops into severe inflammation. If a woman is worried about vaginal odor, she would be well advised to use soap rather than the available sprays (which only mask odor, but do not remove it). The European bathroom fixture called a bidet is specifically designed for genital cleansing and is a much more medically sound answer to the problem. Men who are still uncertain about performing cunnilingus would do well to realize that the bacterial content of their own mouths is generally considerably higher than that of a normal woman's vagina. The danger of infection is probably greater for the woman. So instead of asking a woman to use a vaginal deodorant for his sake, a man would usually be better off using a mouthwash for her sake.

A woman, for her part, may worry about taking a man's semen in her mouth and swallowing it. She may think that this fluid is unclean and harmful to her. In fact, the chemical composition of semen is similar to that of saliva in the mouth. Rather than being harmful, semen is an extremely high-protein, low-calorie substance. The protein content in semen is 30 percent higher than the protein content in cow's milk, for example, while the fat and sugar content of semen are both one ninth as great as in milk.

Oral Sex and VD

Only under special circumstances can oral sex transmit venereal disease. There must be fresh syphilitic sores in or around the mouth for the germs to spread—a condition which is sure to be visible to the sex partner. Gonorrhea cannot survive long in the mouth, but it can survive deep in the throat, so it can be transmitted or contracted during oral sex. In certain rare instances, gonorrhea can spread to the eyes, if the eye comes into close contact with an already infected area. In general, though, oral sex is very unlikely to lead to any kind of infection or disease. It is most likely to result in pleasure.

ANAL SEX

The area around the anus is an important erogenous zone, stimulating to both women and men. A woman often enjoys having a man put his finger in her anus during intercourse and especially just before her orgasm, so that she is twice penetrated. Many men, likewise, enjoy having a woman do this to them. Naturally, a woman with very long fingernails must proceed carefully. A vibrator is also excellent for this purpose.

A couple may start with frequent manual penetration of each other's anuses and decide to try anal intercourse. If a woman has never had anal intercourse before, it will probably be difficult for her to accommodate a man's penis at first. Oral and manual stimulation of the anus before intercourse will help to relax the anal sphincter. Using some lubricant such as K-Y, Vaseline, baby oil, or cold cream, the man should begin to dilate the woman's anus, first with one finger, then two, then three. This is a time for slow, gentle arousal. If the woman is not properly prepared, anal intercourse will be painful. When the woman feels excited and ready, the man can start to enter her gradually with his penis. He should not thrust or move quickly. Both his penis and her anus should be well lubricated. The woman should bear down slightly on her anus to relax it and facilitate initial penetration. Men who enjoy anal intercourse usually like the tight squeeze of the anus around their penises. This tightness also makes penetration more difficult, so the man must not go too quickly, nor penetrate too deeply. He must allow the woman to guide him.

There is, unfortunately, a certain amount of hypocrisy associated with almost all sexual practices and mores. So it is, too, with anal sex. In many religions and societies, anal intercourse is frequently performed just to safeguard the exalted virginity of the women. Since pregnancy is impossible during this practice, some couples use it as a form of birth control. In some societies, anal sex is illegal and referred to as *sodomy*.

Can a Woman Reach Orgasm through Anal Intercourse?

A few women can reach orgasm during anal intercourse, probably as a result of the pulling on the perineum, which is transmitted to the clitoris. Many women do not achieve orgasm, but do enjoy the sensation of anal intercourse. Some women, even after careful, slow arousal and dilation of their anuses, will still experience such pain from anal intercourse that it is not of interest to them. If a woman wishes to try this sexual practice, or has tried it and liked it, she ought to be frank about her desire with her sex partner. If she has tried anal intercourse and found it generally unpleasant, she ought to be equally open about refusing it.

WARNING!

There is one common danger in anal intercourse. If a couple wants to combine both anal and vaginal intercourse, it is important for the man to take the time to wash his penis after he removes it from the woman's anus and before he enters her vagina. The chance of vaginal infection is high if vaginal penetration immediately follows anal, because the *E. coli* bacteria which predominate in the anus will be transferred to the vagina. A man and woman may be reluctant to interrupt their sex play for so mundane a task as hygiene, but the woman must remember that she may pay for her impatience later.

MASTURBATION

For generations and generations, the act of masturbation has been used to scare people. People were told that if they played with their genitals, they would grow hair on the palms of their hands, go blind, grow up crippled or malformed, or eventually go insane. By now, it is hoped that everyone knows the truth, which is that all these horror stories are only repressive scare tactics. Scientific study has long since proven that masturbation is not harmful to any individual in any way.

Sexual responsiveness develops at different rates in different people. Girls are less likely to masturbate than boys, but very young children of both sexes do touch their genitals and masturbate regularly. Many women do not begin to masturbate until they are middle-aged.

Masturbation techniques have been studied in sex clinics, and it has been found that no two women masturbate in the same way. The majority of women do not like to masturbate on the glans of their clitorises, because the concentration of nerve endings is so high that touch can be painful. Women usually masturbate by touching the surrounding area, a gentler stimulation to the clitoris. If a woman masturbates for a long time, she will want to keep her vagina moist with saliva or some other lubricant, such as vaginal secretions. Some women touch their nipples as well during masturbation. This increases the amount and variety of stimulation, and brings a more total sexual experience.

Masturbation and Orgasm

A high percentage of women are able to achieve multiple orgasm by masturbation. Many women bring themselves to three or four orgasms before they feel completely satisfied. The majority of women are multiorgasmic generally, and much more so during masturbation. Some women are happy with a single orgasm; others will continue up to seven or eight or more orgasms until they are exhausted.

Women who have difficulty concentrating on masturbation enough to reach an orgasm should try to fantasize some erotic situation to heighten their excitement. Women usually need to fantasize during masturbation, especially at first. A woman may need to masturbate for an extended period of time before relaxing enough to have an orgasm. Fantasy speeds up the process by creating a more complete sexual situation.

Every woman is capable of achieving orgasm through masturbation. In some difficult cases, a woman must first familiarize herself with a masturbation technique and liberate herself from guilt and other hang-ups. She must be relaxed; she must be *alone*. Initially, she may have to masturbate an hour a day for several weeks before reaching orgasm. Once the first orgasm has been reached, each subsequent orgasm is easier to achieve. If manual masturbation becomes too strenuous, a vibrator can certainly help.

Placing a mirror between her legs allows a woman to watch her masturbation, and this added visual sensation often proves exciting.

Is Masturbation Addictive?

Many women are concerned about masturbation, wondering if it is addictive or if it robs them of the enjoyment of other sexual pleasures. Masturbation is addictive, but in the same way that breathing is habit forming. It is not harmful and it does not prevent you from enjoying any other sexual pleasures. On the contrary, masturbation conditions you in such a way that you more greatly appreciate all other sexual activities.

Masturbation is the ideal solution to the sexual tension of a woman who is alone for any reason—traveling, divorced, isolated. Furthermore, any woman who is familiar enough with her own body to understand exactly what pleases her will also be a more open, responsive sex partner. Masturbation does not have to be practiced alone. Many couples enjoy masturbating themselves and each other, either as a part of sexual foreplay or before continuing to mutual orgasm.

Masturbation presents no problem to the older woman. Women who have begun masturbating in their twenties and thirties usually continue to do so throughout their lives. Older women who are widowed may then begin to practice masturbation, or may return to it after abstaining during marriage.

FANTASIES AND FANCIES

If the sexiest part of a woman is her mind, then the role of imagination in sex is central. One of the biggest sexual stimulants of all is fantasy. People fantasize about making love to people they desire, either people who are known to them or utter strangers. The object of one's fantasy can be a person who is a part of one's everyday life or the misty vision of a favorite movie star. Some people fantasize about watching sexual intercourse, usually between their own sex partners and someone else. Others fantasize that they and their accustomed sex partners are meeting each other as strangers for the first time, or that they are both different people, or in a new location, and so on.

A woman may fantasize while she is alone, masturbating, or while she is having intercourse with a man. She may prefer to keep her fantasies private. Some people can live for years in a world of complete sexual fantasy, and have intercourse with their partners only as a mechanical act. To this degree, fantasizing is certainly destructive to a couple's relationship, because it is being used to substitute or conceal the fact that there is some sexual difficulty. The most successful and enjoyable fantasies are those that are shared.

A couple can use their imaginations in as simple or complex a fashion as they desire. Their fantasies may be unique or regularly continuing, habitual or experimental, consisting of nothing more than a mutually arousing verbal exchange in bed or ranging to epic, costumed dramas.

Telephone Sex

Mutual arousal over the telephone is practiced by couples who are temporarily separated from each other as a means to relieve their sexual tension and can be a perfectly pleasurable experience. Telephone sex is itself a variation of sex talk in general, which many couples enjoy. Sex talk, in bed or over the telephone, can range from tender to coarse, from elegant to vulgar. Two people who are both open about sex can usually improvise a telephone conversation in sex talk that will be exciting enough to bring each other to orgasm with or without simultaneous masturbation.

Sex in Airplanes

Many people feel sexually aroused when they take off in an airplane. The fact is that a person usually becomes more sexually stimulated as the oxygen supply to the brain decreases. This fact has been a part of sexual knowledge for centuries, practiced by heterosexuals and homosexuals alike. Thus, during intercourse, one partner will press forcibly against the arteries of the neck of the other, closing the amount of oxygen-carrying blood to the brain and bringing heightened arousal. People are sometimes strangled to death in the excitement of intercourse by improvised nooses intended for this purpose. The pressure change in the passenger cabin of an airplane produces the same effect.

Underwater Sex

The idea of underwater sex is delightful. The smooth, slippery feel of skin in water, the stimulating coolness of the liquid, and perhaps the setting—a sun-baked ocean beach or a floodlit swimming pool at night. A whirlpool bath offers still another level of sensation, the lovers' bodies being stroked by the swirling water. Whirlpool also offers a pleasant sensation when the genitals are placed in front of the constantly flowing hot-water stream. A soap massage is a pleasant addition to bathtub sex. A hand shower can provide a woman with enough stimulation for many orgasms all by itself.

In reality, though, sexual intercourse underwater is often unsuccessful. Water washes away the very vaginal secretions which serve as lubrication for the man's penis, leaving the vagina dry and tight. This makes penetration by the man more difficult, which in turn is painful to the woman. If, however, the couple is extremely aroused and the man's entry is quick, the water can be an exciting sexual playground.

Vibrators

Women who have difficulty achieving orgasm in intercourse often find that the purchase of a vibrator revolutionizes their lives. A vibrator may be used as an aid to masturbation or as a part of a couple's sex play. Indeed, a vibrator seems to excite both the man who is using it and the woman who is feeling it; to a couple it can be as much a novelty as a new sex position. Also, a woman can use a vibrator to keep herself aroused while the man rests between orgasms.

Vibrators come in many sizes, but one basic shape, which is like a penis. Some women tend to use a vibrator mainly for clitoral stimulation. Most avoid direct contact with the clitoris, choosing instead to place a towel or some other light fabric, like panties, over the clitoris to avoid burning. Other women use the vibrator for deep vaginal penetration, like a dildo. A lubricated vibrator may be used to penetrate a woman anally while she is having vaginal intercourse; the vibrating sensation is in this case felt throughout the pelvic area. A newly marketed vibrator has two extensions for simultaneous penetration of the vagina and anus.

While vibrators have become very popular with women today, artificial penises (dildos) seem to have little appeal. Even among lesbians, manual or oral stimulation is preferred to intercourse with one of these devices. A vibrator does the same, and better.

Medically speaking, vibrators are neither dangerous nor harmful. They are no more or less addicting than manual masturbation.

Gadgets

Artificial vaginas are as available to men in sex shops and by mail order as artificial penises are to women, and the response is about the same. Although a few men buy them, most do not. Younger men may be curious about the various artificial vaginas [from simple soft rubber sheaths to complex suction devices like milking machines]. Most older men prefer massage parlors or prostitutes as a sexual outlet.

A *penis ring* is a rubber or metal band which is placed around the erect penis. By preventing the blood from leaving the penis, it maintains a hard erection as long as it is worn. Certain of these devices have attached rubber knobs which rub against the woman's clitoris during intercourse, giving her extra stimulation which may be either exciting or painful, depending on the woman. The newest-developed penis ring has a miniature vibrator with a battery attachment. This supposedly stimulates both the penis and the clitoris.

Metal penis rings can be extremely dangerous for the man, since the penis can become so swollen that the band can only be removed surgically. The rubber and leather rings are therefore safest. In fact, a simple rubber band can do the job. It's important not to leave a penis ring on more than an hour, since prolonged use can cause damage to the penis. It does not make the penis permanently longer, although the size of the penis may be temporarily increased while a penis ring is worn.

Many sex gadgets are bought for fun as novelty items. People may buy one, take it home, and put it in a drawer, but they'll remember the fun they had buying it. Anything that adds extra enjoyment to one's sex life is welcome. Sex gadgets make provocative presents. But it isn't necessary to visit a sex shop to find sex gadgets, because everyday life is full of possibilities.

As mentioned, certain women find a hand shower attachment to be far more exciting than a vibrator. A woman may lie under a running bathtub faucet and let the water pounding her clitoris bring her to orgasm. Hair dryers and hot combs project a firm jet of hot air which, when trained on the clitoris, arouses some women. Care must be taken in this situation to avoid burning, irritating, or excessively drying the vaginal labia. Many women enjoy masturbating or being penetrated with a bottle, its size and coolness being stimulating. Because the vagina and uterus enlarge as a woman is aroused, there is a suction in the vagina which can draw up smaller items and even beer bottles. If this happens, a woman must have a doctor remove the object before it causes permanent damage. Thus a woman and her partner must be extremely cautious when engaging in such sex play.

With sex gadgets, as with sexual activity in general, the important thing to remember is that there is no perfect way to reach orgasm. There is a vast number of slightly imperfect, giddily exciting ways. Mix them up, and vary your pleasure. There's a lot to choose from.

Group Sex

At one time or another, most people think about group sex. Sex counselors and psychologists are split between those who advocate experimentation with group sex and those who are against it. Since a good sexual relationship is a difficult thing to achieve between even two people, it is still more precarious when a number of people are involved. Obviously, then, the success of a group-sex venture depends on the people.

The essential rule is that no one should be forced to participate. If a couple engages in this activity, it must be at the desire of both partners. The woman and man should consider and discuss how each feels about having sex with others, about watching each other having sex, and about being watched. Reactions should be honest. Although group sex is considered very hip in certain circles, it simply may not appeal to some people.

Once a couple decides to try a sexual experience involving other people, they must consider carefully whom they will choose. Generally, group sex with old friends is difficult, since sexual and social sides develop at a different rate. It's advisable to find new people with whom you can begin a fresh relationship that is both sexual and social. Compatibility is important. Everyone must feel relaxed and comfortable with everyone else. It's better to wait and choose well than to rush into an unpleasant, tense experience.

In a culture still shaped by Puritan tradition, "swingers" (people who enjoy sex with two or more couples) are a threatening subculture with a shared secret. They seek out like-minded people, sometimes sight unseen through advertisements in sex newspapers and magazines. They frequent bars known as swingers' meeting places. Certain sex-therapy centers promote group sex sessions among their patients. All of these situations have the potential for success or failure.

Group sex is a rather epic way to live out a common sexual fantasy. If all the participants possess the two important characteristics of healthy sexuality—that is, openness and imagination—then the reality can be even better than the fantasy.

Threesomes

The simplest form of group sex is the threesome; either two men and one woman, or two women and one man. Given the different orgasmic abilities of women and men, the man with two women may find himself unable to satisfy them continuously, while the woman with two men is likely to satisfy her desire for several orgasms as she alternately fulfills the men. This can be an enormously stimulating experience for a woman. A man with two women will often employ a vibrator on one as he enters the other, in order to keep them both aroused. In many cases, two women will engage in mutual fondling and, perhaps, masturbation while the man rests.

Swinging

In its ordinary usage, the term *swinging* refers to sex between two or more couples. Each person has a partner, which reduces the potential for jealousy, which can be a major problem in threesomes. Each couple will probably engage in sex at their own pace. Sometimes they may combine in larger groups. Couples may be in separate rooms, or all together so that they can watch each other. When a large number of couples are together, spontaneity seems to increase. Some people will be having a lot of sex with a lot of people, some will be having a lot with one person, some will be having a little sex with everybody. You do as you please. It's perfectly all right to refuse, and no hard feelings. It's perfectly all right to *be* refused. In large gatherings, sex may be going on only in one area, with couples joining and leaving continuously; elsewhere people might be conversing, dancing, or whatever. In smaller groups of two or three couples, sex is more intimate and intense, each person being more aware of each of the others. The impersonality of large groups will be exciting to some people; the intimacy of small groups will please others.

Orgies

A session of swinging can be a pleasant, straightforward, shared sexual experience. An orgy, on the other hand, is a frantic, anything-goes situation. There will be lesbian, homosexual, and heterosexual activities, often involving everyone present with or without their consent. A woman having intercourse with a man may find him replaced by another woman with a dildo; a man may find himself fellated by a woman and man in turn. Participation is obligatory, on every level.

Orgies are a much more casual, haphazard sexual environment than swing parties. Swingers tend to gather in homogeneous groups. An orgy involves people of all backgrounds. People rarely know each other at all. The sexual pressure is greater, and it is difficult to refuse anything with anyone. Therefore, there is a very real chance of contracting venereal disease of some kind at an orgy. This is the main physical danger of all group sex experiences, but in the more selective situations of threesomes or swinging, the chance of venereal disease is far less.

Voyeurism and Exhibitionism

With voyeurism and exhibitionism, we have reached the fine line where normal sexual pleasure sometimes shades into perversion. Seeing and being seen are two of the most basic sexual stimulations, for animals and people alike. As a part of sex play with a free, imaginative partner, the display of one's body and the enjoyment of someone else's can become an exquisite erotic delight. But if these fancies are forced on an unwilling stranger or are practiced as a substitute for intercourse, they have clearly crossed the line into sexual aberration.

Can Voyeurism Be Normal?

A *voyeur* is one who gets pleasure from seeing other persons in the nude, undressing, masturbating, or having intercourse. Everyone is, to some extent, a voyeur. Traditionally, men have seemed more inclined to voyeurism than women, but with the freer sexual mores and successful women's movement in today's society, both sexes are now enjoying looking at each other. We have *Playgirl* and *Playboy*. Women are joining men in the audiences of X-rated feature films, and of hard-core porno flicks, too. Many couples having sex like to watch themselves in a mirror. Usually this visual stimulation is a means of arousal leading to orgasm.

In earlier societies, nudity was no cause for shame, either in a woman or a man. Sex was a natural function like eating, and to cover one's sex organ would have been as silly as to cover one's mouth. Indeed, many cultures featured nudity as a proper subject of public appreciation. The Greeks adorned their public squares and buildings with fully nude statues, for example, and fashions for the women of ancient Egypt bared their breasts completely. Then came the long period of sexual gloom brought by Western religions, when nudity was considered savage and immoral. It is against these centuries of inhibition that the sexual energy of modern times is rebelling.

Can Exhibitionism Be Normal?

Exhibitionism, the pleasure of displaying one's body, is the normal complement of voyeurism. Today more and more people, both women and men, realize this. This recognition has rejected generations of shame, and people are again becoming proud of their bodies. The most widespread and obvious example of this is on a beach in summer. Nowadays, both women and men are wearing extremely minimal bathing suits designed to cling to the body and reveal what they must legally cover up. Women are going braless and men are wearing tight pants. The popularity of slenderizing diets and exercise these days undoubtedly has as much to do with the desire to have an attractive body as to have a healthy one.

Thus, in most circumstances, voyeurism and exhibitionism are healthy, natural sexual activities for women and men.

When Does This Behavior Become Abnormal?

Although the women's movement is changing the behavioral patterns of both sexes, men have generally been socially conditioned to be more aggressive in all areas. It is precisely when the pursuit of pleasure from voyeurism and exhibitionism becomes an act of aggression that it becomes a sexual problem. Thus, most cases of this sort involve men either spying on or exposing themselves to women who are usually strangers. These acts generally arise from sexual guilt and/or repression, not sexual freedom. The "peeping Tom" is excited by the forbidden view of nudity or sexual activity; the "flasher" is excited by the forbidden display of his genitals. As with group sex or any other practice, all participants in voyeurism and exhibitionism must be willing, but the women who are the objects of peeping Toms and flashers are in no sense partners in the act. They are victims of it.

Exhibitionism is one of the commonest sex crimes in many countries. In general, an exhibitionist is likely to be harmless and is often impotent. After exposing himself, he will run off and disappear until the next incident. Voyeurs, on the other hand, may become so sexually stimulated by watching a woman that they will try to gain access to the woman and rape her.

Voyeurism, Exhibitionism, and the Law

Although there are no certain cures for peeping Toms or flashers, the social and legal penalties are severe.

This behavior has been condemned since biblical times. Throughout history, the penalties have been stiff. Legend has it that Lady Godiva rode nude through the town of Coventry in protest to a tax levied by her husband against the townspeople. Her husband forbade anyone to watch the ride and all complied with his wishes—all but one. The city tailor, named Tom, secretly watched, or "peeped," through the shutters of his store window. This action made him famous, for the term "peeping Tom" originated with him, but it also provoked Lady Godiva's husband to strike him blind as a punishment.

Today, prison sentences are common penalties. Sadly, this is not the answer, since it does not cure the problem; it just punishes it. Perhaps the solution will come when the sexual revolution has succeeded in instilling in everyone a positive, open view about the nature of the human body.

KINKY SEX

"Kinky" sex is the twilight zone of erotic behavior. Most people would agree, for example, that intercourse is perfectly normal sex and necrophilia (sex with the dead) is downright perverted. But, as in the case of voyeurism and exhibitionism, there is a hazy line between the two obvious extremes. Kinky sex walks that line.

What is considered normal or perverted at any one time and place is largely a matter of fashion. Homosexuality is a good example of this. Other sex practices may be normal or perverted depending on the degree to which they are practiced—if they're indulged in slightly or only occasionally, they're harmless; but if they're regular or extreme acts, they then become dangerous. Voyeurism is one such practice.

A further distinction may be made. All the sex practices discussed so far have been motivated by distinctly sexual stimuli. As one enters the murky gray area of kinky sex, one finds more and more nonsexual causes behind the sexual activities. What is considered sexy has more to do with particular personal associations than with one's general cultural conditioning. Of course, this kind of very personal stimulus is a part of every normal sexual relationship—it's what makes sex different with different people.

The following pages will discuss certain of the more extreme kinds of sexual displacement. These particular pleasures are not for everyone. These are the exotic fruits of kinky sex. In some cases they seem very normal, while other examples seem decidedly less than normal.

Fetishism

Probably the most popularly practiced type of kinky sex is *fetishism*. It is so popular that most people would not consider it kinky —at least, not what *they* do.

A fetishist is a person who receives sexual stimulation from some sexual or nonsexual feature of other people or from some objects. It is most often hair, feet, shoes, or special kinds of clothing that turn such people on, although the list of possible fetish objects is practically endless; some women get pleasure from making love to a partially clothed man; some men get extra kicks from making love to a woman who wears boots or shoes during the sexual act.

Hair—The Most Common Fetish

The most common fetish is hair. From the earliest recorded times, hair has played an important role in sexual stimulation. The story of Samson makes hair the symbol—even the source—of virility. Throughout history, women have had to cover their heads in public. Until recently, the custom of women wearing hats in church was strictly observed, based on the belief that by covering their hair, the women would arouse no lustful thoughts in the men present. Other religions, such as the Jewish Orthodox, forced a woman to shave her head after marriage to deprive her of the means to seduce other men. The tremendous change in men's hairstyles in the last decade is intimately connected with the general social trend toward a more natural, free expression of sensuality and emotion.

Pubic hair has an even more specific sexual connotation. An Arab legend tells that when the Queen of Sheba visited King Solomon, he refused to go to bed with her until she had shaved off all her pubic hair. On the other hand, among certain Oriental peoples, it is considered unlucky for a man to have intercourse with a woman who has shaved her pubic hair. The two different attitudes continue into the present day. Some men like the appearance and scratchy feel when the pubic hair is shaved, others enjoy the sight and pleasant tickle of unshaved pubes. Still others may playfully urge a woman to shave her pubic hair in the form of a heart or other design. It should be pointed out that if a woman does shave her pubic hair for a time, she will find it rather itchy as the hair grows back in.

Women tend not to have such particular feelings about men's pubic hair, but they do have definite preferences about men's body hair. Studies have shown that men with extensive body hair are no sexier or more potent than men with very little hair. The difference is simply genetic. Still, for whatever reason, some women are attracted to men with hairy chests and backs, while others find this type of man unappealing. What's virile to one woman is brutish to another. On the level of pure physical sensation, too, some women like the rough texture of a man's body hair against their naked bodies during sex, while other women like the softer touch of skin against skin.

Smell

Smell can also be a fetish. Many persons get sexual stimulation from different types of smells. Of course, what smells good to one person might not smell good to another. Many European women, for example, do not shave under their arms or use deodorant, because European men are excited by the natural smell of the body. Other smells may be exciting because of personal associations. The smell of horses, for example, could be extremely stimulating to some people. One woman recently admitted that she became sexually aroused at the slightest smell of a horse. This was apparently because her first sexual experience, which still carried a very strong impression, took place in a stable. On the other hand, a particular perfume might remind a man of *his* first intercourse.

A certain amount of fetishism is present in everyone's sexual behavior. Some people, though, are unable to enjoy any sexual activity that does not include their fetishes. They may even withdraw entirely from intercourse and all other mutual sex activities and respond only to the fetishes. There are people who develop a fetish for crippled or deformed partners. In fact, the particular choice of a fetish is probably not as important to one's sexual health as the degree of exclusivity the fetish occupies in one's sex life.

S and M

Sadism and *masochism* are two kinds of kinky sex that are closely related. The essential element in both is a sexual arousal based on pain or suffering. The sadist delights in watching or making other people suffer. The masochist delights in experiencing this suffering. Sadism and masochism have existed since the beginning of human life, but only recently have they been identified and named.

Sadism

Sadism is named for the Marquis de Sade. Born in Paris in 1740, he was enrolled in the French army at the age of fourteen. The extreme daily cruelty he witnessed during his next twelve years as a soldier —beatings, rapes, and torture—undoubtedly colored the rest of his life. De Sade left the army and began hiring prostitutes, with whom he indulged his passion for cruelty. This activity led to his repeated arrest and imprisonment. During his life, de Sade spent a total of twenty-seven years in prisons. He died in a mental hospital at the age of seventy-four.

While he was in prison, he wrote the books for which he is now famous, principally *Juliette* and *Justine*. He described various types of torture that had existed since ancient times, but it was not until de Sade publicized sadistic behavior and its sexual satisfaction that people focused attention on this activity.

In its earliest manifestation, sadism was a feature of religious ceremonies. The infliction of pain was a necessary step in various rites of atonement. The citizens of imperial Rome were extremely enthusiastic about spectacles of human agony, the most obvious example being the gladiatorial shows. Men and women fought each other to the death or faced wild beasts, and the crowds were thrilled. The same sadism underlies the pleasure people have today viewing boxing matches, automobile races, bullfights, or any other sport where the chance of death or mutilation is high. There is a little of the sadist in everyone.

Love and hate are closely linked passions. The desire to cause pain to those we love is normal. In some cases, this duality is reinforced by forgotten childhood incidents. Freud writes of a child who saw his parents having intercourse and imagined that his father was assaulting his mother in a terrible fight. A child frequently beaten severely by his father or mother may associate this pain with the love he feels for them.

The confusion of pain and pleasure may also come from some experience in later life. Men in wartime combat view the killing of their enemy as a positive, rewarding action. For poor or oppressed people, beatings and cruelty are an important means of release from the feeling of powerlessness that fills their lives. There are as many other examples as there are varieties of individual human experience.

CAN SADISM FIT WITHIN NORMAL HUMAN BEHAVIOR? Underlying all forms of sadistic behavior is a completely natural instinct: the instinct to seek dominance over others. It is an instinct which motivates our greatest achievements and all our ambitions, but also our worst atrocities. This is the difficulty with attempting to pinpoint the causes of such particular kinds of behavior as sadism. The texture of human behavior, sexual or otherwise, is a continuous weaving of contrasts. Everything has its cause in everything else.

SNUFF. Sadistic sex can involve nothing worse than a playful spanking given by a man to a woman during foreplay, or it can be as horrifying as the brutalization and sexual murder of children. De Sade himself enjoyed inflicting the torments of whips, knives, and poison on the prostitutes he hired. This extremely sick form of sadism is very much with us today, in the proliferation of the so-called snuff movies. In these films, a woman is shown being dismembered or killed after performing various acts of sex. Many of these films are fakes, but not all. A few women every year are kidnaped and forced to participate unwittingly in these films, losing not only the essence of their human dignity but their lives as well. That there is a definite audience for these films is not only shocking; it illustrates the utter depravity and sickness that is possible in the human condition. It is not only sick sex, it is murder, and anyone who participates on either side of the camera desperately needs urgent psychiatric help. These are potentially the most dangerous people in any society—they have an undeniable attraction to murder and are highly likely one day to satiate this urge directly. If you know anyone involved in any way with the so-called snuff movement, you should report him or her to the police, who can and should monitor their actions. There is, unfortunately, a definite audience for these grotesque spectacles.

Masochism

Just as sadism is basically an act of aggression, masochism is basically an act of submission. Masochism is named for the Austrian writer Leopold von Sacher-Masoch, born in 1838. His father was a local chief of police. He was an exceptionally bright student, a distinguished physician, and a decorated officer in the French-Austrian War. In addition, he wrote several notorious books, in particular *Legacy of Cain* and *Venus in Furs,* in which he vividly portrayed the enjoyment of suffering and pain at the hands of a beautiful woman.

There are three incidents in the life of von Sacher-Masoch which seem to have influenced this behavior. First, it was said that as a child, von Sacher-Masoch was fascinated by stories of the Andean mountain martyrs and their terrible suffering. Then, during puberty, von Sacher-Masoch had a dream which continued to haunt him for the rest of his life. In the dream, he was the slave and victim of a cruel woman. This dream was probably the result of an experience he had as a boy. Lastly, while hiding in a closet in his aunt's bedroom, he witnessed her making love to a strange man and then being caught by her husband, who gave her a beating. Later, when she discovered young Leopold in the closet and realized that he had seen everything, she gave vent to her guilt by beating the boy. Certainly these three incidents in many ways may be responsible for the behavior for which von Sacher-Masoch became known.

Eight years before he died in 1895, France elected him a member of the Legion of Honor, in recognition of his literary achievement in the twenty-four books that were published there.

Masochism has had a significant place in the development of human culture, in the very heart of Western religion. For the glory of God, men and women inflicted upon themselves wounds which they would not allow to heal, but aggravated by rubbing salt into them. They donned hair shirts and slept on beds of thorns. They practiced long periods of thirst, then drank contaminated water to honor God. People tried to outdo each other in the search for ever more horrible methods of self-torture. Christine of St. Troud, for example, fastened herself to a wheel, had herself racked, and was hung on a gallows beside a corpse. Bands of penitents flagellated themselves in public processions for the sins of the world. Many of these men and women were praised for their holiness, and some were canonized as saints. Their example is undoubtedly inspiring—and undeniably masochistic. What are we to think?

The immense popularity of the book and the movie versions of *The Story of O* indicates a current high level of public interest in, and curiosity about, the masochistic experience.

As in the case of sadism, there are a variety of theories which explain the cause of masochistic behavior, but people cannot agree which is right. It is seen as a manifestation of a sense of unworthiness in the individual, as a desire for humiliation. It is seen as an attempt by the individual to absolve her or his own guilt about sadistic tendencies. It is seen as a low-grade death wish. It is the opposite of sadism, and therefore—like love and hate, pain and pleasure—very much like it in many ways—including its elusiveness.

Discipline and Bondage

"D and B" is actually a special kind of "S-M," or sado-masochistic, behavior. The focus in discipline and bondage situations is not the act of sexual intercourse, but the sexual stimulation derived from seeing a woman or man bound in leather harnesses which emphasize and reveal the sexual organs, or tied with ropes or chains, or perhaps gagged with a mask. The idea of being helpless, or of rendering someone else helpless, and thus subject to any whim, is extremely stimulating to some women and men.

A certain level of discipline and bondage is within the scope of normal sexual activity and has recently become popular among both straights and gays, providing their lovemaking with an extra kick.

It is a completely normal fantasy of young girls and women to be bound and raped. Such a fantasy often fulfills their desires to have intercourse without feeling blame or guilt for the act. Many men who seek to be tied and beaten are highly educated and extremely powerful, yet deeply guilty about their success, feeling unworthy of it. They tend to have difficulty expressing this feeling to their wives, and instead seek prostitutes or massage parlors that offer "English therapy"—discipline and bondage.

Some couples are strong enough to be frank about such preferences. Other couples are just curious, or interested in experimenting sexually. Whatever the case, mild forms of discipline and bondage are a frequent spice in many people's sex lives. A woman or man will tie up the other with twine or leather belts or neckties. Another simple form of bondage is blindfolding, which can be accomplished with a mask, or scarf, or even a towel. Blindfolded, a woman or man cannot see and prepare for whatever the other partner is going to do, and sexual stimulation in this situation is heightened for some people.

Also, being blindfolded allows the subject to fantasize freely about the identity of the other partner and/or the setting in which the sexual activity is taking place.

For some people, the enjoyment of discipline and bondage is intimately connected with the sexually stimulating properties of leather, which is often the substance of the variety of available "D and B" accessories. There is nothing more sexy than skin, and leather, of course, is just that. It is not known whether the orgasm is caused by the tightness of the apparel or by the textural quality of the leather; it is probably a little bit of both. Prostitutes have long recognized the attraction of leather boots and garments in plying their trade.

Saliromania

Saliromania, from the French verb *salir,* meaning "to soil," or "to make dirty," is a type of sexual stimulation derived from urine or feces. Some people get excited by urinating or defecating on others; some people get excited being urinated or defecated upon. Obviously, this is another variation of sado-masochistic behavior.

The different forms of saliromania are undoubtedly distasteful to the majority of people. Yet this extremely kinky activity has certainly maintained a steady appeal to people in all periods of history and in all parts of the world.

Necrophilia

This is a practice named from the Greek word *nekros,* which means "dead body," and describes the sexual stimulation some people get from intercourse with a dead person. Even psychiatrists have found it difficult to explain exactly what causes this behavior.

Zoophilia

This is a term describing sexual intercourse with animals. In many cases, this is less a perversion than a need. It is known to be a common practice of farm workers who are isolated from any other sexual outlet, and therefore enter into sexual activities with farm animals. This was confirmed by the Kinsey Report.

Pornographic literature and films often feature a woman having intercourse with a dog, a donkey, a pig, or some other animal. These seem to provide great stimulation to certain voyeurs.

Can an Animal Impregnate a Woman?

There have never been any confirmed reports of pregnancy in women as a result of having sex with dogs or other animals. Nor, in the reverse situation, can a man's semen successfully cause pregnancy in any animal.

Obscenities

Naturally, the potential variety of kinky sex is as unlimited as the human imagination. Many persons get some sexual stimulation from the use of "dirty" words, a practice known as *coprolalia*. The most familiar form of this activity is the obscene telephone call. This can be extremely upsetting and frightening for women who receive such calls. In fact, it is just this sort of response which usually excites and has motivated the caller—a person who is very sick, but is also usually impotent. If you get such a call, do not engage in any conversation. Hang up immediately and report the incident to both the police and the phone company.

Such calls, when unsolicited, are criminal acts; which is one reason, perhaps, that many of these people are now calling prostitutes instead. Other people enjoy screaming dirty words at people they pass on the street; some shout at the height of the sexual act.

Kleptomania

Kleptomania, the persistent impulse to steal, often has a sexual cause. Studies have indicated that a woman's desire to steal actually changes throughout her menstrual cycle, becoming strongest just prior to the onset of her period and also during the time of her menopause. The sexual stimulation which some women feel in kleptomania is thought to be influenced by hormone levels. Every teenage girl who shoplifts a pack of cigarettes for a kick or in rebellion is obviously not a true kleptomaniac, but if the behavior is recurrent, it may indeed have a sexual association. A similar behavioral pattern is pyromania, the enjoyment of setting fires, which is generally considered to have a sexual basis.

The examples proliferate. The fact remains that there's a lot more to sex than just intercourse, and a lot more to sexual arousal than just sex.

HOMOSEXUALITY

The word *homosexual* is not derived, as most people think, from the Latin meaning of *homo*, which is "man," but rather from the Greek *homo*, which means "identical." Thus the term applies to either sex.

Female Homosexuality

Although the written history of female homosexuality (lesbianism) is incomplete—another example of a male-dominated society—it has the same classical roots and historical occurrences as male homosexuality. The word *lesbian* comes from the Greek island of Lesbos. Sappho, who lived on Lesbos in ancient times, opened a school for young women, to whom she taught poetry, music, and dancing. She, who was not married, referred to her pupils as "companions" and fell in love with one after another of these girls, writing several poems about them. This led scholars of antiquity to debate whether these poems were, in fact, expressions of sexual love between women.

Male Homosexuality

The practice of homosexuality has been found in many primitive tribes. The Zunis greatly honored such "men-women." In some regions of the world—Babylonia, Mexico, Peru—it was this group of "men-women" who often made up the tribe's magicians, medicine men, and priests. Certain tribes supplied a man temporarily without a sex partner with a "substitute" female in the form of a boy or young man.

Greek mythology attributed homosexual behavior to some of its gods, including Zeus and Apollo. The Greek civilization valued the nude male figure even more highly than the female, as characterized by the nude male athletes of the Olympic games and the idealized beauty of the prevalent sculptures called *kouros*. The phenomenon of a love relationship between an older, well-educated man (*Erastis,* meaning "lover") who held a prominent place in society and a young boy (*Eromenos,* meaning "beloved person") whom he was to prepare for his future place in that society was very much a part of the ancient Greek culture. Homosexuality was considered a proper aspect of a man's total education. Later, when the boy was older, he himself would take on a younger pupil.

The Romans adopted homosexuality from the Greeks, but debased it into a simple act of pleasure, without the noble aims it had once served. Homosexuality was pervasive throughout Roman society. The elder Curio, a Roman senator, taunted Julius Caesar as "every woman's man and every man's woman."

Religious Disapproval

The Christian religion reacted against the easy vices of the Romans that were everywhere evident. The Bible considered the begetting of children as the only justification for sex. Any other sexual activity was looked upon as an abuse of the worst sort; sex for pleasure was a sin. Homosexuality, according to the Christians, was against God and nature. Christianity has spread throughout the world in the centuries since then, but homosexuality has survived.

Are Homosexuals Different?

Studies indicate that, in general, homosexual individuals do not differ from other people in any physical way. Rather, homosexuality is a pattern of behavior which is very likely established in childhood. Although homosexuality is not inherited, there is probably, in the opinion of most psychologists, a complex interrelation of familial and social factors which develops it.

Kinsey reported in his first study that 37 percent of American men and 20 percent of American women have some kind of homosexual experience at least once in their lives, although the percentage of people who were exclusively homosexual was far smaller. Given the greater sexual freedom and awareness of our contemporary society, these percentages are higher today. Recently it has become a matter of one's "liberation" in certain circles to participate in a homosexual experience. Whether this is an actual trend or simply "bisexual chic" is impossible to determine yet.

Do Homosexuals Marry?

Many homosexuals are married, often for the sake of appearance. Lawyers, doctors, men and women in business, and others in positions of "respectability" in society may be homosexual, yet may marry and have children, maintaining happy family lives and engaging in homosexual activity on the side. It is, of course, impossible to determine the exact frequency of marriage involving homosexuals. Recent research indicates that 35 percent of white women homosexuals and 20 percent of their male counterparts have been married at least once.

Many homosexuals live together as married couples. Some have even secretly performed marriage rites that seem to be as sacred and meaningful to them as marriage is to heterosexuals. Society has not yet fully understood homosexual marriages, and they are not legally binding or governmentally recognized in the United States. Some European countries are more enlightened on the subject and do recognize such marriages.

What Do Homosexuals Do Sexually?

The manner in which homosexuals behave in their sexual relationships does not differ much from the way heterosexuals behave. Homosexuals often maintain that a member of one's own sex is far more capable of understanding one's sexual needs than a member of the opposite sex. Female homosexuals, or lesbians, know exactly how and where to stimulate each other's clitorises, and perform sex at their own proper pace. Touching, caressing, and massaging are important expressions of lesbian love. Lesbians also perform cunnilingus and often engage in mutual vaginal penetration with their fingers. Lesbians may use dildos or vibrators to simulate intercourse.

The most common sexual activity between male homosexuals is oral sex. Anal intercourse is practiced by some male homosexuals, but not all.

Attitudes and Behavior

Homosexuality is more predominant in large cities. Homosexuals find themselves too easily recognizable as "different" in smaller communities, and are usually deprived of easy contact with other homosexuals. Large cities offer an entire homosexual subculture and afford a degree of anonymity which permits the homosexual to live her or his own life free of interference.

With homosexuality becoming more generally accepted, or at least tolerated, in today's society, many lasting long-term homosexual relationships have become possible. Still, the old prejudices live on, and for many homosexuals the usual pattern involves a number of short affairs, perhaps with strangers, in which the threat of exposure is kept to a minimum. Homosexuals tend to be more promiscuous in their sexual activities than most heterosexuals. Therefore the incidence of venereal disease among homosexuals is considerably higher than in the general population.

Many homosexuals are completely happy and fulfilled, particularly when they are younger. However, those who do not have permanent partners will often find themselves lonely as they grow older. This is also true with heterosexuals; it just occurs more frequently with homosexuals and is probably due to the transitory nature of their life.

There is now a nationwide movement toward Gay Liberation—the recognition of the right to live a homosexual life without harassment and disapproval. Homosexual newspapers and magazines are appearing in every major city. The theater, movies, and even TV have begun to treat the topic with seriousness and respect. This new openness among homosexuals and the freedom with which they are voicing their needs is, in a sense, a return to the past—a journey to the days of the ancient Greeks, when homosexuality was not looked upon as scandalous or abnormal, but rather as a particular sexual identity which had its rightful place in the society of mankind.

TRANSVESTISM

Transvestism is derived from the Latin words for "cross clothing," and describes the practice of dressing in the clothes of the opposite sex.

Like most other forms of sexual behavior, transvestism is nothing new. The Greeks spoke of the androgynous nature of human beings and included among their gods Hermaphroditus, who was both man and woman. Transvestism played a part in the fertility rites of the cult of Astarte, where women carried spears and lances and wore false beards, while men wore earrings and other feminine accoutrements.

Although the primary cause of transvestism is no doubt a sexual stimulation, this is not the sole factor responsible for the practice. Wearing the clothes of the opposite sex was thought by early peoples to allow one to assume certain characteristics of that sex. Women facing a situation that demanded they be valorous and brave, for example, might don men's garb to gain a man's strength.

Some women and men feel a great deal of satisfaction in dressing as the opposite sex. Certain people desire to do so only in the privacy of their homes; others want to parade in the streets. This practice has never been confined only to homosexuals, as is often wrongly assumed. A transvestite may be quite happy with her or his sex and dress up as the opposite sex just for fun. Homosexuals, of course, are not unhappy with their present sex, only with the sexual behavior that is expected of them. Thus most homosexuals are as far from wanting to switch clothing as heterosexuals. Other homosexuals, however, enjoy transvestism as a variety of sex play, as an escape from the pressure of socially expected behavior, or as a means to lure "straight" men into a sexual experience with them. It is not uncommon for a man to discover that the woman who has just performed oral sex on him is in fact another man. Other people may feel a tremendous, uncontrollable desire actually to become the opposite sex, and will practice transvestism as a first step toward that end. These people are not true transvestites, but transsexuals, and will be discussed later.

Often a transvestite is simply turned on by the feel of wearing the clothing of the opposite sex. True transvestite women generally achieve a sexual satisfaction by wearing identifiably "male" clothing. This could be due either to the rougher tactile quality of the so-called male fabrics, or to the power transference inherent in such a switch, since society has, up to now, been male dominated. Transvestite men achieve satisfaction wearing women's clothing, which is generally softer in its fabrics than men's and more tightly fitted to the body, another feature of the stimulation.

One of the most visible aspects of the great revolution in manners and morals that has taken place in America over the last decades owes its inspiration to the same pleasure which motivates transvestism. The sight of a woman in pants is now virtually universal in Western society, no matter whether the setting is a business office, a weekend's relaxation, or a formal evening affair. It is increasingly common to see women wearing not only pants of whatever variety, but also man-tailored shirts and suit-coats to go with them. The change in men's fashions is equally great. Flowered shirts with billowing sleeves, tank tops skintight to the body, jackets with shaped waists which give a man an "hourglass" figure, high-heeled shoes, and more are being worn by men of all walks of life. The pleasure these women and men get from crossing the once-rigid sexual barriers to dress in the style of the other is hardly a perverted or abnormal desire. It is a celebration of the freedom to experience all things more fully. Many designers predict that unisex fashions will soon be universal. This will obviously lessen the visibility of transvestism.

THE THIRD SEX

Every human being carries in her or his body vestiges of the opposite sex. A woman has a vestigial penis in her clitoris; a man has rudimentary breasts and nipples. In a like manner, every person produces both female and male hormones.

Under the circumstances, it is not surprising that there exists a significant amount of sexual crossover among women and men of all eras and cultures. Certain individuals find themselves irresistibly attracted to members of their own sex. Still others feel they are, in fact, trapped in the wrong bodies, in the wrong sex, and transform their sexuality entirely through an arduous and complex series of medical procedures.

Whatever the nature or degree of the sexual crossover which occurs in some people, the process is a normal part of the vast sweep of sex and in no way a perversion. This type of sexual crossover is viewed today as a psychologically *special,* not abnormal, form of behavior.

What Does Transsexualism Mean?

The word comes from the Latin, meaning to "cross sexes." Transsexuals define themselves as women or men whose mental representations of themselves—their gender identities—are at odds with their anatomies. A man with an entirely male body believes he is a woman; a woman with a female body believes she is a man. In such cases, one solution is the series of surgical and psychiatric procedures popularly known as a "sex-change" operation. A person who undergoes such a change of gender is called a transsexual.

Are Transsexuals Really Homosexuals?

Emphatically, no. A transsexual lives with the burden of an intense psychological certainty that she or he was "meant" to be the opposite sex.

In homosexuality, the factor which differentiates the homosexual from the heterosexual is the chosen object of sexual desire. A heterosexual chooses someone of the opposite sex and a homosexual chooses someone of the same sex.

In the more complex situation of transsexualism, the differentiating factor is *the person's perception of herself or himself*—that he or she is trapped in a body of the wrong sex.

More explicitly, a homosexual wants to use her or his sex organs with like partners. A transsexual, on the other hand, is usually repulsed by her or his sex organs and does not want to use them. In fact, transsexuals view their natural sex organs as so repulsive that they rid themselves of them.

How Many Transsexuals Are There?

There might be as many as twenty thousand transsexuals living in the United States, but the exact number is unknown. There is great resistance, not only among the public but in the medical community as well, to the procedure, which many consider tampers with God's handiwork. Until recently, most such operations were performed abroad, particularly in Casablanca.

In the last ten years, the operation has become more accepted in the United States, and approximately five thousand sex-change operations have been performed. Still, the prejudice continues both within and without the medical community. That prejudice is, according to most doctors, the chief difficulty every transsexual encounters.

Surgical Preparation

People who want to change their sex should be screened carefully before any irreversible decision is made. In most cases, a complete evaluation from a psychiatrist is required. Counseling about future life and the problems the transsexual will probably encounter should also be a mandatory part of the preparation. Also, a year-long series of hormone treatments is administered. During that time, the person must live, dress, and act as a member of the opposite sex. If, at the end of this year, the person is still certain that she or he wishes to continue, the actual surgery is performed.

The Sex-Change Operation

The man-to-woman procedure is performed approximately ten times more often than the woman-to-man procedure. It is also easier. In this operation, the penis is excised at its base. This exposes the nerves, which become the foundation of the clitoris. Although the new structure is never as sensitive as a woman's clitoris because of the resultant scar tissue, the transsexual can derive pleasure and sensation from the artificial organ. The man is castrated—the testes and some of the scrotal tissue are removed. An artificial vagina is then surgically created an inch or so above the anus, where the tissue is softer and easier to manipulate and where there is no bone structure. An opening is made that is wide enough to admit two fingers and approximately seven to eight inches deep. In order to ensure that this opening does not close, it is lined with a skin graft.

A special machine removes only a superficial layer of skin, usually obtained from the inner thigh. This skin graft is sutured around a plastic rod which has the same dimensions of the new vagina. It is inserted into the surgical opening. The rod remains in the opening until the skin graft has taken in this new location, a process which usually takes three to five weeks. This, of course, creates a great susceptibility to infections, which, in turn, may delay the healing process. When the rod is removed, dilators are used to prevent collapse or closure until complete healing occurs and intercourse is allowed (about six to eight weeks after the operation). Some surgeons use the skin of the excised penis instead, folded inside out around the plastic rod, for the new vaginal lining. A few surgeons even use bowel tissue for this purpose. The remaining scrotal tissue is pulled down and sutured around the edge of the newly created vaginal opening, forming the labia. The breasts, which have already enlarged slightly due to the hormone therapy, can now undergo silastic implantation. Many people choose not to have this performed.

The woman-to-man procedure is considerably more difficult and surgically not as successful. During hormonal therapy, the breasts decrease in size, while the clitoris becomes larger. A total hysterectomy and an oophorectomy (removal of the uterus and ovaries) are performed, in conjunction with a double simple mastectomy. Due to the extent of this procedure, it is often done in several stages. The vaginal mucosa is excised and the vaginal opening is closed. Skin grafts from the clitoral area are implemented to create the penile tissue. The new penis does not contain erectile tissue and silicone rods are inserted inside to provide sufficient stiffness. It is not a true erection, but it is sufficient for intercourse when *manually* inserted into a vagina. The manual insertion is necessary since this constantly stiff penis always hangs down. The main difficulty lies in creating a functional urinary conduit, so the new man can urinate from a standing position. The scrotum is made from labial tissue, and artificial (nonfunctional) testes are implanted inside this newly created scrotum. Since silicone is a body-friendly substance, the artificial testes are made from this material. Sexual activity is usually not possible for at least eight weeks following surgery.

The hospital stay for both operations is usually between one and two weeks. The cost of this operation is minimally around $5,000, although in some instances, insurance may cover a portion of this.

Are Orgasms Possible after This Operation?

The normal male ejaculates during orgasm, but since the penis in a surgical male is nonerectile and no semen is produced in the artificial testes, ejaculation is impossible. Still, the surgical male can achieve *orgasmic sensation*. This sensation is similar to the orgasmic response of the normal woman and focuses in the area of the removed clitoris. Because of this, the surgical male cannot achieve orgasm during intercourse or masturbation which stimulates only the shaft of the penis. Orgasm is, instead, brought about by stimulation to the area of the former clitoris.

The surgical female can achieve orgasm, although many do not. Orgasm in the surgical female is more difficult to achieve than in the normal woman, since no real clitoris exists and some of the nerves are usually damaged during the operation. Orgasm during intercourse

530 IT'S YOUR BODY: A WOMAN'S GUIDE TO GYNECOLOGY

probably occurs as a result of pulling the new vulvar tissue surrounding the artificial clitoris. This pulling stimulates the area of the former penis and orgasmic sensation is achieved.

Are There Any Postoperative Problems?

Of those who have undergone the sex-change operation in controlled conditions, a great number have experienced serious post-op complications. The Stanford University Gender Dysphoria Program in 1974 reported that eighteen of thirty-eight patients—almost *half* —had post-op problems.

In female-to-male surgeries, these problems were broken down to include rejection of testicular implants, infection, and "a desire to take a shotgun and shoot off the genitals of the surgeon."

Are Transsexuals Happier after the Operation?

Happiness is always a difficult quality to measure. With transsexuals, there are many factors affecting happiness—community prejudice, postoperative problems, and the many psychological factors that inevitably arise from any personality change of this magnitude.

According to the Erickson Educational Foundation, a national clearinghouse which disseminates information on the phenomenon of transsexuality, only two out of every ten transsexuals make happy adjustments after the operation. That is a very discouraging number for some, and hopefully society and medical research can effect a change for the better.

Still, the two out of ten who do adjust are supposedly living lives of emotional contentment that were not available to them in their previous genders.

Are Unnecessary Sex-Change Operations Performed?

Without any doubt, too many sex-change operations are performed. In the United States, applicants are carefully screened, and in most cases, from 75 to 90 percent of all applicants are *rejected* for surgery.

Of course, we in the United States cannot control the operations that proliferate outside our country, especially in Casablanca. In many foreign clinics, all a person need do to qualify for the sex-change operation is to show up at the clinic. This is a deplorable situation and one in which even the low twenty-percent success rate is reduced.

Most experts feel that at least ten times as many people apply for the surgery as should have it.

Who Should Have It Done?

Without recommending this arduous procedure, those people who fit the profile for potential success fulfill the following criteria: (1) They are over thirty and under fifty. These people have reached an emotional maturity and still have time to make an adjustment for the rest of their lives. (2) They absolutely hate their natural sex organs, sometimes to the extent of wanting to mutilate them. (3) They see no other viable alternatives to living their lives. The sex-change operation is, in all successful cases, a last-chance procedure.

Societal Benefits of Transsexualism

Many people are extremely prejudiced against transsexuals. Certainly the people who can honestly be defined as transsexuals are extremely rare, and understanding of their dilemma is lacking. But the rarity of this psychological circumstance makes it no less worthy of serious study.

Since Christine Jorgensen became the first "surgical female" in 1952, society has come a long way in accepting these people. Recently, writer Jan Morris and the American tennis-playing doctor Renée Richards have revealed themselves as transsexuals. Their admissions have helped focus public attention on a little-known problem.

It is logical to assume that if modern doctors can change a person's sex by clinical, exterior means—that is, by switching genitalia—there must already be a great similarity between the sexes. If transsexualism forces an examination of this similarity and promotes a greater understanding between all sexes—male, female, and transsexual —then it has been worth the trouble.

RAPE

In the past few years there has been a sharp increase in the number of reported rapes, and rape is now considered one of the fastest growing crimes today. Recent statistics have shown that there is an increase of more than 240 percent in the number of rapists admitted to New York State prisons during the past five years over the previous five years. It cannot be ascertained whether these statistics reflect an increase in the number of rapes committed or an increase in the number of rapes reported. Statistics indicate that 17 percent of reported rapes involve victims below the age of fourteen. Approximately 55,000 rapes are reported annually in the United States.

Physical Trauma during Rape

Women who have borne children or who have had previous intercourse may have minimal physical trauma following rape. However, the physical trauma, such as vaginal lacerations, to a virgin or a child may be severe. As soon as a rape has occurred, a woman should seek medical help either in the emergency room of a local hospital, or from her physician. Vaginal lacerations are occasionally so severe that surgery is necessary to repair the damage and to control bleeding. This vaginal repair should be performed as soon as possible after the assault to prevent infection or extensive blood loss, and to ensure proper healing. If the assault victim is a child, the child must be admitted to a hospital. A child often needs general anesthesia for proper examination and treatment since she may be so frightened that proper examination cannot otherwise be carried out.

What Should a Woman Do While She Is Being Physically Assaulted?

Unfortunately there are no clear gynecological instructions for the woman being raped that will help her avoid either physical or emotional trauma, since each rape case is so completely individual. If escape is not possible and screaming is useless, it might be advisable to let the rapist proceed with the sexual act without physical resistance. Fighting may provoke further violence and physical harm. It has been suggested that as some means of protection, a woman perform some act that might "turn off" her assailant such as vomiting, taking off a wig and throwing it at him, pulling out false teeth, or even urinating. These acts should not anger a potential rapist, but rather shock him.

What Should a Woman Do if She Has Been Raped?

If a woman has been raped she should immediately contact her physician or go to the closest hospital emergency room. She should also contact the police to give a clear description of the assailant and the circumstances of the assault. If there has been trauma to the genital organs, immediate medical aid must be sought. However, even if there is no trauma a woman should seek medical assistance for two important reasons. First, in this emergency situation, if the rape has exposed her to the possibility of pregnancy she can receive DES, "the morning-after pill" (see Chapter 9, Modern Methods of Contraception) to prevent conception, and secondly she should be tested for VD. If there is any suspicion of venereal disease, antibiotics should be administered. Another important reason for the examination by a physician is to obtain physical evidence of the rape such as vaginal smears of sperm or a description of any genital laceration.

Since rape victims have often been mistreated and humiliated by the very people who are supposed to help them—the physicians and the police—women are often ashamed to seek medical and legal help. Because of this, many rapes go unreported. Luckily, attitudes are changing and rape victims are given priority treatment in many emergency rooms and psychological assistance is readily available.

Psychological Trauma after Rape

Even when there is minimal physical trauma, there is often severe psychological trauma following a rape. This psychological trauma can be so severe that it will permanently influence a woman's view of sex, men, and herself. Women are often shocked and fearful that this crime might happen again. Voluntary intercourse with a desired partner can be disturbed by the fear of the past rape and even vaginismus may develop. A number of counseling services are available throughout the country to help women over the shock of rape. NOW, the National Organization for Women, has set up a number of such centers and may be contacted by telephone in case of rape for reference to the appropriate counseling organization.

How to Prevent Rape

It is as difficult to prevent rape as it is to prevent many other crimes; and you take the same precautions to avoid being raped as you would to avoid being mugged or having your home burglarized. A woman alone should avoid deserted streets at night. If she is followed by a car, she should reverse direction and run. If attacked in a building it is far better to scream FIRE than to scream RAPE to get doors open. Locks on windows and doors should be adequate, and unidentified strangers should never be let in. The list of warnings could go on and on; the major warning is simply to be careful and prudent and to avoid, rather than confront, the dangerous situation. Parents should always know the whereabouts of their children and warn them against strangers.

PROSTITUTION

A prostitute is a person, usually a woman, who engages in sexual activity in exchange for money. A prostitute is also referred to as a hooker, a call girl, a working girl, a party girl, a whore, or a street walker.

The practice of prostitution has existed for centuries but today it is more openly talked about. One of the main problems related to prostitution is the spread of venereal disease, and this has been minimized in countries where prostitution is legalized. Governmental regulations there require prostitutes to have frequent physical examinations to check for VD. The legalization of prostitution has allegedly reduced sex-related crimes in these countries also. In most of these countries, women must work in so-called red light districts and must constantly carry a health certificate indicating the date of their last medical check-up.

In countries including the United States in which prostitution is not legal, it is too often carried out in back streets and in high crime areas. Prostitution in the United States is therefore often associated with muggings, assaults, and murders, in addition to a higher incidence of VD than in countries where prostitution is legal.

What Do Prostitutes Do?

The sexual services offered by a prostitute often depend on her status in the profession. Many "call girls" have relations only with a limited number of regular clients whom they see on an established basis. The range of sexual practices available in brothels and so-called massage parlors depends on the predisposition and the wallet of the client.

There is a growing demand for exotic sex, and some brothels specialize entirely in sadomasochistic practices. "English therapy" and other S-M activities seem to be in demand particularly among well-educated, successful executives.

Massage parlors offer a variety of services with international designations. The least expensive service is manual masturbation. The French massage is oral sex. Swedish massage usually refers to penile massage between the woman's breasts. Danish massage, also referred to as "straight," is vaginal intercourse without manual stimulation. Greek massage is the professional term for anal intercourse. The most common practice is the so-called "half & half." During this practice the prostitute initially stimulates the client manually, then orally, and finishes with vaginal intercourse.

Since call girls are usually sophisticated professionals sexual relations with them are usually safe and rarely associated with real criminality. They will inspect new clients carefully for any obvious signs of VD prior to indulging in sex.

Brothels and massage parlors are so concerned about the spread of VD that often two women will at the outset inspect a client for any syphilitic sores, then milk the penis to make sure that there is no discharge that indicates gonorrhea. The women will then carefully wash the man's genitalia as well as their own before indulging in any sexual practices. Intercourse is only carried out with the aid of a condom.

The most dangerous prostitutes are the so-called "street walkers" or the women picked up on street corners. Many of these women offer their services in high crime areas. They are often involved with drugs and may be addicts or former addicts. They are usually under the control of pimps and are not careful about their bodies to prevent the spread of VD.

The Profession

There is a lot of money to be made in this profession and it is hard to judge those women who cannot find other suitable or well-paying jobs. It is, however, not as easy to earn money as one might think, and many professionals are unhappy and depressed. The happiest women in the profession seem to be those who have steady relationships or marriages in which their partners accept their work completely.

The women who are usually most satisfied with their jobs are those who have a steady clientele and thus a steady income. The most unhappy are probably those women who are drug addicts and who had to resort to prostitution to maintain their habits. There is, furthermore, a great psychological pressure inherent in working as a prostitute, since they must indulge in sexual relationships with many unappealing men. Any worker who feels this stress should immediately find a new profession.

Before any woman works as a prostitute she should be sure that she is familiar with all the signs and symptoms of venereal disease. She should know how to examine a man properly for VD and should wash both the man and herself with soap and water prior to intercourse. She should, furthermore, never indulge with any stranger without the use of a condom. Above all she should have regular medical examinations.

chapter 22

SEXUAL DYSFUNCTIONS

Many sexual problems are a result of lack of information and understanding and can be solved with nothing more than a greater awareness and openness between the two partners in a sexual relationship. The colorful variety of sexuality already presented has been, it is hoped, a step in that direction.

Despite all the openness and understanding in the world, there are sexual problems, or *dysfunctions*—such as frigidity, vaginismus, impotence, premature ejaculation—for which professional help is usually needed. These problems have many complex causes rooted in more serious psychological factors or marital problems which may result in a complete failure to enjoy, or even experience, sex. If a couple finds themselves with a major sexual problem of this type which cannot be improved by discussion and understanding and freedom between the two individuals, and which does not in the opinion of a gynecologist or urologist stem from any physical malfunction, the couple should seek counseling at a reputable sex clinic.

It is important that good professional help be obtained. This is not always easy. In recent years, there has been a burgeoning number of sex therapists to meet the public demand for this kind of treatment. Unfortunately, a great number of these physicians are not qualified to act as sex therapists, and may do more harm than good. Unless a doctor has participated in postgraduate study and training in the specific area of sexual dysfunction, he does not have adequate knowledge to treat sexual problems. This is equally true of general practitioners, urologists, and gynecologists and also of marriage counselors and psychiatrists. A doctor may be highly skilled in one of these related fields, yet be incompetent as a sex counselor. Today we believe completely in medical specialization: If one has heart trouble, one goes to a cardiologist; if one has sexual problems, one should go only to a reputable, trained sex therapist.

People often suppose that a doctor's knowledge of sex must be greater than the layperson's, and that doctors generally have more open, balanced attitudes toward sex in their own lives. This isn't necessarily true. Quite often medical students are so busy studying and specializing that they themselves have little specific sex education and perhaps only minimal sex lives. Sexual problems abound as much among physicians as among people of other professions. Doctors are not immune to the social pressures which produce guilt in so many people. Indeed, a physician may acquire a feeling of hostility toward sex as easily as anyone. There are many cases of gynecologists who are reluctant to treat women with venereal infections because this is "proof" that the woman has a promiscuous sex life in the eyes of the doctor.

Doctors who are uninformed or guilt-ridden about sex present an obvious problem to a couple seeking sexual therapy. An even more serious problem is the proliferation of downright quacks who infest the field of sex counseling, especially since the success of Masters and Johnson's groundbreaking clinic in St. Louis. It has been widely advertised, for example, that hypnosis is being used to treat sexual dysfunctions in certain clinics, although most responsible sex counselors say there is no proof that this has ever been successful.

Therefore, a couple seeking help for a sexual dysfunction would do best to consult one of the organizations listed below for referral to a reputable, effective sex clinic in their area. These organizations are the recognized leaders in the field:

Masters and Johnson, in St. Louis, were, as mentioned, the first physicians to study expertly and report on human sexual behavior. They have personally trained numbers of other physicians in this field.

Dr. Helen Kaplan, associate professor of psychiatry at Cornell University and head of the sex therapy program at the Payne-Whitney Clinic of New York Hospital in New York City, is another acknowledged expert in human sexuality.

Dr. Harold Lief, director of the Marriage Council of Philadelphia.

In addition, most U.S. medical schools and university centers now have, or are in the process of establishing, human sexuality programs which treat patients and train professionals. Therefore, the best way to find a well-trained sex therapist in your area is to contact your local medical school's hospital facility. But good qualifications are not enough. The same rules apply in choosing your sex therapist as in choosing your gynecologist: he or she must have good training, but, most importantly, you should feel good and comfortable and "right" with him or her or them.

Competent sex clinics deal with several major kinds of sexual dysfunction. The remainder of this chapter involves the most common of these dysfunctions—what they are and what they aren't, how a couple can recognize and deal with a big sexual problem at the outset, and what to expect if you decide to seek help at a sex clinic.

FRIGIDITY

A woman's orgasm can fall anywhere along a wide spectrum of sensation. Some women can reach orgasm simply by fantasizing. Some reach orgasm just by squeezing their thighs together. Some can reach orgasm if only their breasts are stroked. Some reach orgasm being penetrated by a man's penis. Some need direct clitoral stimulation.

Other women can become aroused during sex play and intercourse, and yet are unable to reach orgasm. Some women do not respond to any form of sexual stimulation and have a total inhibition of orgasm.

Although sex therapists still have no single, widely accepted definition of frigidity, it is certainly safe to say that women who fall into the last two categories of sexual response may be considered frigid.

Frigidity is a term that is used loosely by many people. If a couple is having a fight, the man may accuse the woman of being frigid. A woman who has never been as excited about sex as she thinks she should be may think she is frigid. These are usually cases of sexual disappointment, not sexual dysfunction. Sexual disappointment between two people can almost always be cured by better information and greater openness.

What Is Frigidity?

True frigidity, by contrast, is a serious sexual impairment for a woman. If a woman is capable of being aroused at all, there is a good chance she can be brought to orgasm. A woman whose sexuality is totally inhibited is in the more complex situation of having actually to relearn her sensual awareness before she can enjoy any sexual experience whatsoever. .

In the first case—that of a woman who gets aroused but no more —the usual culprit is fear. The woman is nervous about letting go, either physically or emotionally. Her feelings about the act of sex are probably ambivalent, and therefore her feelings about her sex partner or partners are also ambivalent. She may be uncomfortable about showing affection toward a man. She may be afraid of crying out during her orgasm, or of losing control of herself in front of someone else. She may be afraid of what she might say. She may want to keep her sex life superficial, without realizing that this condemns it to being unsatisfactory. Perhaps she wants to enjoy sex, yet punishes herself at the same time for enjoying it. Or she may simply have an excessive fear of pregnancy.

The second kind of frigidity—total sexual inhibition—is an extreme form of the first. At least 10 percent of all women have this problem. The reasons are many—often a combination of factors such as family and religious upbringing, childhood trauma (rape, for example), severe depression, and so on.

Mutual Responsibility

Sexual problems are private failures that a person is reluctant to admit, even to a spouse. This can start a pattern of snowballing misery for a couple. A frigid woman may let her husband have intercourse with her just to avoid a fight. She may even fake orgasm. But her continuous lack of pleasure will drive her further and further into resentment. She begins to make excuses: She's sick, she's tired. She may start a fight to avoid having intercourse. The couple has less and less sex. They withdraw from each other, making discussion of their problem impossible.

According to Masters and Johnson, there can be no uninvolved person in a sexual relationship. Both members of the relationship bear equal responsibility for its success or failure. Nearly every reputable sex clinic, therefore, requires both partners to undergo treatment for any type of sexual dysfunction. Once a couple realizes this, they should be able to confront each other about their sexual behavior without any feelings of hostility on one side or embarrassment on the other.

If a woman finds herself unable to achieve orgasm, there are certain immediate measures she and her sex partner can take. She must be sure the man knows exactly what pleases her. The man should be careful to arouse her slowly and at length, with a variety of foreplay. During intercourse, she may wish to take the superior position. The man might stimulate her clitoris with his fingers or a vibrator. New kinds of sex can be tried. In some cases, the problem can be solved by honesty, openness, and understanding.

Professional Treatment

If the problem persists, the couple should seek help at a sex clinic. There are several schools of thought about the treatment of frigidity, but all of them in one way or another emphasize the retraining of the woman's body to its natural sensuality.

The most frequently employed treatment is that which Masters and Johnson developed during their research on human sexuality. The couple is examined to be certain there are no physical causes for the sexual problem and interviewed together to discuss the situation. The couple is not allowed any sexual activity for a few days prior to beginning the treatment. The treatment begins with the couple clothed or unclothed, engaging in mild kissing and touching. The woman plays with the man, and the man with the woman, first by gentle body caresses and then, eventually, by direct genital stimulation. Intercourse is not permitted until the woman is ready for it, aroused by the sex play. Then the woman usually takes the superior position, accepting the man's penis only as little or as much, as slowly or as fast, as she wants. As the woman progresses from being tense and afraid to accepting and enjoying sexual activity, she is carefully guided closer and closer to orgasm, until it is finally achieved. This treatment may at first seem uncomfortable or upsetting to the woman, but if she has the encouragement and support of her partner, she has an excellent chance of reaching the satisfaction that has been so long absent from her life.

Treatment by Masturbation Training

A newer theory prevails in some sex clinics, where the treatment for frigidity involves counseling for the woman alone, followed by masturbation training. Proponents of this type of therapy maintain that a woman must first be capable of exciting herself and bringing herself to orgasm before she can expect to be excited by anyone else. The women being treated will meet as a group to discuss their individual versions of the common problem. Then they will be given thorough instruction on techniques of masturbation. They will be told about the different erogenous zones of their bodies and how to stimulate each one. Usually they will be told to fantasize while masturbating, to create a total sexual environment for themselves. The women then meet once or twice a week in a group to discuss their progress and share experiences. Many women find they are not alone in needing to masturbate for an hour or more before becoming excited. One by one, the women will find themselves at last reaching orgasms, and helping each other to find the way in their discussions. After a woman has been able to stimulate herself successfully, she will in turn teach her sex partner how to masturbate her.

IMPOTENCE

Impotence is the approximate male equivalent of frigidity. It is an inhibition of the man's erectile reflex.

Impotence can occur in teenagers just beginning to experience sex, in men at their peak of sexual vigor, and in older men who feel their age is showing. In fact, it is estimated that about one half of all men have known an occasional incident of impotence. Impotence, furthermore, crosses all racial and socioeconomic lines. It occurs among whites, blacks, and Chinese and from the ghetto to Beverly Hills.

What Is Impotence?

Some men have such severe impotence that they have never been able to achieve an erection with a woman, although they may when they are alone. Other men experience more limited, particular kinds of impotence in certain situations.

An impotent man might feel aroused by and want to have intercourse with a woman, yet still be unable to get an erection. Some men get erections during foreplay but lose them as they are about to enter the woman's vagina. Some men are impotent in intercourse, but can maintain an erection during manual stimulation or oral sex. Some men can only achieve erections when they are clothed, and fall soft as soon as their penises are exposed to view. Some men have erections when they are in a situation where intercourse is impossible, but lose their potency when intercourse is feasible and expected. Some men can only get erections when the woman is dominating the sexual activity; others become impotent whenever their partners try to take control. Some men get erections when they are with a prostitute but not when they are with their wives. Other men couldn't be unfaithful to their wives if they tried—with anyone else, they are impotent. Some men are impotent with their wives but respond to homosexual experiences.

Causes of Impotence

There are as many kinds of impotence, and as many causes for them as there are different circumstances in different men's lives.

Impotence can have a variety of purely physical causes, too. Chronic hormone imbalance, or the natural decrease in testosterone that occurs in a man's later life, can cause impotence. It can occur after the man has suffered an accident or disease in which the nerves involved in the erectile reflex are damaged. In severe cases of diabetes, for example, the high blood-sugar level will damage these nerves and make a man impotent. Habitual, excessive use of alcohol or barbiturates can damage the body and lead to impotence. Men who have cancer of the prostate and are treated with estrogen compounds, or men who are given medications to combat high blood pressure, might experience an adverse effect from these substances on their erectile reflex.

Therefore, if a man begins to experience recurring impotence, he should have a complete physical examination to determine whether there is some neurological or physiological explanation. In each of the situations mentioned above, there is a specific course of treatment that can be prescribed by a doctor to eliminate the man's sexual dysfunction.

Most often, though, the causes are emotional or psychological and related, in some way, to anxiety. The anxiety may have roots in the childhood conflicts of the Oedipal (mother-son relationship) period of development. It might have to do with the indelible anxiety of a man's first sexual experience. It might reflect a man's worry about proving himself through his sexual performance. The anxiety may result from a man's rigid moral upbringing: he wants to have "dirty" sex with his "nice" wife, and can't reconcile the two. The anxiety can be of a completely nonsexual kind, as well. A man's nervousness or depression over his job, his marriage, or a problem can produce a sufficient psychological pressure on him to make him impotent. No relationship between impotence and any single psychodynamic pattern has been established; it is a serious sexual problem precisely because it is such a complex one.

Impotence does not mean sterility. A man can become aroused and ejaculate with a soft penis. Men suffering from impotence have been able to impregnate their wives, but this is only the most fundamental, reproductive level of sex. Impotence affects myriad other functions of sexual activity—pleasure, relaxation, and love, both given and received.

Professional Treatment

A man who experiences severe impotence and has been examined and found in good health should seek help from a sex clinic. As in the case of frigidity, both partners will usually be required to participate in the treatment.

Most treatment follows the basic principles developed by Masters and Johnson to diminish a man's sexual anxiety and restore his positive view of himself. The immediate goal is one successful act of intercourse, on the assumption that this success will give the man confidence and break the block to his sexual pleasure, although treatment may be continued beyond this point.

Again, as in the case of frigidity, the treatment must be preceded by several days of sexual abstinence. Then the couple is told to engage in mutual caressing, both bodily and genitally. The man is told not to *expect* to get an erection, not to *try* to get an erection, and not to worry about *losing* his erection if one does occur. Thus the man is under no pressure. He is permitted to remain clothed at first if he so desires. The situation is made as comfortable as possible for him. When, with continued mutual stimulation, the man does achieve an erection, he is told not to have intercourse until he is ready for it.

The "Squeeze" Technique

Some men are tremendously encouraged when they discover they can have erections, and promptly undermine the therapeutic gain by becoming obsessively concerned with whether they can keep it, and if, once lost, it will ever happen again. This is a fairly common, understandable reaction, and Masters and Johnson chose to meet it directly by forcing the man to lose his erection and regain it several times before allowing him to continue into intercourse. This is accomplished with what they term the "squeeze technique." At the height of the man's erection, his partner is instructed to squeeze his penis tightly just under the head, which causes his erection to weaken and disappear. He is then stimulated by the woman to achieve another erection, and squeezed again until he loses it. Once the man becomes confident of his ability to continue to have erections, he is guided into the act of intercourse.

Final Treatment Stage

At this time, the man lies on his back and the woman mounts him. The couple then separates without building toward orgasm. The important step is that the man now knows he can maintain an erection and penetrate the woman, yet he does not have to perform or satisfy her. This is repeated until the man is confident that he can maintain his erection inside her. In subsequent acts of intercourse, the man proceeds at his own rate toward orgasm until he has finally achieved it. The initial coital experience is a critical landmark in the treatment of impotence. Further treatment focuses on making the sexual act ever more pleasant and mutually satisfying for both partners.

DYSPAREUNIA

Dyspareunia means "badly mated" in Greek, but what it means medically to a woman is *painful sexual intercourse*. This is one of the most common sexual dysfunctions affecting women. If a woman experiences regular pain during sex, she should see a physician—a gynecologist, however, since the majority of cases fall into the category of pelvic diseases.

Causes of Dyspareunia

Unlike frigidity and impotence, dyspareunia is often a result of one of several physical causes. Yet, as in any sexual problem, there may be psychological factors as well.

An inconsiderate or clumsy sex partner, for example, may fail to arouse a woman sufficiently before having intercourse with her. Since she is not excited, her vagina might not have gone through the changes necessary to accommodate a man's penis—that is, lubrication and enlargement. The friction of the man's penis against the dry, relaxed tissues of her vagina will be painful for the woman.

Psychological factors involved in situations of dyspareunia include a woman's own personal history of sexual trauma, misinformation, or simple embarrassment. Indeed, a woman's embarrassment is one of the chief obstacles to her successful treatment for dyspareunia, since many women are extremely reticent about discussing painful intercourse with their doctors and often invent other, less intimate, complaints instead.

There are a variety of physical conditions that may produce dyspareunia. One of the most common is infection. If a woman has contracted a venereal or other pelvic infection, and if the infection has traveled up through the uterus and into the fallopian tubes or the abdominal cavity, it can cause tremendous pain to her during intercourse. One trouble with such disease is that a woman can have a severe infection in her pelvic organs without having a significant temperature elevation, so self-diagnosis is not always easy.

Painful intercourse can also be due to adhesions—the phenomenon of unconnected tissues growing together—after an operation. During intercourse, there will be a pulling on those tissues which causes tension and pain. Similarly, if a woman has a fibroid tumor in her uterus, intercourse could cause a pressure on the tumor which might be painful.

Another reason for dyspareunia is the condition known as endometriosis, in which the tissue lining the uterus which is usually passed in the blood flow of menstruation, has instead spread up into the fallopian tubes and the abdominal cavity, where it grows like a foreign body. Some women can have such severe pain from endometriosis that sexual intercourse is impossible. A tilted uterus or other uterine abnormalities may also be at fault.

Treatments

There are effective, specific medical treatments for each of the physical problems mentioned above. The benefit is a double one: relief from the physical abnormality, and an end to painful sex.

A partially intact hymen, for instance, may require several acts of sexual intercourse to open a woman's vagina fully, and until this happens, intercourse may be painful. A woman with a *tipped uterus* often experiences pain when the man's penis strikes her uterus during sex. Vaginal or abdominal operations—the most common of these is the *episiotomy*, an incision made at childbirth to enlarge the vaginal opening—may leave scar tissue or may heal so that the vagina is smaller, thus causing a structural change in the woman which makes sex painful for her. In the case of organic defects such as these, doctors recommend that each woman experiment with different coital positions to find one that changes the angle or lessens the depth of the man's penetration. A woman with a tipped uterus, for example, may find that by lying on her back and pulling her knees to her chest, she can enjoy full vaginal penetration without pain.

If no physical causes are found for dyspareunia, it is probably caused by deeper psychological problems. In this case, a sex therapist or psychiatrist should be consulted.

VAGINISMUS

Vaginismus is the involuntary spasm of the muscles surrounding the vaginal opening which causes the vagina to close so tightly that it is impossible for a man to enter. This can occur in women who are organically normal and sexually active.

Vaginismus often serves as a woman's unconscious reaction against fear of vaginal pain. This may stem from an incident of infection or painful medical treatment that the woman experienced as a child. It may be a fear of the pain of pregnancy and childbirth. It may be a reaction against the pain of intercourse with a brutal, incompatible, or insensitive sex partner.

Causes of Vaginismus

This tight closing of the vaginal opening makes penile entry extremely painful, if not impossible. Thus vaginismus can lead to dyspareunia. And in the reverse situation, dyspareunia can lead to vaginismus. The painful intercourse that results from some internal physical problem can so frighten a woman that she develops vaginismus in reaction to it.

Masters and Johnson have discovered that one main cause of vaginismus is an impotent sex partner. The man's continual failure to enjoy sex will affect the woman so that she will want to avoid his problem and protect herself from further frustration. She can do this by, literally, closing herself off from sex.

Vaginismus can be the result of a deep-seated hostility the woman has toward men in general or her man in particular. The hostility may not be specifically toward men, but toward the sexual act itself, because of a woman's stern moral upbringing. If her distaste for sex or her sex partner causes her unresolvable conflicts, her subconscious may react and her vagina close.

A Myth Regarding Vaginismus

One of the most widespread and persistent of all sexual myths relates to vaginismus. This is the myth of *penis captivus*—the situation in which, during intercourse, the woman's vagina snaps so tightly around the man's penis that he is unable to withdraw it. Supposedly, the couple is taken by surprise while having sex, and must go, with the man still firmly clutched inside the woman, to a hospital, where they are separated either surgically or by being doused with a bucket of cold water. It is a fascinating picture, no doubt, but not true. Although it has occurred in animals, no medically recorded instance of such *penis captivus* exists in humans.

Treatment of Vaginismus

Treatment for vaginismus focuses first on finding the underlying psychological problem and dealing with it through appropriate counseling. Thereafter, the mechanics are dealt with. The woman is placed in a relaxing situation and her vagina is progressively dilated with dilators of increasing diameters. Then she attempts to penetrate herself with a lubricated finger. When this is successful, the same procedure is performed in a relaxed atmosphere with her sex partner. One lubricated finger is tried first—gently. Then two fingers (other therapists prefer the use of vaginal dilators). If this direct manual stimulation does not make the woman nervous or fearful, the couple will be guided into simple penile penetration, and finally into intercourse.

PREMATURE EJACULATION

This is probably the most common sexual problem in men. The exact definition of premature ejaculation differs from authority to authority. One textbook defines it as a male orgasm occurring within thirty seconds of vaginal entry. Kinsey defined it as ejaculation within two minutes of stimulation. Some clinicians accept the criterion of ejaculation in less than ten penile thrusts. Masters and Johnson diagnosed premature ejaculation if a man reached orgasm ahead of his wife more than fifty percent of the time.

Perhaps the best basic definition of premature ejaculation is orgasm happening before the man wants it.

A man's ability to control his ejaculation is vital to good sexual relations and his own self-confidence. The effective lover must be able to continue sex play even after he has become highly aroused, so that the woman, who will take longer to respond, can be satisfied. Also, if a man is secure about his ability to control his orgasm, lengthy foreplay gives the couple an opportunity to explore and extend their range of sexual activities and pleasures. This is why boys and young men, although more sexually energetic than older men, are poorer lovers—they do not know how to control their reflexes and usually, in their excitement, reach orgasm too quickly.

A man who knows he cannot control himself will feel depressed and incompetent, an attitude which may carry into other areas of his life. In bed, it is impossible for him to be sensitive and responsive to his partner while he is worried about becoming too aroused himself. A woman will usually be unaware of her partner's effort to restrain his excitement and interpret his behavior as cool and uninterested instead. While he tries to hold himself back to please her more, she feels rejected. Premature ejaculation is a serious sexual dysfunction which can ruin a couple's sex life and maybe their relationship as well.

Causes of Premature Ejaculation

There are a number of psychological factors that may contribute to, or cause, premature ejaculation. Many times premature ejaculation is almost like a habit for a man whose first sexual experiences were sneaky, speedy gropings for pleasure with the dire threat of discovery always imminent. Masters and Johnson stated that when a man's first sexual experience occurs with a prostitute who imposes time restrictions on him, premature ejaculation sometimes becomes a problem in later life because of the time associations he places on the act. Premature ejaculation may also be a response to some unresolved psychological problem that exists between a couple. A husband who no longer desires his wife will dutifully have intercourse with her, yet want to get it out of the way as fast as possible. A husband who is angry at his wife may try to punish her by ejaculating quickly and denying her her orgasm.

There are also physical abnormalities that can cause premature ejaculation. A man might have some infection of his urethra or prostate which causes this problem. It can be associated with some diseases of the nervous system.

Home Remedies

The great majority of men who seek treatment for premature ejaculation are involved in friendly or loving relationships and are in good health. Often these men have already tried to deal with their problem at home, perhaps by desensitizing their penises in some way —like rubbing powdered aspirin, Novocain jelly, or cocaine on the tip —or by treating the penis with a substance which reduces friction —oil, Vaseline, or a lubricated condom. Some try taking their minds off sex by thinking of other things while arousing their partners. This last home remedy is, admittedly, difficult. Home remedies can help in cases of minor dysfunction, but more profound problems require professional aid.

Professional Treatment

The prevailing opinion among sex clinicians is that most cases of premature ejaculation are caused by a state of excessive sensitivity in the man, which leads to an overly active ejaculatory reflex. Dr. James Semans, a urologist, developed the basic elements of the treatment procedure that is now widely used for this problem. The general therapeutic approach consists, initially, of several days of discussion and counseling. Episodes of mutual man-woman arousal and sensual-focus exercises, during which intercourse is prohibited, are then employed. The woman is directed to stimulate the man's penis manually or orally until the man feels close to ejaculation. At this time, the stimulation is stopped until his excitement decreases. Then she begins stimulating again. This "stop-start" technique is repeated over and over so that the man can become accustomed to the sensation of sexual pleasure over a long period.

Masters and Johnson advocate a slight variation of Dr. Semans's technique. When the woman has stimulated the man's penis just short of bringing him to orgasm, he will tell her to stop, at which point she squeezes his penis just below the head, which makes it impossible for him to ejaculate. Then he will lose his erection and be restimulated back to arousal, and squeezed again. This "squeeze technique" can be used by any man to retard his orgasm in any situation.

After the man has been manually stimulated a given number of times, he is directed to lie down and the woman directed to take his penis into her vagina. When he feels close to orgasm, she stops moving completely and sits with his penis in her until he begins to lose his erection. Then the woman begins to move again to excite him. It is important for the man to remain passive during this initial intercourse and allow the woman to do the moving. Also, the woman must be in the superior position, because the male-superior position provides too much stimulation for the man. In the case of a man with premature ejaculation, this extreme sensation can be too much.

It is possible for a man with clinical supervision to reach ejaculatory control using the female-superior position in intercourse within a month. Once a man learns this control, it is usually permanent, although complete control in missionary intercourse may take somewhat longer.

RETARDED EJACULATION

This is a much less common problem among men than premature ejaculation. Many men may experience occasional incidents when they have difficulty coming to orgasm, or may not be able to reach orgasm. This can be due to any of a variety of minor temporary upsets or illnesses, or simple fatigue.

The man who cannot ejaculate after extended periods of stimulation, intercourse, or fantasy, or the man who must withdraw from the woman and masturbate in order to reach an orgasm, suffers from a much more serious degree of retarded ejaculation. The cause of the problem may be a chronic illness, such as diabetes, or a long-term physical condition, such as alcoholism, or a persistent psychological block of some type. Whatever the cause, the man constantly finds that he does not experience sufficient sensation to ejaculate.

Treatment of Retarded Ejaculation

Except in situations in which the man suffers from the effect of damage to his nervous reflex system, the treatment for retarded ejaculation involves providing a heightened level of stimulation to the man during intercourse. The woman is directed to reach down and grasp the man's penis while he is penetrating her, stroking it with her fingers near the base of the shaft, an action which is very stimulating for her partner. She is also directed to cup and caress, gently and lightly, the man's testicles. These techniques provide the man with greatly increased sensation. A woman may excite a man this way during oral sex if she desires to bring him to ejaculation in her mouth. The extra excitement is a good bet to bring an end to a man's difficulties with retarded ejaculation.

CONCLUSION

Sex and sexual problems used to be "private" matters fraught with unspoken fears and angers. Modern women and men should realize that major advances have been made—and continue to be made—in our understanding of the complex physical and psychological mechanisms which control sexual response. Reputable sex clinics are often able to pinpoint a problem and proceed with a specific program of effective treatment, as thousands of happy couples can testify. There is no longer any reason for anyone to suffer in private misery about a bad sex life.

chapter 23

SEX THROUGHOUT YOUR LIFETIME

Everybody has a sex life. A kid has one and Granny does, too. Good or bad, sex is with you your whole life long. This is the most urgent reason for having the most rewarding sex life possible.

Because of our cultural conditioning, we tend to forget or ignore how really sexy we all are. Yet self-denial is a more twisted form of behavior than any act of sex. Sex is our connection with the processes of the universe and nature, with the history of our people and our planet, with the deepest sensibilities of others and of ourselves. Our sex lives begin near birth and end near death.

FREUD'S THREE STAGES OF PSYCHOLOGICAL DEVELOPMENT

According to Freud, children move through three stages of psycho-sexual development. The first is the *oral stage,* from birth to about eighteen months of age. During this stage, the infant's main pleasure is oral: the purely selfish delight in feeling and tasting with the mouth. This is followed by the *anal stage,* from eighteen months to four years old. This is the toilet-training period, when the infant must learn to control and direct a free, natural bodily function to conform to an external authority. The final stage is the *genital stage,* from age four to about six, when the child's pleasure becomes erotically located in the genitals. This is the period in which children pass through their Oedipal or Electral conflicts, which complicate their sexual feelings forever afterward. The child chooses the parent of the opposite sex as the object of her or his erotic focus; necessarily, this attraction brings frustration, anxiety, and guilt and, frequently, a conflict with the parent of the same sex. As the child grows older, these dilemmas usually disappear.

PARENTS' ROLE IN SEX EDUCATION

Children should be exposed to the truths of sex at every age. Children living in the country will routinely observe sexual activity between animals, and this is a good, natural time for parents to put in a few words of explanation. A pregnant mother has another perfect opportunity to mention sex in a comfortable, conversational way. A couple's own sexual behavior with each other will fix a strong image, for better or worse, in a child's mind. A wife and husband ought to be equally natural about nudity and privacy alike, because both are parts of healthy sexuality. What a child sees is what becomes "normal" for that child. A child should see Mommy and Daddy happy together, kissing and touching affectionately.

On the other hand, exposure to overly explicit sex is probably more confusing than helpful to a child. What may register on the child's mind is not the specific details of what it sees, but only the sheer intensity of the physical act. For children, intensity is usually a hostile feeling and a little frightening.

The most important thing to remember about a child's sexual education is *not to wait*. Parents may be tempted to put it off, assuming that school will take care of it. The act of *not* telling a child about sex in itself tells the child a lot about sex. In fact, sex education ought to be a simple, fundamental part of a child's family life.

The Language Barrier

One of the problems with discussing sex with a child is the language barrier. The child is exposed to words like *fuck, cunt,* and *cock,* yet parents and sex educators teach words like *intercourse, vagina,* and *penis* for the same function or genital parts. What the child is being taught is not the same as what the child hears on the street. Thus sex begins to have a dual existence in the child's mind: the split personality of sex and Official Sex. One of them comes to have an importance it doesn't deserve. Sex is too much fun ever to have to be Official. Some societies already realize this problem. In the Scandinavian countries, sex educators use both sets of words when teaching children.

Many cities have clinics which recognize the problems and dispense both information and methods of contraception to minors without parental consent.

TEENAGE SEX

Teenage pregnancy has been called the No. 1 population problem and it is estimated that more than 11 million teenagers are sexually active. Many teenagers have more sex than their parents. This is usually astonishing and threatening to the parents. Yet while teenagers may be having a lot of sex, they don't know a lot about it. The average teenager is likely to be only vaguely informed about orgasm, menstruation, contraception, childbirth, and venereal disease. Parents are (or ought to be) wiser than their children and ought to help them adapt to their new sexual expression, rather than hinder it. Punishment doesn't hinder, anyway; it only drives it out of sight.

In adolescence, as in adulthood, a person's motives for sexual activity reflect the full spectrum of human needs, from purely erotic sensation to completely nonsexual factors. Sexual activity, for example, might be a teenager's attempt to gain peer approval and popularity by doing the "in" thing. It might be a means of rebellion from a blatant expression of hostility to the teenager's parents. Those parents who are uneasy, anxious, and threatened by their children's sexuality are the most vulnerable to its effect as a weapon. Sexual activity may be a teenager's means of forcing a marriage to escape from the home environment. Children from cold, hostile families may try to produce babies to have something to love.

Recent studies show that more than 30 percent of teenagers who engage in sexual intercourse do not use any form of contraception, because they don't dare try to get it. In some instances, it is easier for a girl to get an abortion than a contraceptive. This is a shocking fact. Among other people standing in the way are physicians, who are often unwilling to supply a minor with any means of birth control without her parents' consent. The dilemma here is that a girl may know that her parents don't, and won't, approve. It should be pointed out that parental disapproval is unlikely to keep a girl from having sex if she wants it; but disapproval might keep her from having it safely. Many parents worry that if they make birth control available to their children, they are encouraging their children's promiscuity. Studies have proven that a teenager's rate of sexual activity *does not change after beginning use of contraceptives*. It is also interesting to note that a majority of gynecologists give their own daughters some form of contraceptive as soon as the girls become sexually active.

There has been a statistically enormous increase in the number of childbirths among girls under the age of seventeen, even with birth control and abortion becoming more readily available.

It is estimated that there are one million teenage pregnancies per year and two-thirds of these are unwanted. A teenage girl should know that both she and her boyfriend are in the most fertile period of their lives, and she should get contraceptive advice. In order to avoid the physical and emotional trauma of teenage pregnancy, it is strongly advised that contraception be available when wanted and needed.

VD and Teenagers

Another large problem in the sex lives of teenagers is venereal disease. Most teenagers are virtually ignorant of the symptoms, transmission, and treatment of gonorrhea and syphilis. Because adolescence is, in every area, an age of experimentation, teenagers often engage in sex with an enthusiasm that blinds them to practical concerns. This is another area in which parents can help a great deal by informing—not lecturing—their children on the subject. Parents who care about their children, and not just about a social code, will do this. A girl ought to know that a boy who has a discharge from his penis may have gonorrhea. She should realize that if she finds a sore on her vagina, she may have syphilis. These diseases can be treated effectively if they are caught at the beginning. But if, for reasons of embarrassment or ignorance, a teenager waits too long to see a doctor, the consequences can be far-reaching, and can include sterility.

THE TWENTIES AND THIRTIES

After the primitive conflicts of childhood and the psychological holocaust of adolescence, the twenties and thirties are a time of comparative sexual fulfillment for most people. People in this age group are at their most physically fit and attractive. Whatever problems occur sexually have usually been at least identified, and perhaps dealt with, by most people. The chances of a successful sexual life are good.

During their thirties, women usually start to find themselves. They have finally begun to overcome their inhibitions, they know their own bodies enough to know how they want to be satisfied, they know enough about men to be able to be satisfying sex partners, and they are close to their peak of sexual response. A man's sexual peak occurs earlier, in his twenties. At this time, the man's testosterone level, as well as his sperm production, is at its highest and he is able to reach an orgasm with minimal stimulation and with only a short pause between orgasms. As the man moves into his thirties, his sexual capacity gradually begins to decline.

It is for these reasons that a woman may take a younger man as a lover at this time in her life. The match is ideal, sexually speaking. Both partners are in the primes of their sex lives and have the capacity for extended sessions of intercourse, with multiple orgasms for woman and man alike.

On the other hand, a younger man may not satisfy a woman in other areas; he may very well be far less sophisticated and sensitive than she. His great sexual energy means the younger man has less control over his orgasm than an older man, and may not be as skillful a sex partner for a mature woman.

THE FORTIES

A woman and a man are most similar sexually in their teens and most different at about forty. Many women feel that their sexuality is heightened and their need increased as they get older. This is because of the removal by that time of the majority of psychological blocks the woman has about sex. She wants sex more because she has fewer inhibitions about it. She is inclined to try oral and anal sex if she has been reluctant to have these experiences before. As a woman enters menopause, her hormone level usually decreases, making her vagina drier during intercourse, but this minor problem can be treated effectively with a medically-supervised regimen of anti-aging substances. A woman's sex life can continue to improve right through menopause.

A man in his forties is in the male menopause and usually experiences some decrease in his sexual desire. This is caused by a combination of factors. There is a decrease in his hormone level, although the decrease is small for most men. Testosterone treatments can quickly restore a proper balance. A man at this time in his life is often devoting the greater amount of his energy to his work or business and has little left over for sex. Family responsibilities are at their most burdensome, with children to put through school or college, house or car payments to be met, and so on, so the potential for worry and depression is very high for the middle-aged man. His physical condition may not be the best.

It is a fact that overweight people of any age experience a change of body metabolism which produces a decreased interest in sexual activity. In the middle-aged man, this weight problem is often combined with a general loss of strength and youthful vigor, which renders him less capable of sustaining what sexual activity he does desire. Other medical factors associated with middle age can affect sexual performance: overuse of alcohol or drugs, for example, or diabetes.

Thus, just as a woman is experiencing increased desire in her forties, a man is experiencing a decrease. The difference can make a man temporarily impotent. A woman's newfound sexual appetite and freedom are threatening to a man who finds his erections coming more slowly than they used to, and not as firmly, and who needs more direct stimulation to become aroused—especially when once a mere fantasy was enough. This is a time for understanding all around. The man in his forties usually has overcome his inhibitions and is more sensitive to women from experience. Thus he will be a skillful, thrilling lover, if a somewhat slower one.

THE FIFTIES AND SIXTIES

A woman's sexuality decreases to a slight degree in her fifties and sixties, which brings women and men back to a state of sexual compatibility at this age. One of the main problems now likely to affect a couple's sex life is the real possibility of the man suffering a heart attack. The new medical opinion on treatment of coronary disease recommends a speedy return to all kinds of physical activity as a way to strengthen the heart and prevent recurrence of the problem. A patient will be advised to begin walking as soon as possible, and a program of daily exercise will be prescribed for him. Once a doctor has indicated that a man can resume a relatively normal degree of exercise, it means he can usually resume sexual relations as well. Naturally the man must be careful not to overdo it. A heart attack is a warning signal. But it need not be a stoplight to a couple's future sexual pleasure.

SEX AND THE ELDERLY

Our youth-oriented society has shrouded most of the processes of aging with a veil of embarrassment, discomfort, and ignorance. The gradual deterioration of body and mind which occurs in the elderly is frightening to those still in the flush of good health. We don't want it to happen to us. It is, of course, inevitable. A lot of the fear and distaste we feel about aging might be dispelled if we could realize that old people do just about the same things everybody else does. Age makes things take longer (and more difficult to do), but age does not necessarily rob us of our joys. That most emphatically includes sex.

Sexual activity, particularly among happily married couples, continues through the sixties and seventies and even into the eighties.

Studies have found that this activity is somewhat higher among elderly blacks than among elderly whites, somewhat higher among men than women, and somewhat higher among lower socioeconomic groups than among the more well-to-do. More than 60 percent of couples over the age of sixty enjoy regular sexual intercourse. By the age of eighty-five, the incidence of sexual activity drops to about 10 percent of couples studied. In short, older people may well enjoy the varieties of sexual delights until the day they die.

This lovely truth ought to be a source of hope and delight for us all. Yet many people are upset at the idea of elderly women and men engaging in sex. Some middle-aged couples have tried to commit their aged relatives to mental institutions when the old people struck up lively romances instead of behaving "properly" and fading away. There are actually people who think that sex among the elderly is a sign of insanity, but if you think about it at all, what could be more sane?

SEX AND THE UNIVERSE

Sex is the proof that the natural—which is to say the universal—will prevail. From the minute we gain consciousness until the minute we lose it, we are affected by conflicts, inhibitions, and repressions about our sex lives by the entire panoply of dark forces spawned by our Puritanical heritage. Thus it has been for ages. Yet we cannot keep the unwitting infant from gleefully masturbating at any time; we cannot keep the adolescent from plunging into the glorious fun of unmasking sexual secrets; we cannot any of us resist having sex for more reasons than simple reproduction; we cannot and will not give up the good feeling of sex, even in our last years on earth. For all the mighty foes it faces, sex just keeps winning.

We began with the question: What is "normal" sex? We end by saying that sex is what keeps us normal.

INDEX

References to illustrations are in italics.

A

Abscesses: of Bartholin's glands, 142; ovarian, 175; vaginal, 55

Abdominal organs: examination of, 47, 52–53

Abnormal bleeding, *see* Bleeding

Abortions, 33, 101, 193, 282–300; choosing method of, 299–300; effects of, on labia minora, 19; effects of late, 298–99; fetal sex determination and, 102; gynecologist's position on, 30, 31, 39; history of modern, 282–84; with IUDs, 233; IUDs following, 224; methods of, 285–99; PID and, 175; and recognizing first signs of pregnancy, 284–85; teenage, 553; *See also* Miscarriages

Acne, 182–83; the Pill and, 255; premenstrual, 106; vitamin B$_6$ for, 86, 247

Acute cervicitis, 135, 136

Adenomas: serous and mucinous cyst, 361–62

Adenomatous hyperplasia, 465

Adenomyosis, 356

Adenosine 5'-monophosphate (AMP), 172

Age: adenomatous hyperplasia and, 465; and breast cancer, 416, 457; cervical cancer and, 461; of circumcision, 404–5; and corrective

breast surgery, 426–27; effects of, on immune system, 473; effects of, on labia majora, 17; of gynecologists, 29, 31; and heart attacks, 253; infertility and, 304; and irregular menstruation, 114–15; of IUD users, 234; and masturbation, 506; menstrual cramps and, 109; oophorectomy and, 388; oral contraceptives and, 243–44; ovarian cysts and, 361, 362; pregnancy and, 101; and prolapsed uterus, 351, 353; sex and, 552–57; TSS and, 149; uterine cancer development and, 463–64; vulvar cancer and, 467

Alcohol: cancer and, 453; impotence and, 542; infertility and, 302, 305; metronidazole and, 132; sex and, 491–93, 555

Alkaline douches: for infertility, 320

Alkaline phosphatase, 98

Allergies: to sperm, 317

Amenorrhea, 89, 112–13; danazol for, 356; Depo-Provera for, 257; infections due to, 318–19; infertility and, 302; the Pill and, 250

Amniocentesis, 101–2, 293

AMP (adenosine 5'-monophosphate), 172

Amphetamines: sex and, 493

Amyl nitrate: sex and, 493

Fetal effects: of metronidazole, 132; of phenylmercuric acetate, 146; of the Pill, 254; of spermicides, 199; of VD, 156, 161

Fertilization, 97

Fetishism, 514–16

Fever blisters, 184

Fibrocystic breast disease, 254, 422–24

Fibroid tumors (myomas; leiomyomas), 336–50; bleeding due to, 117; contraception and, 344–45; definition and origin of, 337–38; diagnosis of, 342–44; and dysmenorrhea, 111; hormonal stimulation of, 338–39; hysterectomy for, 345–47, 349–50, 384–85; infertility and, 345; laparoscopy for, 394; malignant, 347; and menstrual blood flow, 84; and menstrual pain, 109; myomectomy for, 348–49, 385–87; the Pill and, 243; protection against, 347–48; types and characteristics of, 339–42, 340–41; what to do about, 343–44

First-trimester abortions, 282–83; by suction, 285–87, 288, 289–90

5-Fluorouracil, 460

Foaming tablets (contraceptives), 197–99

Foams, contraceptive, see Spermicides

Follicle-stimulating hormone (FSH), 95–96, 99, 113, 261; danazol effects on, 259, 356, 424; effects of oral contraceptives on, 237; infertility and, 306, 308, 318–21; menopause and, 119; and menstruation, 89, 91; vaccination against, 260; vasectomy and, 279

Follicle-stimulating hormone-releasing hormone (FSH-RH), 306

Follicular cysts, 358

Follicular syphilides, 160

Forward uterus, 64, 65

Frigidity, 538–41

FSH, see Follicle-stimulating hormone

FSH-RH (follicle-stimulating hormone-releasing hormone), 306

Fumigation: as contraceptive method, 187

Functional ovarian cysts, 358–60

G

G spot (Grafenberg spot), 489–90

Gallbladder disease: the Pill and, 253–54

Gantrisin, 140

GC, see Gonorrhea

Genetic factors, 101–2; cancer and, 449–50, 457–58; 469–70; in fibroid tumor development, 337–39; tilted uterus and, 64; See also Congenital abnormalities and malformations

Gentian violet, 129

Goiter, 51

Gonadotropins, 50, 119, 303; See also Follicle-stimulating hormone; Human chorionic gonadotropin; Luteinizing hormone

Gonorrhea (GC), 56, 60–61, 137, 151, 163–68, 502; advanced stage of, 164–65; asymptomatic, 152; with atrophic vaginitis, 138; and Bartholin's gland abscesses, 142; examination for, 56, 60; history of, 154–55, 163–64; incidence, diagnosis and treatment of, 166–68; PID and, 173; prevention of, 165; symptoms of, 164; among teenagers, 554

Gossypol, 262

Graafian follicle, 89–90, 96, 118, 237

Grafenberg spot (G spot), 489–90

Granuloma inguinale, 151, 172

Gray zone: abortions in, 290–92

Group medical practice, 32

Group sex, 474, 509–11

Growth and development: effects of oral contraceptives on, 244

Industrial pollutants: cancer and, 456

Infections: Bartholin's glands clogged by, 56; and menstrual irregularities, 89; pain as symptom of, 66; and uterine congenital malformations, 330–31; See also specific types of infections

Infertility, 32, 301–29; and adenomyosis, 356; artificial insemination for, 323–25, *326*, 327–28; causes of, 302–3; consulting with specialist for, 303–5; diagnosis of female, 305–7, *308–10*, 311–12, *313*, 314–18; diagnosis of male, 321–22; and endometriosis, 302, 317–18, 355; and fibroid tumors, 345; gonorrhea and, 164; hysterectomy and (see Hysterectomies); IUDs and, 234; jogging and, 303; laparoscopy for, 394; and ovarian cysts, 359; and test-tube babies, 328–29; thyroid function and, 50; tilted uterus and, 335; treatment of female, 318–21; treatment of male, 322–23

Infundibulation, *190*, 192

Intercourse, see Sex

Intermenstrual pain (*Mittelschmerz*), 98–99, 112

Internal pelvic examination, 60–61, *62*, 63–64, *65*, 66–68

Intraamniotic instillation: abortions by, 292–94, *295*, 296–97, 299–300

Intramural (interstitial) fibroid tumors, 340, 342, *340–41*

Intrauterine devices (IUDs), 24, 25, 61, *62*, 64–66, 194, 199, 219–35, 243; advantages and disadvantages of, 227–28; bleeding due to, 115–19, 228–29, 376; cancer and, 233–34; condoms compared with, 211; diaphragms compared with, 206, 207; effectiveness of, 265; effects of, on menstrual blood flow, 84; expulsion of, 229–30; fibroid tumors and, 344; GC and, 165; history of, 220; indications for, 223–24; insertion of, 224, *225*, 226, 290; mechanism of action of, 221; and menorrhagia, 114; pelvic infections and, 175, 230–31; perforation by, 231, *232*; and polycystic ovaries, 114; postcoital insertion of, 256; postinsertion period, 227–28; pregnancy and, 232–33; removal of, 234–35; with spermicides, 198; and synechia, 317; types of, 219–21, *222*, 223; vaginal secretions and, 124; while breast feeding, 257

Inverted nipples, 424–25

Iodine, 51

Iron, 228; and menopause, 120; menstruation and, 87; the Pill and, 246–48

Irregular bleeding, see Oligomenorrhea

IUDs, see Intrauterine devices

J

Jellies, contraceptive, see Spermicides

Jogging: infertility and, 303

K

Kanamycin, 167
Kegel exercise, 479
Keloids, 401
Kidney examination, 53
Kinky sex, 514–21
Kleptomania, 521
Knee-chest position, 25
Koromex, 205
Kwell lotion, 180, 181

L

Labia majora, *20*, *483*; examination of, 55; self-examination of, *13*, 15, 17, *18*, 19

Labia minora, *13*, *20*, *483*; self-examination of, 15, 17, *18*, 19

Labor: menstrual cramps compared with contractions of, 107; orgasm and initiation of, 488–89; *See also* Childbirth

Lactation: following midtrimester abortions, 297; *See also* Breast feeding

Lactic dehydrogenase (LDH-X), 261

Laetrile (vitamin B_{17}), 471, 472

Laparoscopy (band-aid procedure), 390, 393–95; for congenital uterine malformations, 331, 332; for fibroid tumor diagnosis, 343; for infertility diagnosis, 314; for ovarian cysts, 359; sterilization by, 269, *270*, 271, 394

Laparotomy: for ovarian cancer diagnosis, 466; for ovarian cysts, 360–61; tubal ligation during, 268

Latent syphilis, 160

Law, the: oral sex and, 474–75, 500; voyeurism, exhibitionism and, 513

LDH-X (lactic dehydrogenase), 261

Leiomyomas, *see* Fibroid tumors

Leiomyosarcomas (malignant fibroid tumors), 347

Leukemia, 50, 450

Leukorrhea, 124–25, 249

LH, *see* Luteinizing hormone

Libido: effects of the Pill on, 250; testosterone level and, 260

Lippes Loop-D, 219, 221, *222*, *225*

Liver: examination of, 52; the Pill and impaired function of, 242; the Pill and tumors of, 254; *See also* Hepatitis

LSD (lysergic acid diethylamide), 495

Lung cancer, 368

Lungs: examination of, 47, 51

Luteinizing hormone (LH), 99, 113, 261; danazol effects on, 259, 356, 424; infertility and, 306, 317, 319–21; menopause and, 119; menstruation and, 88, *91*; vaccination against, 260; vasectomies and, 278

Luteinizing hormone-releasing hormone (LH-RH), 306

Lymph glands: examination of, 50

Lymph nodes, 54, 173

Lymphogranuloma venereum, 151, 172–73

Lysergic acid diethylamide (LSD), 495

M

Macrophages, 221

Macular syphilides, 157

Males: circumcision of, 402–3, *404*, *405*, 406; as gynecologists, 33–35; homosexual, 522; infertility among, 302–3; pills for, 261–62; sterilization of, 189, *190*, 192, 264, 276–81, 323, 327; temperature cycle of, 94–95

Malignant cysts, 360–62, 387

Malignant fibroid tumors (myosarcomas, leiomyosarcomas), 347

Malignant ovarian cysts, 360–62

Mammography, 415–16, *417*, 421

Marijuana: sex and, 491–92

Marsupialization, 143

Masochism, 518–19

Mastectomies, 395–97, *398*, 399–400, 421–22; radical, 396–97, *398*, 399–400, 442, 459–60; reconstruction following, 441–44; simple, 396, 399–400

Mastitis, *see* Cystic mastitis

Masturbation, 18, 75, 504–6; clitoral, 20–21; as crime, 474–75; effects of, on labia minora, 19; for frigidity, 540–41; and vaginal discharge, 139

Medical history, 45

Melanomas, 457

567

Nausea and vomiting: the Pill and, 249

Necrophilia, 520

Neisseria gonorrhea, 151, 164

Nipples: inverted, 424–25; reconstruction of, following mastectomy, 442

Nitrosamines, 452

Nongonorrheal methritis, 179

Nonspecific vaginitis, 134

Nonvenereal warts, 182

Novocaine, 286, 548

Nutrition, *see* Diet

O

Obesity: cancer and, 470; and menstrual blood flow, 84; the Pill and, 252; postmenopausal, 120; and uterine cancer, 464; vaginitis and, 125, 127

Obscenities: sexual, 521

Oligomenorrhea (irregular bleeding), 113–15, 359; the Pill and, 250, 251

Omentum, 64–65

Once-a-month suppositories, 258–59

Oophorectomies, 119, 387–88; for endometrial cancer, 465; *See also* Salpingo-oophorectomies

Oophoritis, *174*

Oral contraceptives, 93, 94, 194, 199, 235–38, 263; acne and, 183; advantages and disadvantages of, 247–48; and amenorrhea, 113, 319; bleeding associated with, 116–17; for bleeding due to IUDs, 117; breast feeding and, 257; and breast growth, 428; cancer and, 233, 241, 242, 248, 254–55, 454, 458; cervicitis and, 61; condoms compared with, 211; contraindications for, 52, 241–43; diaphragm with, 206; diaphragm compared with, 206, 207; duration of use of, 246; effects of, on uterus size, 224; for fibrocystic disease, 423; and fibroid tumors, 339, 344, 349; forgetting to take, 245–46; GC and, 165; history of, 235, 237; indications for, 241–42; and infertility, 304; with IUDs, 228; mechanism of action of, *236*, 237–38; menorrhagia and, 114; for menstrual cramps; 110–11; for ovarian cysts, 358; for polycystic ovaries, 114; side effects of, 106, 248–55; smoking and, 243–45, 252, 263; with spermicides, 198; synechia and, 317; TSS and, 149; types of, 238–40; and vaginitis, 124, 127; vitamins, iron and, 246–47

Oral sex (cunnilingus, fellatio), 499–502; as crime, 474–75, 500; hepatitis B transmission and, 178; technique of, 500–1; VD and, 164, 168, 502

Orgasm, 482–87; and anal sex, 503–4; clitoral, 21; and dysmenorrhea, 110; excitement phase of, 482–84; following transsexual operation, 529–30; and Grafenberg spot, 489–90; hysterectomy and, 382; and labor initiation, 488–89; masturbation and, 505; multiple, 488; oral sex and, 501; orgasm phase of, 484, *485*, *486*; and pelvic congestion, 487–88; during pelvic examination, 67–68; plateau phase of, 484; for premenstrual tension, 107; resolution phase of, 487; status orgasmus, 488; for tension relief, 140

Orgies, 511

Ortho-All-Flex, 205

Osteoporosis, 119, 120

Ovarian abscesses, 175

Ovarian cancer, 121, 248, 361, 362, 387, 466–67

Ovarian cysts, 390; benign, 357–60; and infertility, 302; malignant, 360–62; rare, 363; *See also* Polycystic ovarian syndrome

Ovarian stroma, 118

Ovaries, *23*, *26*, *85*, *100*; examina-